TEXTBOOK OF MEDICINE
WITH RELEVANT PHYSIOLOGY
AND ANATOMY

MODERN NURSING SERIES

A SELECTION OF TITLES
AVAILABLE AS PAPERBACKS

General Editors
A. J. HARDING RAINS M.S., F.R.C.S.
MISS VALERIE HUNT S.R.N., S.C.M., R.N.T.

Anaesthesia, Recovery and Intensive Care
D. A. BUXTON HOPKIN F.F.A., M.D., M.R.C.S.

Obstetrics and Gynaecology
JOAN M. E. QUIXLEY S.R.N., R.N.T.
MICHAEL D. CAMERON M.A., M.B., B.Chir., F.R.C.S., F.R.C.O.G.

Ophthalmology
I. M. DUGUID M.D., Ph.D., F.R.C.S., D.O.
A. A. BERRY S.R.N., O.N.D., BTA Cert., C.M.B. Part I Middle Management Cert.

Principles of Medicine and Medical Nursing
J. C. HOUSTON M.D., F.R.C.P.
MARION STOCKDALE S.R.N.
HILARY HYDE WHITE S.R.N.

Principles of Surgery and Surgical Nursing
SELWYN TAYLOR D.M., M.Ch., F.R.C.S.

Neurology
EDWIN R. BICKERSTAFF M.D., F.R.C.P.

Venereology and Genito-Urinary Medicine
R. D. CATTERALL F.R.C.P.(Edin.)

Psychology and Psychiatry for Nurses
PETER DALLY M.B., F.R.C.P., D.P.M.
HEATHER HARRINGTON S.R.N., R.M.N.

Emergency and Acute Care
A. J. HARDING RAINS M.S., F.R.C.S.
VALERIE HUNT S.R.N., S.C.M., R.N.T.
KEITH REYNOLDS M.S., F.R.C.S.

Community Health and Social Services
J. B. MEREDITH DAVIES M.D.(London), D.P.H.

Therapeutics
J. G. LEWIS M.D., F.R.C.P.

Microbiology in Patient Care
H. I. WINNER M.D., M.R.C.P., F.R.C.Path.

Pathology
C. P. MAYERS M.R.C.Path.

TEXTBOOK OF MEDICINE
WITH RELEVANT PHYSIOLOGY AND ANATOMY

Second Edition

R. J. HARRISON
Ch.B., M.D.
Lecturer in Medicine for the St Helens and Knowsley
Area Health Authority;
Examiner for the General Nursing Council for England
and Wales 1961–1970

HODDER AND STOUGHTON
LONDON SYDNEY AUCKLAND TORONTO

EDITORS' FOREWORD

The scope of this series has increased since it was first established, and it now serves a wide range of medical, nursing and ancillary professions, in line with the present trend towards the belief that all who care for patients in a clinical context have an increasing amount in common.

The texts are carefully prepared and organised so that they may be readily kept up to date as the rapid developments of medical science demand. The series already includes many popular books on various aspects of medical and nursing care, and reflects the increased emphasis on community care.

The increasing specialisation in the medical profession is fully appreciated and the books are often written by Physicians or Surgeons in conjunction with specialist nurses. For this reason, they will not only cover the syllabus of training of the General Nursing Council, but will be designed to meet the needs of those undertaking trainings controlled by the Joint Board of Clinical Studies set up in 1970.

PREFACE TO THE FIRST EDITION

The aim of this book is to provide a comprehensive text of medicine which is set out in a manner which helps the reader to understand and assimilate facts and to be able to revise the subject either for review in a clinical situation or for examination purposes.

An ideal comprehensive medical text is one which contains more than the conventional subjects of the standard textbook. Those subjects omitted by convention have been included here, subjects such as geriatrics, ionising radiations, psychiatry, skin diseases, infectious diseases, medical disorders of the eye and ear, and therapeutics. The reader is thereby helped to see medicine as a whole and, where interest is stimulated or special information is required, reference may be made to larger and more specialised texts.

Physiology, anatomy and some pathology applied to symptoms, signs and treatment are included in this text, as they form an integral part of our knowledge in clinical practice today. Indeed, physiology and anatomy, as a basis for explaining disease, is now a requirement of the General Nursing Council.

Standard International (S.I.) units are coming into use throughout much of the world and these, with the old units in parentheses, have been incorporated in the text.

PREFACE TO THE SECOND EDITION

This textbook has proven to be so overwhelmingly popular, both with students and amongst those who have qualified, that the first edition sold out in approximately 30 months, and a reprint was necessary in order to cope with the demand.

In view of the rapid changes in medicine, rather than merely reprint the first edition again, it was decided that a second edition should be prepared.

The book, therefore, has been thoroughly revised throughout and brought up to date. Drowning, electrical shock, the method of venepuncture, schistosomiasis (bilharziasis), many new drugs, and the treatment of poisoning by paracetamol, paraquat, and heavy metals have been added. The glossary and the chapter on geriatrics have been enlarged.

R. J. Harrison

CONTENTS

COMMON NURSING PROCEDURES

In order to avoid repetition, common nursing procedures are described once in the appropriate chapter, as follows. Other procedures are described under the system or disease concerned.

GLOSSARY

The index should be referred to for words not given in the glossary.

A-, an-	negative; e.g. anuria, no urine formed
Abduction	to move away from the midline of the body
Achlorhydria	lack of gastric hydrochloric acid
Acholuric	no bile in the urine
Acro-	an extremity
Acromegaly	large hands and feet
Adduction	to move towards the midline
Adenitis	inflammation of a gland
Aden(o)-	gland
Adenoma	tumour of a gland
-aemia	blood
Aerophagy	swallowing air
Aetiology	causation
Agnosia	inability to recognise the meaning of sensory perceptions
Agranulocytosis	no (or few) granular leucocytes (polymorphs)
Albumin	a blood protein
-algia	pain
Allele	the alternative form of a gene
Allergen	a substance provoking allergy
Allergy	hypersensitivity, abnormal response to a substance
Alopecia	baldness
Alpha, α	Greek letter *a*
Amnesia	loss of memory
Anaemia	deficiency of red blood cells or haemoglobin
Anaerobic	life without air
Anaphylaxis	acute severe allergy
Anarthric	disjointed
Angio-	vessel
Angiogram	radiography of vessels injected with radio–opaque material
Angioma	tumour of blood or lymphatic vessel
Anion	an ion with a negative electrical charge
Anopia	without vision
Anorexia	loss of appetite
Anoxia	lack of oxygen
Ante–	before
Ant(i)-	against
Antibody	a substance antagonising injurious particles
Antigen	a substance causing the production of antibody or antitoxin

Antitoxin	a substance antagonising injurious soluble material
Aphasia	loss of speech due to brain disease
Aphonia	loss of voice (due to laryngeal disease)
Apraxia	inability to understand the use of things, due to brain damage
Arthr(o)–	joint
Arthropathy	joint disease
Ascites	fluid in the peritoneal cavity
–ase	enzyme
Ataxia	inco-ordination of muscular action
Atopy	inherited hypersensitivity
Atrophy	wasting
Attenuated	reduced in force
Aur–	ear
Autism	morbid day-dreaming with failure of social contact and language
Auto–	self
Auto-immunity	the presence of an immune reaction against one's own tissues
Bacillus	rod-shaped bacterium
Bacterium	a unicellular micro-organism
Base	a substance neutralising an acid
Beta, β	Greek letter b
Blepharitis	inflamed margin of the eyelid
Bronchiolitis	inflamed bronchioles
Bronchitis	inflamed bronchi
Bruit	a noise
Cachexia	malnutrition
Carcinoma	cancer of epithelial tissue
Cardiac	pertaining to, or near, the heart
Casts	small protein bodies formed in renal tubules
Cataract	opacity of the lens of the eye
Cation	an ion with a positive electrical charge
Cephal–	head
Chelating agent	a drug combining with, and detoxifying, a metal
Cholangitis	inflamed bile ducts
Chole–	bile
Chromosomes	structures in cell nuclei which carry genes, the units of heredity
Claudication	limping
Coagulate	clot
Coarctation	narrowing
Collagen	the main constituent of connective tissue
Congenital	present at birth
Contagious	disease spread by contact
Coombs test	a test which detects antibody attached to red cells
Cost(al)–	rib

Crepitus	crackling
Cyanosis	blueness
Cyst	sac containing fluid
Cyt(e)	cell
Cytotoxic	cell–damaging
Delirium	temporary mental disturbance
Delta, δ	Greek letter *d*
Delusion	false belief
Dementia	lack of coherent thought
Derm(is)	skin
Dermatitis	inflamed skin
Desquamation	scaling
Diabetes	to pass through
Dialysis	separation of substances in solution using membranes
Diastole	relaxation of the heart between beats
Dilatation	expansion of a hollow organ or part
Diplopia	double vision
Dys-	bad, painful, difficult
Dysarthria	faulty articulation
Dyscrasia	a fault
Dysgenic	faulty genes, causing hereditary abnormality
Dyskinesia	faulty movement
Dyslexia	inability to read due to brain damage
Dysmenorrhoea	painful menstruation
Dyspepsia	painful digestion
Dysphagia	difficult swallowing
Dysphasia	difficulty in speaking due to brain disease
Dysphonia	defective voice (as in laryngeal disease)
Dyspnoea	difficult breathing
Dystrophy	defective nutrition
Dysuria	difficult or painful urination
-ectomy	cutting out
Eczema	allergic inflammation of the skin
Effusion	the pouring out, usually of fluid from the blood into the tissues or body cavities
Electrolyte	a substance which, in solution, forms ions and conducts electricity
Embolism	a circulating substance which may obstruct a blood vessel
Emesis	vomiting
Emphysema	puffed up (with air)
Empyema	a collection of pus
Encephal(on)	brain
Encephalitis	inflamed brain
Endo-	within
Endocardium	inner lining of the heart

Endotoxin	toxin liberated by degenerating bacteria
Enter(on)	intestine
Enterology	study of the intestine
Enzyme	a substance which speeds a biochemical reaction
Eosinophilia	an increased number of eosinophils in the blood
Epistaxis	nose-bleed
Eryth(ro)-	red
Erythema	redness
Erythrocyte	red blood cell
Euphoria	sense of well-being
Ex(o)-	out, outside
Exostosis	bony outgrowth
Exotoxin	toxin released by live bacteria
Fibroma	tumour of fibrous tissue
Fistula	a tube joining two epithelial surfaces
Flaccid	limp
Fusiform	spindle-shaped
Gamete	ovum or sperm
Gamma, γ	Greek letter g
Gamma globulin	protein in the blood consisting of antibodies
Gangrene	death of tissue due to loss of its blood supply
Gast(ric)	stomach
Gastritis	inflamed stomach
Gene	the carrier of an hereditary characteristic
Gland	specialised epithelium with secretory action
Glossal	pertaining to the tongue
Gluco-, glyco	glucose
Glycosuria	glucose in the urine
Goitre	a swelling in the neck
Granulation	new tissue formed in healing wounds
Granulocyte	polymorph leucocyte
Granuloma	tumour of granulation tissue
Haem	blood
Haematemesis	vomiting blood
Haematocrit	red cell volume as a percentage of whole blood
Haematuria	blood in the urine
Haemodialysis	dialysis of blood
Haemoglobin	the red protein, in the red blood cell, which carries oxygen
Haemolytic	blood dissolving
Haemoptysis	coughing up blood
Haemostasis	prevention of haemorrhage
Halitosis	foul breath
Hallucination	a perception without any external object

Hapten	a substance which is antigenic only when combined with protein
Hemi-, semi	half
Hemianopia	loss of sight in half the visual field
Hemiparesis	partial paralysis of one side of the body
Hemiplegia	paralysis of one side of the body
Hepatic	pertaining to the liver
Hepatomegaly	enlarged liver
Hereditary	passed on by an ancestor
Hetero-	other, different
Hidrosis	sweating
Hilum	a fissure where vessels, nerves and ducts enter or leave an organ
Hirsute	hairy
Homo	same
Hormone	a substance secreted directly into the blood by an endocrine gland
Hydro-	water
Hydrocephalus	water head, i.e. excessive cerebrospinal fluid in the skull
Hyper-	over-, excess
Hyperglycaemia	high blood sugar
Hyperkalaemia	high blood potassium
Hypersensitivity	oversensitive; allergic
Hypertension	high blood pressure
Hypo-	under, less
Hypochromia	low colour (haemoglobin)
Hypoglycaemia	low blood glucose
Hypokalaemia	low potassium level in the blood plasma
Hyponatraemia	low sodium level in the blood plasma
Hypotension	low blood pressure
Hypothermia	low body temperature
Hypotonia	reduced muscle tone
Hypovolaemia	low blood volume
Ichthyosis	dry and scaly
Idiopathic	without apparent cause
Illusion	false perception
Immunise	produce immunity
Immunity	exemption from burden or disease
Immunogenesis	production of immunity
Immunology	the science of immunity
Infarct	death of tissue due to loss of its blood supply
Inflammation	heat, swelling, redness and pain
Infra-	below
Innate	inborn
Inter-	between

Intra-	within
Ion	an electrically charged particle
Iritis	inflammation of the iris of the eye
Ischaemia	lack of blood supply
Iso-	same
Isotonic	same strength
-itis	inflammation
Jaundice	yellowness
Kernicterus	bile-staining of the basal ganglia in the brain
Kernig's sign	pain on extending the leg with the thigh flexed to a right angle
Ketosis	presence of excessive ketones
Kinesis	movement
Koilonychia	hollow nail
Kyphosis	humpback
Larynx	voice box
Leuc(o)-	white
Leucocyte	white blood cell
Leucocytosis	increased numbers of normal white cells in the blood
Leucopenia	low numbers of white cells in the blood
Leukaemia	excessive and abnormal white cells in the blood
Lipoma	a benign tumour of fat
Lith(os)	stone
Lumbago	backache
Lumen	the cavity inside a tube or sac
Lymphoma	tumour of lymphoid tissue
Lysis	breaking down
Macro-	large
Macule	a flat spot
Mal-	bad, ill
Mediastinum	the part of the chest between the two pleurae
Melaena	black stools due to blood
Melanoma	tumour pigmented with melanin
Mellitus	honey
Meninges	the membranes covering the brain and spinal cord
Meningioma	a benign tumour of the meninges
Metabolism	the physical and chemical processes constantly taking place in a living organism
Metabolite	a chemical product of metabolism
Metastasis	spread of disease from one part of the body to another
Micro-	small
Microcyte	small cell

Mono	one
Monoplegia	paralysis of one part of the body
Morph	shape
Mural	pertaining to a wall
Mutation	heritable change in gene(s)
Myalgia	painful muscle
Myasthenia	weak muscle
Mydriatic	drug which dilates the pupil
Myelin	fatty sheath surrounding medullated nerve fibres
Myelitis	inflammation of the spinal cord
Myeloid	pertaining to the marrow or spinal cord
Myeloma	tumour of plasma cells
Myo-	muscle
Myocarditis	inflamed heart muscle
Myocardium	heart muscle
Myopia	short sightedness
Myositis	inflamed muscle
Myotic	drug which contracts the pupil
Myxoedema	hypothyroidism
Naevus	a congenital mole (birthmark)
Necrosis	death of tissue
Neo-	new
Neoplasm	abnormal tissue growth, tumour
Nephr(ic)	kidney
Nephritis	inflammation of the kidney
Nephropathy	any disease of the kidney
Neuralgia	painful nerve
Neur(o)-	nerve
Neurofibroma	fibrous tumour of a nerve
Neuroma	nerve tumour
Neuropathy	any disease of nerves
Neurosis	mental disorder without physical disease of nerves
Occlude	close, shut
Ocular	relating to the eye
Odontoid	tooth-like
Oedema	excess of fluid in the extracellular tissue
Oligo-	few, scanty
Oliguria	scanty urine formation
-ology	knowledge, study of
-oma	tumour
Oophoritis	inflamed ovary
Ophthalmic	pertaining to the eye
Opsonins	substances in plasma which prepare bacteria for phagocytosis

Optic disc	the optic nerve where it enters the retina
Orchis	testis
Orchitis	inflamed testis
Ortho-	straight, upright
Orthopnoea	upright breathing, i.e. difficult breathing on lying down, relieved by sitting up
-osis	a state or condition
Osteitis	inflamed bone
Oste(o)-	bone
Osteoma	benign tumour of bone
Osteoporosis	reduced density of bone due to loss of calcium
-ostomy, otomy	cutting an opening
Pachy-	thick
Pan-	all, total
Papilloedema	swelling of the optic disc
Papule	pimple
Para-	around
Paraesthesia	abnormal sensation; e.g. tingling, burning
Paraplegia	paralysis of the lower part of the body, especially the lower limbs
Parasite	an organism that lives on, and obtains nourishment from, another
Paresis	partial paralysis
Parotitis	inflamed parotid gland
Patho-	disease
Pathogenic	disease-producing
Pathology	the science of disease
Paul-Bunnell test	a blood test for glandular fever
Pedunculated	having a stalk
Pellagra	a disease due to nicotinamide deficiency
Per-	through
Peri-, circum-	around
Pes	foot
pH	an expression (the negative logarithm) of the hydrogen ion concentration. The pH of water is 7 (neutral), above 7 is alkaline, below 7 is acid.
Phleb(o)-	vein
Photophobia	dislike of light
-plegia	paralysis
Pleura	the serous membrane covering the lungs, thorax and upper surface of the diaphragm
Pleurisy	inflamed pleura
Plexus	a network
Plumbism	chronic lead poisoning
Pneumon	lung
Pneumonitis	infection of lung

-pnoea	breath
Poly-	many
Polyarthritis	many joints inflamed
Polymorph	granulocyte, one type of leucocyte
Polyp, polypus	a tumour
Post-	after
Pre-	before
Pre-natal	before birth
Presbycusis	impaired hearing due to old age
Presbyopia	long-sightedness
Pro-	before
Proct(o)-	rectum
Proctitis	inflamed rectum
Prodromal	before the onset of symptoms and signs
Prothrombin	a blood-clotting factor
Protozoa	small unicellular organisms
Pruritus	itching
Ptosis	drooping upper eyelid
Purpura	purple spots in the skin due to extravasated blood
Pustule	pimple containing pus
Putrefy	to decay with foetid odour
Pyel(os)	renal pelvis
Pyelitis	inflamed renal pelvis and calyces
Pyo-	pus
Pyrexia	fever
Quinsy	peritonsillar abscess
Reticulocyte	young red blood cell
Retro-	behind
Rhesus factor	a blood group factor
Rhin-	nose
Rigor	stiffness, shivering
-rrhoea	discharge, flow
Sarcoma	malignant tumour of connective tissue
Sclerosis	hardening
Splenomegaly	enlarged spleen
Spondyl(os)	vertebra
Spondylitis	inflamed vertebrae
Steatorrhoea	fatty stools
Stenosis	narrowing
Stoma	mouth
Stupor	stunned mental faculties
Stools	faeces
Sub-	under

Submental	below the chin
Suppurate	to generate pus
Supra-, super-	above
Suprarenal	above the kidney, adrenal
Symptom	what the patient complains of
Syncope	faint
Syndrome	a group of symptoms and signs having more than one cause
Synovitis	inflamed synovium
Synovium	the membrane lining the joints
Systole	the contraction phase of the heartbeat
Tachy-	swift
Tachycardia	rapid heartbeat
Tachypnoea	rapid respirations
Tela	web
Tele	at a distance
Theca	a sheath
Thrombocyte	platelet
Thrombocytopenia	a low blood-platelet count
Thrombus	clot of blood
Thrush	Monilia (Candida) fungus infection
Tic	spasmodic twitching
Toxic	poisonous
Trait	a special characteristic
Trans-	across
Transplant	to remove and plant in another place
Tremor	tremble
Tumour	a swelling
Ulcer	sore, local loss of surface tissue
Ultra-	beyond
Ultrasound	sound waves having a frequency above audibility
Uraemia	excess urea and other urinary constituents in the blood
-uria	urine
Urobilin	a brownish pigment in the urine, derived from bilirubin in the gut
Urticaria	nettle rash, itching wheals in the skin
Uvea	the pigmented layer of the eye
Uveitis	inflamed uvea
Vaccine	an inoculable immunising agent
Varices	dilated tortuous (varicose) veins
Vas(o)	vessel or duct
Ventricle	a cavity in the body, as in brain and heart
Viable	able to live
Viscera	internal organs
Vital capacity	the maximum amount of air that can be inhaled in one breath

1 INTRODUCTION

Medicine is the study of disease, its cause, effects and treatment. Diseases have many causes:

1. Heredity, due to genes inherited from parents, e.g. haemophilia.
2. Trauma (injury), e.g. mechanical, chemical, thermal (burns, scalds, frostbite), electrical, radiations.
3. Inflammation, due to infection (e.g. mumps) or allergy (e.g. eczema, urticaria, asthma).
4. Neoplasm (growth, tumour), an overgrowth of tissue cells.
5. Malnutrition, such as deficiency of vitamin D causing rickets.
6. Degeneration, e.g. due to wear (osteoarthrosis), ischaemia (deficient blood supply), poisons.
7. Metabolic defects may cause the accumulation of unwanted metabolites, e.g. uric acid which causes gout.
8. Endocrine, due to undersecretion or oversecretion of hormones by the endocrine glands, e.g. overproduction of thyroxine by the thyroid gland causes thyrotoxicosis.
9. Congenital abnormalities are present at birth. They may be hereditary and due to abnormal genes, e.g. mongolism, or acquired in the uterus, e.g. rubella (German measles) in the mother may damage the fetus and cause congenital heart disease and cataract.
10. Psychological. Few diseases are due to psychological factors but emotional stress, e.g. anxiety, may cause diarrhoea or the taking of an overdose of drugs. Many mental diseases have a physical cause, e.g. dementia may be due to atherosclerosis, myxoedema, or vitamin B deficiency; depression occurs in many illnesses, e.g. influenza, cancer.
11. Poisons. Industrial accidents, accidental ingestion or inhalation of insecticide, chronic alcoholism.

Many diseases have more than one cause, often an hereditary predisposition plus an environmental precipitating cause, e.g. the predisposition to one form of diabetes mellitus is inherited but the disease often does not appear unless the subject over-eats (environmental) and becomes obese. Infectious disease, e.g. tuberculosis, is predisposed by malnutrition.

Iatrogenic disease is illness due to treatment, e.g. infection due to corticosteroid therapy, anaemia due to phenylbutazone or chloramphenicol, rashes due to one of many drugs.

Heredity, the environment and neoplasms are now discussed. Details of trauma may be obtained from surgical books. The other causes of disease mentioned above are dealt with in the appropriate chapters.

HEREDITY

A cell consists of a nucleus surrounded by cytoplasm, all contained within the cell membrane (*Fig. 1.1*). The cytoplasm contains numerous tiny structures (mitochondria, endoplasmic reticulum and ribosomes) required in cellular metabolism.

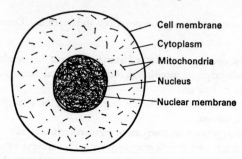

FIG. 1.1 A cell

The nucleus contains chromosomes consisting of deoxyribonucleic acid (D.N.A.), and in humans there are 46 chromosomes. Half the chromosomes are inherited from each parent, thus there are 23 pairs of chromosomes. Twenty-two pairs are autosomes, one pair are the sex chromosomes. In the female this pair is XX, in the male it is XY.

The female egg cell (ovum) and the male germ cell (spermatozoon) have only 23 single (unpaired) chromosomes, all the ova contain an X chromosome, but half the spermatozoa have an X and half have a Y chromosome. During the division of the primary germ cells from 46 to 23 chromosomes some genetic material may interchange between a pair of chromosomes. This is one form of mutation and results in a difference in the offspring. During conception the 22 X ovum may be fertilised by a 22 X sperm producing a 44 XX (= female) offspring, or by a 22 Y sperm, producing a 44 XY (= male) offspring.

On each chromosome there are about 100,000 genes and since the chromosomes are in pairs the genes are also paired. Each gene pair is responsible for the production of one enzyme (an enzyme is a protein which has one specific chemical action).

Inheritance may be: (1) dominant or (2) recessive, and (3) sex-linked or (4) autosomal. If one gene of a pair has a stronger influence than the other it is termed 'dominant', the less effective gene being 'recessive'. Thus if one gene of a pair determines blue and the other brown eyes the eyes will be brown since brown is dominant. The inheritance of characteristics due to genes on the sex chromosomes is sex-linked, and on one of the other 44 chromosomes is autosomal.

Inherited diseases are the results of abnormalities of genes. Genetic faults are known to be caused by ionising radiation such as X-rays, certain viruses, and chemicals. The chromosome containing the abnormal gene usually appears normal under the microscope; e.g. in renal rickets and phenylketonuria, but sometimes is visibly abnormal and shows:

1   Too few chromosomes, for example 44 XO i.e. there is only one X chromosome instead of two, and this causes Turner's syndrome—women who are short in height, have 'webbing' of the skin of the neck, and whose ovaries do not develop.

2   Too many chromosomes. A woman with an extra X chromosome has 44 XXX (= triple X syndrome) and is likely to be mentally retarded.

In the male an extra X chromosome produces 44 XXY, Klinefelter's syndrome—thin infertile men with small testes and female breasts. In mongolism (Down's syndrome) there are either 47 chromosomes due to an extra chromosome number 21 (i.e. triple-21), or 46 chromosomes, but with a portion of an extra number 21 attached to another chromosome (translocation). 25% of spontaneous abortions are due to severe chromosomal abnormalities.

If one of the 44 autosomal chromosomes of either parent contains a gene which causes a dominant abnormality, the abnormal gene is transmitted to one in two of their children who will be affected (Fig. 1.2) and who in turn will transmit the

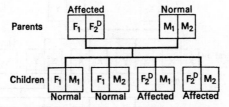

FIG. 1.2   Autosomal dominant inheritance. F_1 and F_2 = female genes; M_1 and M_2 = male genes, D or r = Dominant or recessive inheritance

disorder to half of their children; e.g. Huntington's chorea, Marfan's syndrome, multiple polyposis of the colon.

If the gene causes a recessive abnormality and only one parent is carrying it (Fig 1.3), their children will appear normal but one in two children will be carriers.

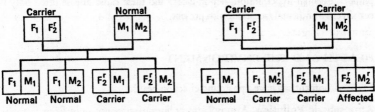

FIG. 1.3   Autosomal recessive inheritance; one parent a carrier

FIG. 1.4   Autosomal recessive inheritance; both parents carriers

If both parents are recessive carriers then one in four children will show the disorder, one in four will be normal, and the other two will be carriers (Fig. 1.4), e.g. cystic fibrosis (fibrocystic disease) and sickle-cell anaemia. If one parent is affected by a recessive disorder (i.e. both genes of a pair are abnormal) and the other parent is normal, then all children will be carriers but will not show the disease (Fig. 1.5).

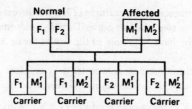

FIG. 1.5   Autosomal recessive inheritance; one parent affected

If the abnormal gene is on the X chromosome (= X-linked) in a female, half the male children will be affected and half the female children will be carriers, e.g. haemophilia (*Fig. 1.6*, generation A). If the abnormal gene is on the X chromosome in the male the boys are normal but all the daughters are carriers (*Fig. 1.6*, generation B).

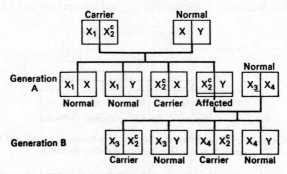

FIG. 1.6   Sex-linked inheritance; female carrier

Many disorders which run in families are due to several abnormal genes on different chromosomes (multifactorial inheritance); e.g. diabetes mellitus, schizophrenia, essential hypertension, peptic ulcer; and these cause disease often only if certain environmental factors are also present.

HEALTH AND THE ENVIRONMENT

The environment can have a profound effect on health.

Atmospheric Pollution. Atmospheric pollution arises not only from factories and vehicles but also from houses, and smokeless fuels produce invisible pollutants (sulphur oxides, nitrogen oxides, carbon oxides), although they do not emit soot particles. The lungs of city-dwellers are a mottled black due to dusts inhaled from the contaminated atmosphere, whereas those in country-dwellers and infants are a bright pink. Chronic bronchitis is a disease of industrial countries such as Britain and is almost unknown where the air is clear (Spain, Africa, India, Middle East), except in smokers. Smoking produces a locally high concentration of pollutants;

both irritants, causing chronic bronchitis, and carcinogens, causing cancer of the bronchus. The incidence of cancer of the lung rises in proportion to the number of cigarettes smoked. Vehicle exhaust fumes emit 6 million tons of carbon monoxide a year in the U.K. and 66 million tons a year in the U.S.A. They also emit nitrous oxides and lead. Exhaust fumes cause headache and irritability, and traffic noise reduces the efficiency of workers. Burnt tetraethyl lead may have more serious effects.

The atmosphere in the U.K. is also polluted with 6 million tons yearly of sulphur oxides which form sulphuric acid in the atmosphere, injuring the respiratory tract, corroding £500 million worth of metal each year, and damaging limestone buildings and clothing. Numerous other chemicals contaminate the atmosphere, including hydrocarbons which cause cancer, and nitric oxide which predisposes to pneumonia.

Local pollution varies from occupational diseases to odours which may be a social nuisance; e.g. odours from tanneries, chemical and plastics factories, motor exhausts, sewage, power stations and the local bonfire. Occupational diseases include miners' pneumoconiosis due to coal and silica dusts; byssinosis due to cotton dust; and asbestosis due to asbestos. Many infectious diseases are airborne; e.g. influenza, common cold, tuberculosis and psittacosis, and are spread by droplets or by dried particles suspended in the air.

Pollution of Water. A person drinks 1·5 litres (about 3 pints) of fluid daily to replace water losses from the body, but uses 230 litres (50 gallons) a day for washing, flushing toilets etc. in the U.K., and twice this in the U.S.A. Water for drinking has to be pure but may become contaminated by chemicals (carbonates, sulphates, nitrates) which it dissolves from the ground, and by mosses and flatworms if the water is open, as in reservoirs. Water is therefore purified before being piped to consumers, but contamination may occur by excreta containing pathogens (dysentery, salmonellae, leptospira) if there is poor sanitation, as in less advanced countries, leaking sewage pipes, or earthquake fracture of pipes.

Enormous amounts of sewage and industrial wastes are poured into the rivers each day, including alkalis, metals, mercury, oily wastes, sludges and detergents. Diseases caused by swimming in infected waters include conjunctivitis, otitis, skin diseases, verrucae and intestinal infections. The water in swimming baths commonly contains organisms such as *E. coli* and has to be filtered and chlorinated for disinfection. Bathers should take a shower before using swimming baths.

Food. Chemicals are added to food for colouring, flavour, thickening, emulsifying, anticaking, stabilising, sequestrating, acidifying, sweetening and preservation. A few food additives are beneficial to health, e.g. chalk added to flour to provide calcium, vitamins added to margarine, but there are over 300 additives permitted which have no value to health and may be harmful, e.g. nitrite is added to most preserved meats to retain their colour and act as preservative. Nitrite can form nitrosamines which are powerful carcinogens (cancer-producers); it combines with haemoglobin to form methaemoglobin which does not transport oxygen; and may cause headache ('hot-dog headache'). Food additives also cause 'Chinese-restaurant headache'. Skin rashes may be due to antibiotics fed to animals, e.g. pigs, to increase their weight.

Other hazards include injury from accidents, deafness due to noise, and anxiety caused by pressure of work or difficult relationships with other people. Deafness due to noise is well known in boiler-makers and gun-firers, and is also occurring in those who attend discotheques frequently. *Drowning* causes either spasm of the glottis and asphyxia (dry drowning) or inhalation of water into the lungs. Fresh water is absorbed into the circulation causing haemolysis of red blood cells. Salt water in the lungs attracts water from the circulation by osmosis, causing haemoconcentration. Those who survive are liable to pneumonia. Treatment includes clearing the airway, resuscitation with mouth-to-mouth respiration, and cardiac massage. *Electric shock* may cause burns, haemorrhage into the brain, temporary paralysis, apnoea, or ventricular fibrillation—the usual cause of death. Treat by disconnecting the source, resuscitation and defibrillation.

Population. The increase in population is altering the environment. More land is used up for buildings and less is available for growing food, grazing animals and recreation. The world population in 6000 BC was 5 million, by AD 1000 it was 180 million; by 1950 it was 2500 million and it is now over 4000 million. Further increase may be limited by the amount of food that can be grown.

Climate has an effect on the distribution of certain diseases. Malaria, leprosy, cholera, typhoid and other diseases occur in the tropics and subtropics but are rare in temperate climates. Respiratory infections, apart from tuberculosis, are commoner in moist temperate climates than elsewhere.

NEOPLASMS (New growths, Tumours)

Neoplasms are new growths of tissue which are independent of bodily control and needs, unlike normal tissue undergoing repair which stops growing when the repair is complete. A tumour is a local swelling. Strictly speaking abscesses and aneurysms are tumours, but they are not neoplasms.

Note: Hypertrophy is increase in the size of a tissue without increase in the number of cells; e.g. muscular hypertrophy with exercise. Hyperplasia is an increase in the number of cells; e.g. fibroadenosis of the breast.

Causes. Neoplasia has multiple causes:

1   *Radiation.* Radiation acts by altering the genes and chromosomes of cell nuclei. Leukaemia was particularly common in radiologists and in atom-bomb survivors in Japan. Osteosarcoma developed in painters using radium for luminous watch-dials. White people exposed for years to sunlight (farmers, sailors, Australians) have a high incidence of skin tumours.

2 *Viruses* cause warts in man and cancers in mice, rabbits, cats and chickens, and probably some malignant diseases in man.

3 *Parasites*. Schistosomiasis causes nodules in the bladder which become carcinomas.

4 *Carcinogenic chemicals*. Those in cigarette smoke cause carcinoma of the bronchus, and those in coal tar and oil cause skin cancer. Aniline dyes cause carcinoma of the bladder; another dye ('butter yellow') which was used to colour edible fats causes carcinoma of the liver. Carcinoma of the liver may also be due to aflatoxins which may contaminate certain foods. Asbestos causes tumours of the pleura.

5 *Hormones*. Carcinoma of the prostate and breast require sex hormones for their growth. Fibroids of the uterus are related to oestrogen abnormality. (Hormone dependency is used as a basis for treatment; e.g. oestrogens destroy carcinoma of the prostate, the anti-hormone 'nafoxidine' inhibits some carcinomas of the breast.)

6 *Heredity*. Some tumours run in families; e.g. polyposis of the colon, neurofibroma, retinoblastoma. Susceptibility to other cancers is probably due to hereditary factors.

7 *Chronic irritation*. A chronic ulcer of the leg may become malignant (epithelioma); natives of Kashmir who carry baskets of hot charcoal on a pad on the abdomen develop carcinoma of the abdominal wall.

8 *Defective immunity*. Deficiency of 'antibodies' and cell-mediated immunity predispose to malignancy, e.g. of the lymphoreticular system, which may be due to failure of the body to recognise the malignant antigen, or to an inadequate immune response.

TABLE 1.1 *Types of Tumours*

Tissue of origin	Benign tumour	Malignant tumour
Surface epithelium	papilloma, melanoma	epithelioma, rodent ulcer, malignant melanoma
Glandular epithelium	adenoma	adenocarcinoma
Fibrous tissue	fibroma ⎱ fibromyoma	fibrosarcoma
Muscle	myoma ⎰ (fibroid)	myosarcoma
Vessels—blood	haemangioma	haemangiosarcoma
—lymph	lymphangioma	lymphangiosarcoma
Bone	osteoma	osteosarcoma
Cartilage	chondroma	chondrosarcoma
Fat	lipoma	liposarcoma
Nerve	neuroma, neurofibroma, glioma	neuroblastoma, glioblastoma
Testis		seminoma, teratoma
Ovary	dermoid cyst	
Lymphoreticuloendothelial system	Lymphoma is a general term which includes benign and malignant growths of lymphoid tissue	Hodgkin's disease, leukaemia, lymphosarcoma

Mechanism. Chemicals, viruses and radiations cause tumours probably by altering the genetic nucleic acid (D.N.A.) in the cell nuclei, and this causes abnormal multiplication of cells. The mechanism of the other causes is uncertain.

Types (*Table 1.1*)

1 *Benign.* These grow slowly, resemble the tissue of origin, are often surrounded by a capsule and do not spread but may cause symptoms due to pressure on adjacent parts; e.g. dyspnoea due to a large thyroid adenoma.
2 *Malignant* (cancers) grow rapidly, are more primitive cells than their tissues of origin, invade surrounding tissues and spread elsewhere (metastasise); e.g. carcinoma of the bronchus metastasises to brain, bone, adrenal glands and liver. Carcinomas spread especially along lymphatics to lymph nodes and across body cavities. Sarcomas spread via the blood stream.

Tumours are named after their tissue of origin and end in 'oma'; e.g. fibroma from fibrous tissue.

Treatment

General: good nutrition, vitamin C, rehydration, treatment of anaemia.

Specific:

1 Surgical removal of the malignant tissue and any affected lymph nodes draining lymph (and detached malignant cells) from the growth.
2 Irradiation to destroy the neoplasm. Deep X-ray therapy is the use of a beam of X-rays focussed onto the tumour in such a way that the least possible damage is caused to nearby normal tissues. Radioactive isotopes may be used instead. Certain isotopes are taken up by particular tissues and thus destroy the tissue; e.g. radioiodine is concentrated in the thyroid and in active thyroid tumours. Radiation acts by disrupting the cell protein. Alteration of nucleoprotein (chromosomes) of cell nuclei prevents cellular reproduction. Damage to the protein of enzymes prevents cellular metabolism, thus the cells die. Cells with the highest degree of metabolism and reproduction, such as tumour cells, are the most easily destroyed. Radiations, therefore, may be able to cause or to cure tumours, depending on the quantity of radiation received. Small amounts cause changes in small numbers of chromosomes only, and may result in malignant reproduction of the cell without damaging the cell sufficiently to kill it. Large doses of radiation kill the cell by causing widespread damage not only to the nuclei but also to the cytoplasm.

    The use and disposal of radioisotopes and the care of patients treated with them is described in Chapter 21.
3 Chemotherapy is the use of drugs. The drugs used in malignant diseases are antimetabolites, cytotoxins and hormones. Antimetabolites and cytotoxins interfere with the division of cells and therefore have the greatest effect on cells which are dividing rapidly, such as tumour cells. The blood-forming cells in the bone marrow are also rapidly dividing and these drugs unfortunately tend to cause leucopenia (a low white-cell count), anaemia (a low haemoglobin and red-cell count) and thrombocytopenia (a low

platelet count), and the dose of drug has to be adjusted to provide the maximum effect against the tumour while having only a slight effect on the marrow.

Antimetabolites, e.g. methotrexate, mercaptopurine and fluorouracil, are chemically so similar to a normal metabolite that they are taken up by the growth, but are sufficiently different to block its metabolism (competitive inhibition); e.g. folic acid is required in nucleic acid synthesis, the methotrexate, being of a similar structure, is taken into the cell and prevents the formation of nucleic acid and therefore of nuclei.

Cytotoxins, e.g. nitrogen mustard, vincristine, chlorambucil and cyclophosphamide, directly attack and damage nucleoprotein, so that the cell cannot divide.

Hormones act differently; e.g. in carcinoma of the prostate the cancer requires the presence of androgens (male sex hormones) for its growth. Oestrogens counteract the androgens and prevent the tumour from growing. Corticosteroids are active against acute lymphoblastic leukaemia by an unknown mechanism.

4 Reagents such as radioisotopes, enzymes and cytotoxins, chemically combined with antibody to cancer tissue. The antibody, being specific for the malignant tissue, attaches only to the growth, the reagent then attacks the malignant tissue with minimum damage to normal tissues.

2 NUTRITION AND MALNUTRITION

An optimum diet should contain adequate water, calories, carbohydrate, protein, fat, vitamins and minerals.

Calories (Joules)

The energy value of food is measured in calories (cal.) or Joules (J). One million joules = 1 MJ. A calorie is the amount of heat required to raise the temperature of 1 g of water by 1°C. 1 calorie = 4·186 J. A basal amount of energy is used in maintaining the body temperature, circulation, respiration, peristalsis and muscle tone. The basal need is 6·3–8·4 MJ (1500 to 2000 kcal.) in 24 hours. An additional 2·1–10·5 MJ (500–2500 kcal.) are needed for muscular activity, growth in children, and pregnancy. The average adult in Britain uses about 10·5 MJ (2500 kcal.) a day, although 12·6 MJ (3000 kcal.) of food are actually sold in the shops, 2·1 MJ (500 kcal.) being wasted. A coal miner uses 16·8 MJ (4000 kcal.) a day, a moderately active woman 9·2 MJ (2200 kcal.). Sitting uses only 0·06 MJ (15 kcal.), walking 14·7 MJ (350 kcal.), and rowing 5 MJ (1200 kcal.) an hour. Energy is obtained from carbohydrate (the cheapest), protein and fat.

Carbohydrate

The average daily intake is 400 g (6 MJ = 1640 kcal.). Some is stored in the liver and muscles as glycogen; any excess is stored as fat. Sugars (sucrose, glucose, lactose) and starches (in cereals and potatoes) are carbohydrates.

Protein

A minimum of 40 g a day is required for health, although 70 g is usually recommended and provides 1·1 MJ (290 kcal.). Protein is obtained from meat, fish, eggs, milk, peas and beans and is broken down in the intestine into amino acids which are absorbed to be made into the protein of the plasma and tissues of the body. Eight amino acids are essential; i.e. they must be present in the diet because the body is unable to make them. Protein is not stored and any extra is burnt up for energy or changed into fat; in the liver its nitrogen is metabolised to urea which is then excreted in the urine. Protein contains sulphur and phosphorus.

Fat (Lipid)

Fat contains fatty acids, some of which are essential for health. The average daily intake is 70 g which provides 2·6 MJ (650 kcal.). Fats are present in large amounts in the nervous system and in cell membranes, some are attached to protein (= lipoprotein); e.g. in the plasma. The steroids are a group of fats made from cholesterol and include bile salts and steroid hormones (hydrocortisone, aldosterone, sex hormones). Fat deposits protect certain organs, e.g. the kidneys, and act as an energy store. Fat is needed in the secretions of the sebaceous glands in the skin and for storage and absorption of fat-soluble vitamins.

Types of Nutritional Disorder

1 *Insufficient food*, causing undernutrition or starvation. Starvation in infants is called marasmus.
2 *Excess food*, causing obesity; excess vitamin A and D causing toxicity.
3 *Wrong (unbalanced) diet*, causing malnutrition such as adequate carbohydrate with low protein causing kwashiorkor; vitamin deficiencies causing rickets and scurvy.

Causes of Malnutrition

1 *Social*. Even when adequate food can be obtained, prejudice, ignorance and bad housekeeping often cause malnutrition; i.e. the diet fails to contain a proper balance of the various foods.
2 *Economic*. Poverty is common in the underdeveloped countries but true poverty no longer exists in Britain. (Malnutrition exists but this is due to social factors, particularly ignorance and bad housekeeping; i.e. many 'poor' families spend several pounds each week on cigarettes, beer and gambling rather than on proper food for their malnourished children.) On the other hand many people in Asia, Africa and South America die of starvation from real poverty.
3 *Pathological*
   (*a*) Anorexia (loss of appetite) due, e.g., to mental depression.
   (*b*) Persistent vomiting; e.g. due to pyloric stenosis.
   (*c*) Chronic alcoholism, which provides energy but not vitamins or proteins.
   (*d*) Food fads; e.g. vegetarians have a poor intake of vitamin B_{12}.
   (*e*) Malabsorption; e.g. coeliac disease, chronic pancreatitis.
   (*f*) Excessive menstrual bleeding (menorrhagia) causing iron deficiency.

Protein–Calorie Malnutrition

1 **Marasmus** is malnutrition in infants due to deficiency of both protein and energy (calories). Vitamin and mineral deficiency is also present. The child is wasted, thin and wizened and growth is retarded. Diarrhoea is common. There is no oedema, unlike kwashiorkor.

   Treatment: improved diet, beginning with skimmed milk (protein and calcium) and bananas (potassium), increasing gradually as the digestive tract improves its digestive ability.
2 **Kwashiorkor** is common in Asia, Africa and South America and is due to protein deficiency with an adequate intake of total calories, the diet usually consisting of starchy gruels. Protein deficiency causes retardation of growth, hypoproteinaemia (low blood proteins) and anaemia. Low plasma-protein levels cause oedema which may hide the wasting. The child's liver is enlarged by an excess of fat, and vitamin deficiencies and diarrhoea are usual.

Treatment is to give adequate protein, beginning with skimmed milk, vitamins and minerals, especially iron.

3 **Elderly People** often suffer from a moderate protein deficiency, partly due to the high cost of protein and partly due to apathy and neglect. Protein deficiency may also occur in ulcerative colitis, chronic suppurative infection, and chronic gastric ulcer, especially if the ulcer is bleeding. These patients therefore need a high protein intake.

4 **Obesity** is the commonest form of malnutrition in the prosperous countries.

Cause

This is due to a greater intake of food, whether carbohydrate, protein or fat, than is burnt up as energy. The familial tendency to obesity is usually not due to genetic factors but to faulty eating habits acquired by example from parents. The 'middle-aged spread' is due to decreased physical activity (relax more, sit more, sleep more) while the appetite remains unaltered. Increased weight restricts exercise and this sets up a vicious circle. If a 70 kg (11 stone) person walks for 20 minutes each day this uses only 0·4 MJ (100 kcal.), i.e. 11 g (0·3 oz.) of fat. This is a tiny amount, but in one year it amounts to 4 kg (9 lb)! Some obese people eat more for psychological reasons (frustration, unhappiness). Endocrine factors are often blamed for obesity but these are seldom the cause, although obesity very rarely may be due to a lesion of the appetite centre in the hypothalamus or to Cushing's syndrome.

Complications

1 Psychological. Patients may become unhappy from aching joints and tiredness due to their obesity, and eat more, creating a vicious circle.
2 Mechanical. Osteoarthrosis of the lumbar spine, hips, knees and ankles, and flat feet, are due to the extra weight carried by the joints and feet. Abdominal herniae, including hiatus hernia, and varicose veins are due to increased intra-abdominal pressure due to fat. Accidents are common—the obese easily trip and are unable to save themselves from falling, and slowness causes difficulty in avoiding accidents.
3 Metabolic. Atheroma, gallstones (cholesterol) and adult-onset diabetes mellitus are commoner in the obese.
4 Cardiovascular. Hypertension and strokes are commoner in the obese than in those of normal weight. Angina and cardiac failure are both due to the increased work of the heart moving the overweight body, and are associated with coronary atheroma.
5 Skin. Maceration and infection occurs at the flexures.
6 Life expectancy is reduced by 10 years for every 5 kg (11 lb) overweight.
7 Surgical. Operations are difficult, and there is a risk of incisional hernia.

Treatment

1 Explanation of the cause and complications.
2 Teach the patient the caloric value of foods and make it clear that the

only 'slimming' foods are those low in calories, whatever the adver-
tisements claim. Most lagers and beers contain 0·8 MJ (200 kcal.) in
0·57 l (1 pint). Two heaped spoonfuls of sugar in each cup of tea for
7 cups a day equals 100 g sugar daily or 36 kg in a year.

3 Strict diet of, e.g. 4 MJ (1000 kcal.) a day (see Appendix) will lose 1 kg
(2·2 lb) a week. A 2·4 MJ (600 kcal.) diet may be used and is more
encouraging to the patient since 1·8 kg (4 lb) weekly will be lost. A diet
of 4 MJ should contain fat 40 g, protein 50 g and carbohydrate 100 g,
including fruit and vegetables for vitamins and the prevention of
constipation, and 0·3 l (½ pt) skimmed milk to provide calcium. Signs
of anaemia should be watched for and iron given if necessary. Water is
not restricted but sweetened juices and alcohol are avoided or counted
as calories. The patient is weighed weekly. Numerous 'diets' are on the
market but have no advantage over carefully balanced meals.

4 Anorectic drugs depress the appetite but may cause addiction and are
better avoided, although a short course (3 weeks) may be given if a
patient is dieting and genuinely feels hungry, e.g. fenfluramine
(Ponderax) 20 mg one to four times daily. Methylcellulose 1·5–6 g may
be used to provide bulk to reduce the feeling of hunger and prevent
constipation.

5 Regular exercise should be encouraged.

Minerals

Essential elements are sodium, potassium, chloride, calcium, phosphorus, sulphur,
iron, iodine, fluorine, magnesium, copper, cobalt, zinc and manganese.

Sodium Chloride (common salt) is needed by all tissues, especially the extracellular tissues. It is present in large quantities in cheese, milk, cereal foods (to which
it is added, e.g. bread, cornflakes), and in canned and salted meats. It is present in
most food in smaller amounts. The daily intake is an excessive 10–15 g. The excess
is excreted in the urine unless there is cardiac or renal failure, when its retention
causes oedema.

Potassium is mostly intracellular (within cells). It is therefore present in all food
except glucose, white sugar and some oils. The body needs 1 g daily and the
average intake is 3 g daily. The excess is excreted by the kidneys. Potassium
accumulates in the body in acute renal failure.

Calcium is needed in bones and teeth, the clotting of blood, and muscular contraction. The best sources are milk, cheese and bread—3 g of chalk (calcium
carbonate) is added to each 1 kg of bread. Calcium is absorbed only under the
influence of vitamin D. Hypocalcaemia (low blood calcium) causes tetany (muscle
spasm). Hypercalcaemia (high blood calcium) causes calcification of tissues and
renal calculi. Calcium balance is controlled by vitamin D metabolites, parathormone, and calcitonin.

Phosphorus and Sulphur are present in nearly all food and are needed in all tissues; phosphorus is particularly needed in bone.

Iron is required in haemoglobin and in all cells for their respiratory metabolism. The best sources are liver, meat, eggs and vegetables. The normal diet contains 15 mg daily but the amount absorbed is adjusted to equal the losses and is normally 0·6 mg in men to 1·5 mg in women. Excess of iron causes haemochromatosis or haemosiderosis. Deficiency of iron causes hypochromic anaemia.

Iodine is needed by the thyroid gland for the formation of thyroxine (thyroid hormone). It is present in sea fish and in traces in most food but is deficient in the soil (and therefore in the food grown) in mountainous areas. Deficiency causes simple goitre (swelling of the thyroid) and potassium iodide should be added to table salt to prevent this.

Fluorine. Traces are taken up by growing bones and teeth and in dental enamel it may help to prevent dental caries (decay) in children. One milligram is added to each 1 l of drinking water; 0·2 mmol/l (4 mg/l) may damage the teeth, which become rough, pitted and mottled; 0·5 mmol/l (10 mg/l) damages bones. Many people object to mass fluoridation of drinking water since fluorine is a poison and does not prevent dental decay in adults. Fluoride toothpaste is available to those who want it.

The Other Minerals are present in many foods and dietary deficiency is unknown.

Vitamins
Vitamins are organic substances in the diet and are required for normal metabolism but do not supply energy.

Vitamin A (retinol) is needed in rhodopsin in the visual cells of the retina for vision in dim light ('night' vision); for the health of all epithelium and for bone growth. The vitamin or its precursor is present in liver, fish liver oils (halibut, cod), carrots, spinach and butter. An excess is toxic. Deficiency first causes night blindness, then damages epithelium which blocks the ducts of the tear glands causing a dry eye (xerophthalmia) and corneal damage (keratomalacia) leading to opacity of the cornea and blindness. Sebaceous ducts are also blocked, causing a dry skin.

Vitamin B complex is a group of vitamins which are required in the enzyme systems in all the tissues. It includes thiamine, riboflavine, biotin, nicotinic acid, pyridoxine, pantothenic acid, folic acid and cobalamin.

Vitamin B$_1$ (thiamine, aneuryn) deficiency occurs in the far east in those whose diet consists largely of polished rice, the husk containing the vitamin having been lost by polishing. Deficiency also occurs in chronic alcoholics and food faddists. Whole cereals, e.g. wholemeal bread, yeast, liver, broad beans, peas and nuts, are good sources. Thiamine is essential for carbohydrate metabolism and the function of the nervous system. Deficiency causes beri-beri in which there is polyneuritis (paraesthesiae, anaesthesia, muscle-wasting and weakness) and mental change, and/ or congestive cardiac failure with severe oedema.

Vitamin B$_2$ (riboflavine). Good sources are yeast, liver, egg yolk, whole cereals, cheese, milk, peas and broad beans. Deficiency causes swollen and cracked lips (cheilosis) and angles of the mouth (angular stomatitis), glossitis (tender magenta tongue), dermatitis and corneal damage.

Nicotinic acid (nicotinamide, niacin) is present in yeast, liver, whole cereals (but that in maize cannot be utilised), and meat. Deficiency causes pellagra—dermatitis, glossitis, diarrhoea and mental disturbance.

Pyridoxine (vitamin B$_6$). Yeast, whole cereals, liver, eggs and vegetables are good sources. Deficiency may be caused by certain drugs, e.g. isoniazid (used in tuberculosis), and penicillamine, and oral contraceptives increase the need for pyridoxine. Deficiency causes polyneuritis and hypochromic anaemia.

Folic acid is found in leafy green vegetables. It is synthesised by the bacteria in the large intestine but is not absorbed from there (dietary folic acid is absorbed from the small intestine). It is necessary for blood formation, and deficiency causes macrocytic anaemia and leucopenia (low white-cell count in the blood).

Vitamin B$_{12}$ (cobalamin). Good sources are liver, meat, eggs, milk. It is needed by all tissues, especially by the nervous system and blood. Deficiency causes macrocytic anaemia (e.g. pernicious anaemia), leucopenia, and neuropathy (damage to the nervous system).

Vitamin C (ascorbic acid) is found in citrus fruits, blackcurrants, tomatoes, green vegetables, and rose hips. It is needed for the formation of fibrous tissue, blood and antibodies, and for healthy capillaries. Deficiency (scurvy) occurs in infants fed on dried, tinned or boiled milk unless fruit juice is also given, and in the elderly living alone who do not eat fresh fruit and vegetables.

Scurvy was known in sailors in 1497 (when 100 out of 160 died on one ship) since they travelled on long voyages without fresh food. Deficiency causes capillary fragility, and the capillaries rupture easily causing haemorrhages into the skin and joints; children develop pain and tenderness in bones due to subperiosteal haemorrhages. There is anaemia, fatigue, and bleeding and infection of the gums, except in the edentulous (toothless). Wounds are slow to heal.

Prevention: fruit juice for infants; fresh fruit and vegetables for the elderly. Patients with burns or having extensive operations need vitamin C to promote the healing of wounds.

Investigations: blood plasma or leucocyte vitamin C levels. Urine vitamin C excretion test.

Treatment: vitamin C 200 mg q.i.d. for 7 days then 25–50 mg daily.

Vitamin D (calciferol). Vitamin D$_3$ (cholecalciferol) is made in the skin by the action of ultraviolet light. After absorption it is changed into the active hormone by the liver and kidneys. It is needed for the absorption of calcium and in the calcification of bone. Most food has a low content of vitamin D, but good sources are fish-liver oils, egg yolk, butter and vitaminised margarine. Deficiency causes rickets in children and osteomalacia in adults. In temperate climates coloured people may not obtain sufficient ultraviolet light, and hence develop vitamin D deficiency.

Rickets. Rickets is due to lack of vitamin D or of calcium in the diet, malabsorption of calcium, phosphate or vitamin D (e.g. coeliac disease), lack of sunshine or failure of the kidney to activate vitamin D. Rickets develops during the period of most active growth, i.e. between three months and three years of age. The child is restless, irritable, and anorectic, with weak flabby muscles and anaemia. The epiphyses of bones enlarge causing 'beading' of the ribs ('rickety rosary') and enlargement of the lower end of the radius. The long bones bend producing bow legs or knock knees, the spine curves (kyphosis, scoliosis), the sternum becomes prominent ('pigeon-chest') and the skull enlarges producing prominence of the forehead ('bossing') and parietal bones, causing a 'hot-cross-bun' appearance. The fontanelle, which normally closes at 18 months, remains open. The teeth are delayed in erupting, they are soft and decay easily. Convulsions and tetany may occur, due to the low serum calcium (hypocalcaemia). There is susceptibility to infection, e.g. bronchitis.

Treatment:
1 Vitamin D 25 to 125 μg (1000–5000 i.u.) daily as cod liver oil, halibut liver oil, or calcium with vitamin D tablets B.P.C. which contain 12·5 μg of calciferol, one or two daily, crushed. *Note:* These tablets must not be confused with calciferol tab.strong (B.P.) which contain 1·25 mg (= 50,000 i.u.) vitamin D used in hypoparathyroidism. Excess of vitamin D is toxic.
2 Fruit juice for vitamin C.
3 Orthopaedic correction of deformities, e.g. light splints, operation.

Prevention: sunlight, vitamin D—a few drops of cod liver oil with feeds each day.

Osteomalacia. This is defective calcification of bone in the adult. It is due to vitamin D deficiency and calcium deficiency in the diet, malabsorption, or frequent pregnancies, the fetus using maternal calcium. There is fatigue, muscular weakness, pain and tenderness in bones, bones are deformed and easily fracture.

Treatment: vitamin D 25 to 125 μg daily or 1α-hydroxyvitamin D_3.

Excess of vitamin D causes nausea, vomiting, diarrhoea, hypercalcaemia (high blood calcium), calcification of tissues and colic due to renal calculi.

Vitamin E (tocopherol) is present in milk, eggs, meat and leafy vegetables. It is needed in the metabolism of most tissues. Deficiency is not known in man.

Vitamin K is required by the liver for the formation of prothrombin and other clotting factors. The best sources are green vegetables (vitamin K_1, phytomenadione), e.g. spinach, cabbage, kale. Vitamin K_2 is synthesised by the bacteria in the gut. Deficiency causes a bleeding tendency and occurs in liver disease or obstructive jaundice. A damaged liver is unable to make prothrombin from vitamin K. Obstructive jaundice prevents the release of bile into the gut thus preventing fat absorption. Vitamins A, D, E and K are soluble in fat and are normally absorbed with it. Vitamin K_3 (menaphthone) is synthetic and fat-soluble.

3 WATER, ELECTROLYTES AND ACID–BASE BALANCE

WATER AND ELECTROLYTES

Definition

Electrolytes are substances which dissolve in water to form electrically charged particles named ions; e.g. sodium chloride in water forms positively charged sodium ions (Na^+) and negatively charged chloride ions (Cl^-).

An **ion** with a positive electrical charge is a *cation*; e.g. sodium (Na^+), hydrogen (H^+), potassium (K^+), calcium (Ca^{++}) and magnesium (Mg^{++}). Calcium and magnesium have two positive charges each.

An ion with a negative electrical charge is an *anion*; e.g. bicarbonate (HCO_3^-), chloride (Cl^-), sulphate $(SO_4^=)$ which has a double charge, and phosphate $(PO_4^{\equiv})$ which has a triple charge.

Filtration (*Fig. 3.1*) is the forcing of fluid through a barrier due to differences in the hydrostatic ('mechanical') pressures on the two sides of the barrier; e.g. blood plasma, except its protein, is forced out of the arterial end of the blood capillaries, through the capillary wall into the interstitial tissues, by the blood pressure. (The interstitial tissues are those surrounding and supporting the cells.)

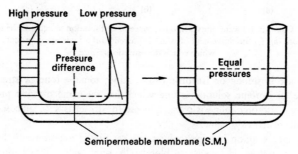

FIG. 3.1   Filtration

Diffusion ('spreading out') is the transfer of a substance from a region of higher concentration to a lower one (*Fig. 3.2*). Substances diffuse through a membrane if the pores in the membrane are large enough. Water diffuses freely through the capillary membranes between the blood and the interstitial fluid, but proteins, which are large molecules, do not.

Osmosis is the transfer of fluid across a membrane into the compartment that contains the highest concentration of dissolved substances or particles (*Fig. 3.3*).

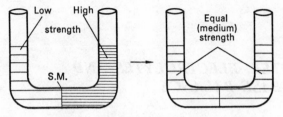

FIG. 3.2   Diffusion

The osmotic pressure (osmolarity or osmolality) of a solution may be thought of as a suction pressure which can draw water into it. All the particles in a liquid contribute to the osmotic pressure, but electrolytes in the body diffuse readily between the plasma and the interstitial fluid; thus their osmotic pressures balance, and any osmotic difference between the plasma and the interstitial fluid has to be provided by molecules which do not diffuse, such as protein. Solutions with the same osmotic

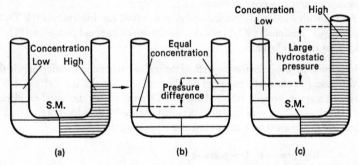

FIG. 3.3   Osmosis: (*a*) water moves into the concentrated solution to equalise the strength of the solutions (*b*); (*c*) the movement of water is prevented if a hydrostatic pressure is applied which equals the osmotic pressure

pressure are isosmotic or **isotonic** (iso = same; tonic = tone or strength). In medicine an isotonic solution is one which has the same osmotic pressure as plasma; e.g. isotonic saline is 0·9%, glucose (dextrose) is 5%, glucose–saline is 4·3% glucose in 0·18% saline.

A stronger solution is hypertonic; a weaker one is hypotonic. A hypotonic solution haemolyses (destroys) red blood cells, since water diffuses into the cell which swells and bursts. Solutions given intravenously must be isotonic, except in special circumstances.

Distribution

The body of a normal 70 kg (11 stone) man contains 62% of water (= 43 litres). Of this, 29 l is intracellular (within the cells) and 14 l is extracellular (outside the cells). Part of the extracellular fluid (e.c.f.) is in the plasma (3 l); the remainder (11 l) is interstitial (between the cells) and in the cerebrospinal fluid and body 'cavities'. Water distributes readily throughout the body.

Sodium and chloride are concentrated mainly in the extracellular fluid, whereas potassium, magnesium, phosphate,and sulphate are in highest concentration inside the cells (*Table 3.1*). Because electrolytes easily pass through the capillary walls their concentration is similar in the plasma and in the interstitial fluid. Since there

TABLE 3.1   *Normal electrolyte composition of body fluids.*

| | Venous plasma | | | Cells |
	(mmol/l)	(mEq/l)	(mg/100 ml)	(mmol/l)
Bicarbonate	27±3	27±3	—	10
Calcium	2·4±0·2	5±0·5	9 to 10·5	—
Chloride	102±4	102±4	—	10
Magnesium	0·8±0·2	2±0·4	1·8 to 2·4	15
Phosphate	1·1±0·3	2±0·5	2·5 to 4·5	90
Potassium	4·7±0·8	4·7±0·8	18 to 20	150
Sodium	141±5	141±5	—	4
Sulphate	1	1	—	15

is a high concentration of sodium in the e.c.f. and of potassium in the cells, there is a tendency for sodium to diffuse into the cells and potassium out of them. This would soon stop the cell from functioning, so the cell continuously has to pump out sodium in exchange for essential potassium. This is called the 'sodium pump'.

Function
Water provides the medium in which all the metabolic (chemical and enzyme) reactions of the body take place. The plasma (and red cell) is the transport system of the body, carrying oxygen, nutrients and water to all the tissues; and carbon dioxide, waste products and excess of water for disposal by the lungs, liver, skin and kidneys. The interstitial fluid bathes the cells and supplies them with nutrients from the blood; it also delivers waste products from the cells to the blood. It contains considerably less protein, and therefore has a lower osmotic pressure, than the plasma. This causes a rapid interchange of water and its dissolved substances to take place between the plasma and the interstitial fluid by osmosis, thus rapidly removing unwanted materials thrown out of the cells and keeping the cells in a 'clean', as well as a nutritious, environment. The intracellular fluid allows cellular metabolism to proceed. The cells continuously pump out, into the interstitial fluid, unwanted substances such as sodium and chloride. They also eject manufactured substances (e.g. hormones from endocrine cells), for transport by plasma to other parts of the body.Electrolytes have various functions: sodium and potassium provide an electrical charge across the cell membrane, calcium and magnesium are required in muscular contraction (calcium is also needed in blood clotting and bone), and zinc, magnesium and iron are essential in many enzyme systems. Electrolytes affect osmosis since all particles have an osmotic pressure, and they, especially bicarbonate, also aid in buffering the body against changes in 'acidity'.

Control of the Water and Electrolyte Content of the Body

The volume of fluid and the concentration of salts in the body have to be kept constant for the proper function of the tissues. Since there are considerable hourly variations in the intake of fluid and electrolytes the kidneys excrete any excesses or excrete less if there are deficiencies (see 'renal function', Chapter 10).

The total amount of water in the body is regulated by the osmolality of the plasma via the osmoreceptors in the hypothalamus. Osmoreceptors are cells sensitive to changes in osmotic pressure. They control the release of antidiuretic hormone (A.D.H.) from the posterior part of the pituitary gland, and A.D.H. controls the reabsorption of water from the renal tubules. The sodium content of the body is controlled by groups of cells (the juxtaglomerular apparatus) near the glomeruli in the kidneys. These cells are sensitive to blood pressure and blood flow through the kidneys, and control the secretion of aldosterone by the adrenal cortex. Aldosterone stimulates the kidney to reabsorb sodium. For example, a fall in plasma volume reduces the blood pressure and blood flow to the juxtaglomerular cells which release renin. Renin stimulates the secretion of aldosterone by the adrenals and this causes the kidney to retain sodium. The increased sodium increases the osmotic pressure of the plasma and this stimulates the osmoreceptors in the hypothalamus to release A.D.H. from the pituitary. A.D.H. circulates to the kidneys which then retain more water. Thus both salt and water are retained to restore the plasma volume (*Fig. 3.4*).

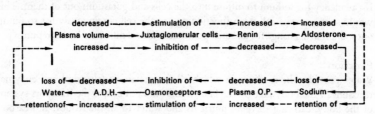

FIG. 3.4 Control of water and salt balance. A.D.H. = antidiuretic hormone; O.P. = osmotic pressure

Since water diffuses freely throughout the intracellular and extracellular fluid the volumes of these fluids depend on osmotic and hydrostatic pressures. Although the osmotic pressure of a fluid is due to its total concentration of electrolytes, protein and other molecules, the major influence on osmotic pressure in the e.c.f. is by sodium and chloride, and in the cells is by potassium and phosphate. The plasma proteins contribute slightly to the osmotic pressure of the plasma, but the protein level of the interstitial fluid is so low as to have a negligible effect on its osmotic pressure.

The Mechanism of Fluid Exchange

The mechanism of fluid exchange between the blood and the interstitial fluid is based on this slight difference of osmotic pressure. The blood (hydrostatic) pressure, by the time it has reached the arteriolar end of a capillary, has fallen to 4·3 kPa (32 mmHg). The pressure falls further along the capillary until at the venular end it is 1·6 kPa (12 mmHg). The hydrostatic pressure of 4·3 kPa (32 mmHg) is greater than the osmotic 'suction' pressure of the plasma proteins (which is 3·3 kPa = 25 mmHg), therefore fluid is forced out of the arteriolar end of the capillary into the interstitial fluid, providing the interstitial fluid with nutrients, oxygen and water. At the venous end of the capillary the osmotic pressure of the plasma proteins is greater than the 1·6 kPa (12 mmHg) hydrostatic venous pressure, therefore fluid is withdrawn from the interstitial fluid into the capillary. This produces a continuous circulation of fluid from the arterial blood into the tissues and back into the venous blood (*Fig. 3.5*).

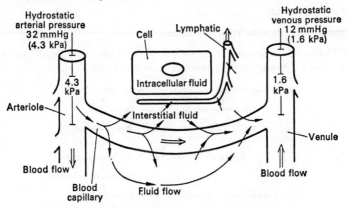

FIG. 3.5   The mechanism of plasma and tissue fluid exchange

The Normal Balance of Water and Electrolytes

The normal intake of water in 24 hours is 2·5 l (4·5 pints) and comprises the fluid drunk (1·5–2·5 l), the water in the food eaten (400 ml) and the water formed metabolically in the body by the oxidation of food (400 ml). The normal output of water in 24 hours in a temperate climate is 350 ml expired as water vapour from the lungs, 500 ml evaporated from the skin, 150 ml excreted in the faeces, and 1500 ml excreted in the urine, totalling 2·5 l. The fluid drunk is approximately equal to the urinary output. The *minimum* urinary volume required to excrete wastes is 500 ml in 24 hours. Normally the average amount of sodium lost daily is 5 g. This is replaced by giving 550 ml isotonic saline i.v. if the patient is unable to take fluid or food by mouth. The remaining 2 l of water required is given as 5% dextrose i.v., or the total fluid and salt required is provided in 2·5 l of dextrose-saline. 2·5 l of isotonic saline contains too much salt and may cause fatal pulmonary oedema, or general oedema. More salt or water, and possibly potassium, may be needed if there is any disturbance of water and electrolyte balance, hence the importance of a fluid balance chart.

DISTURBANCES OF WATER AND ELECTROLYTE BALANCE

Dehydration

This may be due to pure water deficiency or to sodium depletion.

Water Deficiency is due to an insufficient intake of water due to coma; inability to swallow (dysphagia); apathy, e.g. elderly; or if there is no water available, as in a desert. Renal water loss is due to diabetes insipidus or hypokalaemia. Dehydration is made worse if there is an increased loss of water from the lungs, due to tachypnoea, or skin, as occurs in pyrexia.

Clinically: the concentration of the e.c.f. rises and increases its osmotic pressure, therefore water passes from the cells into the extracellular fluid by osmosis, thus the cells also become dehydrated. There is haemoconcentration, producing a rise in haemoglobin and serum sodium; and dehydration causes thirst, dry mouth, confusion and coma.

Treatment: water by mouth or 5% dextrose i.v.

Salt Deficiency automatically means loss of water also, since water cannot be retained by the kidneys in the absence of sufficient salt (*Fig. 3.6*).

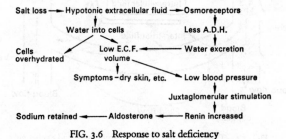

FIG. 3.6   Response to salt deficiency

Causes:

1   Gastro-intestinal disorders—diarrhoea, vomiting, intestinal fistulae, intestinal obstruction.

2   Excessive sweating—stokers, tropical countries—if there is an inadequate salt intake.

3   Burns. Serum oozes from the damaged surface.

4   Failure of the kidneys to conserve salt because of renal disease, deficiency of salt-retaining hormones, e.g. Addison's disease, the osmotic diuresis of diabetes mellitus, or excessive use of diuretic drugs.

Clinically: since sodium is mostly extracellular its deficiency results in a reduced e.c.f. volume which causes weakness, a dry tongue, loss of elasticity of the dry skin, increased pulse rate, low plasma volume and blood pressure and reduced renal blood flow which causes oliguria. Oliguria prevents the excretion of waste products, and uraemia (renal failure) follows. There is compensatory vasoconstriction of the skin which becomes pale and cold. Plasma sodium and chloride are low, but the serum proteins and the haemoglobin are increased due to haemoconcentration.

Treatment: salt and water orally or isotonic saline i.v. or p.r. Fluid balance chart. Giving water alone makes the e.c.f. hypotonic and water passes into the cells, the e.c.f. being no better off. The water is soon excreted since it is not retained in the absence of sufficient salt.

Overhydration

Water Intoxication. It is difficult for the normal person to overload the body with water since moderate excesses of water are excreted by the kidneys, but mentally disturbed people may drink large amounts of water, which the kidneys are unable to excrete, and this causes water intoxication. It also occurs if there is oversecretion of antidiuretic hormone by the pituitary, and in patients given an excess of fluid by i.v. drip, e.g. 5% dextrose.

Clinically there is headache, nausea, confusion, convulsions, coma, and death. The water is distributed throughout both the extracellular fluid and the cells, so that oedema is slight.

Treatment is of the cause.

Salt retention results in water retention in the e.c.f. and causes oedema.

Oedema is the collection of fluid in the interstitial tissues.
Causes (Figs. 3.7 and 3.8):

1. Increased venous pressure increases the hydrostatic pressure in the capillaries and prevents the reabsorption of fluid from the interstitial tissue, as in congestive cardiac failure and constrictive pericarditis. Local oedema is due to local venous obstruction, as in venous thrombosis, or to pressure on a vein by a tumour.

2. Failure of the kidneys to excrete sodium and water, as in nephritis, or when there is a poor renal blood flow as in cardiac failure, or increased renal reabsorption of sodium and water due to corticosteroid drug therapy or Cushing's syndrome.

3. A decreased osmotic pressure of the plasma due to a low concentration of plasma proteins (hypoproteinaemia), which is due to loss of albumin in the

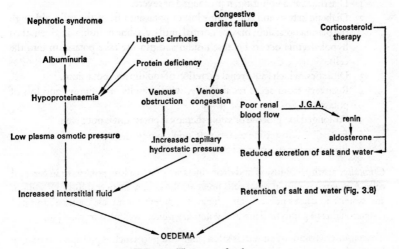

FIG. 3.7   The cause of oedema

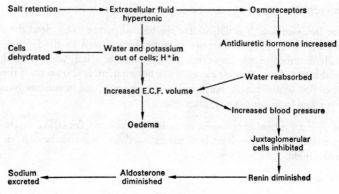

FIG. 3.8   Effects of salt retention

urine (nephrotic syndrome), impaired production of albumin by the liver in cirrhosis, or protein malnutrition (dietary deficiency of protein or protein-losing enteropathy).

4   Lymphatic obstruction by tumour, inflammation or parasites.
5   Increased capillary permeability due to inflammation.
6   Excessive i.v. saline.

Treatment: restriction of salt intake, increase salt excretion with a diuretic. Acupuncture (acu = needle, puncture = prick) in resistant cardiac oedema (p. 144). Treatment of the cause.

Hypokalaemia is a low concentration of potassium in the plasma, and is always associated with a low cellular potassium.
Causes:
1   Diarrhoea and vomiting, if prolonged or severe.
2   Diabetic ketosis and coma cause loss of potassium from the cells, although the plasma potassium may be normal until i.v. saline or insulin is given, then hypokalaemia occurs because insulin and glucose take potassium into the cells.
3   Diuretics, which cause renal excretion of sodium and potassium.
4   Recovery from acute renal failure, which results in a diuresis and loss of potassium.
5   Prolonged i.v. glucose or saline therapy if potassium is not given.
6   Excessive aldosterone secretion (Conn's syndrome).
7   Prolonged corticosteroid therapy.

Clinically: apathy, confusion and drowsiness are due to a low potassium in cerebral cells. A low potassium in renal cells prevents the kidney from reabsorbing sodium and water and causes polyuria and thirst. A low level in muscle causes abdominal distension due to paralytic ileus, and voluntary muscle weakness or paralysis.

Treatment: potassium by mouth is safest; e.g. fruit juices such as pineapple or orange juice, which contain a high concentration of potassium, or potassium chloride or effervescent potassium 0·5–2 g t.d.s. Potassium chloride in glucose may be given i.v. if the rate of infusion is controlled by E.C.G. and blood and urine electrolyte levels.

Hyperkalaemia is a high concentration of potassium in the plasma. Cellular potassium may be low.

Causes:
1 Acute renal failure (the kidneys normally excrete any excess of potassium).
2 Addison's disease. Deficiency of adrenocorticosteroids causes retention of potassium by the kidneys.
3 Circulatory failure, causing a poor renal blood flow.
4 A **falsely** raised level may be due to slight haemolysis of the blood taken for potassium estimation (the red cells contain thirty times the level in the plasma, so slight haemolysis releases much potassium).

Clinically: lethargy, confusion, muscular weakness, irregular slow pulse. Cardiac arrest occurs if the plasma potassium exceeds 10 mmol/l (10 mEq/l).

Treatment is of the cause. In an emergency 10% dextrose and insulin i.v. returns potassium into the cells.

Magnesium Deficiency is due to prolonged diarrhoea or vomiting which has been treated with fluid but not magnesium, prolonged diuretic therapy, or severe undernutrition (malabsorption syndrome, kwashiorkor). It causes mental depression, confusion, convulsions and tremor. The plasma magnesium is below 0·6 mmol/l (1·2 mEq/l). Treatment is with 75 mmol (150 mEq) of magnesium chloride or hydroxide orally daily.

Hypermagnesaemia occurs in renal failure.

Treatment is of the cause.

The Administration of Fluid

Routes:
1 Oral in mild dehydration if the patient can swallow and retain the fluid.
2 Rectal drip may be used.
3 Intravenously in severe dehydration or vomiting. A 'cut down' and cannulation of a vein may be necessary, or in infants a drip into a scalp vein. A catheter passed into the vena cava may be used for concentrated solutions since the solution is less likely to cause thrombosis of the large veins where the blood flow is more rapid.
4 Subcutaneously with hyaluronidase (this process is seldom used now).

Intravenous Infusion. The patient is made comfortable. The procedure and the reason for it is explained. The bedding is protected with a plastic sheet. A vein in the arm is usually used. Clothing is removed from the arm, a sphygmomanometer cuff is applied and inflated to distend the vein so that the needle enters more easily. The cuff is then deflated and removed. Air is removed from the drip tubing by running fluid through it into a receiver, before attaching it to the needle. The drip is usually run at 40–60 drops a minute. The arm is splinted and the lower part of the drip tubing taped to the splint to prevent the patient from pulling out the needle.

Rectal Infusion. Up to 2·5 l (5 pts) of water or one-fifth strength isotonic saline may be absorbed from the rectum in 24 hours. Isotonic saline and dextrose are not as well absorbed. The bowels and bladder are emptied. The patient lies in the left lateral position or on his back. To remove air, liquid is run through the tubing which is then clipped. The lubricated catheter is passed 10 cm (4 in.) into the rectum, The catheter is secured to the skin with tape, and the fluid run in at 37°C at 40–60 drops a minute.

Types of Fluid:

1　Isotonic saline (0·9% sodium chloride). This was incorrectly called normal saline. If several litres are to be given 500 ml of M/6 sodium lactate should be given for every litre of isotonic saline in order to provide the normal ratio of 140 sodium to 100 chloride, as in plasma.

2　5% dextrose (glucose) replaces water without giving salt, and also provides 880 kJ (210 kcal.) per litre.

3　0·18% saline in 4·3% dextrose is isotonic. A normal daily salt and water intake consists of 2–3 l.

4　Sodium lactate M/6 is used to correct metabolic acidosis.

5　Sodium bicarbonate 1·4% is also used to correct metabolic acidosis and is preferable to lactate if there is shock, since lactate may not be metabolised.

6　Potassium chloride 0·3% in dextrose or saline solution is used in hypo-kalaemia. It must not be infused too quickly (1 l must take at least 2 hours to be infused) since there is a danger of hyperkalaemia, which is toxic.

7　Plasma volume expanders such as dextran may be used in an emergency for shock due to burns or haemorrhage, but interferes with blood grouping and cross-matching.

Quantity of Fluid. The normal body loses 2·5 l of fluid and 5 g of salt every 24 hours. More is lost if there is pyrexia or tachypnoea. Therefore 600 ml saline plus 2400 ml 5% dextrose are given if the patient is not dehydrated. If there is dehydration or fluid losses are abnormal (e.g. due to vomiting), then more fluid is needed and the amount is based on a **fluid balance record.** This should state:

1　Intake, by mouth, gastric drip, i.v., rectal, s.c. or intraperitoneal drip.

2　Output in the urine, vomit, faeces, discharges, aspirations, and an allowance made for excessive sweating, burns or haemorrhage.

In each 24-hour period intake should balance output.

ACID–BASE BALANCE

The acidity or alkalinity of a solution depends on how many hydrogen (H) ions it contains, and pH is a measure of this. A neutral substance, such as water, contains $1/10,000,000 (= 1/10^7 = 10^{-7})$ of a gram of H ions in 1 litre, and this is a pH of 7 (neutrality). Acids contain more hydrogen ions and have a pH below 7; e.g. gastric acid (hydrochloric acid) has a pH of 2, which is very acidic. Bases ('alkalis') have fewer hydrogen ions and a pH above 7.

The pH of plasma is normally $7·4 \pm 0·05$ which is slightly alkaline. Under abnormal conditions the pH of the plasma may lie between 7·0 and 7·6, but death is likely outside these limits. Acid is constantly being produced by the body's metabolism and this must be temporarily neutralised (buffered) while it is in the tissues and plasma, and then excreted. A **buffer** is a mixture of acid and base which can neutralise acid *or* base and thus prevent change in pH, e.g. hydrochloric acid (HCl), a strong acid, added to carbonic acid–bicarbonate buffer, forms carbonic acid which is only a weak acid; the acidity is therefore reduced from strong to weak although not eliminated altogether. This reaction can be written as:

$$H^+ \qquad HCO_3^- \qquad H_2CO_3 \text{ carbonic acid}$$
$$+ \qquad = \qquad +$$
$$Cl^- \qquad Na^+ \qquad NaCl \text{ salt}$$

hydrochloric acid   sodium bicarbonate

Other buffers are phosphate and protein.

Excretion of acid is by:

1 The lungs, which excrete carbonic acid as carbon dioxide (CO_2) and water vapour ($H_2CO_3 \rightleftharpoons CO_2 + H_2O$).

2 The kidneys which excrete H ions into the urine as sulphuric acid, phosphoric acid and hydrochloric acid. The kidneys normally reabsorb bicarbonate, but can excrete it if necessary.

Acidosis

Acidosis is the presence of excess of acid in the extracellular fluid. Moderate amounts of acid are buffered and the pH remains in the normal range, but large amounts of acid reduce the plasma pH. A reduced plasma pH is called acidaemia.

Causes are respiratory or metabolic:

A. *Respiratory acidosis* is acidosis due to failure of the lungs to excrete carbon dioxide. The retained CO_2 in solution becomes carbonic acid. This situation occurs when there is inadequate ventilation of the lungs, as in chronic bronchitis and emphysema; asthma; paralysis of respiratory muscles, e.g. poliomyelitis; morphine or barbiturate poisoning. The kidneys compensate to some extent by excreting more acid (H^+ ions) and retaining bicarbonate.

Symptoms are of the cause, e.g. dyspnoea, cyanosis, confusion, and coma due to chronic bronchitis and emphysema.

Treatment is of the cause.

B. *Metabolic acidosis* is acidosis due to:

1 Diabetic acidosis, due to incomplete metabolism of fats with the production of keto-acids, or sometimes to excess of lactic acid.

2 Renal failure, in which there is failure to excrete acid.

3 Inadequate oxidation of pyruvic and lactic acids as in cardiac arrest or hard physical exercise.

4 Ureterocolostomy (transplantation of the ureters into the colon). Urine, and therefore acid, is partly reabsorbed from the colon.

5 Loss of bicarbonate as in severe diarrhoea or renal tubular acidosis; the tubules are abnormal and fail to reabsorb bicarbonate.

6 Salicylate poisoning.

Clinically: hyperpnoea (deep and rapid breathing) is compensatory and removes carbon dioxide. Lethargy, weakness, vomiting, coma.

Treatment is of the cause, and the correction of water and electrolyte imbalance. Isotonic saline is effective since, although it is neutral, the kidney retains the sodium but excretes the chloride in exchange for bicarbonate which is reabsorbed. Sodium bicarbonate may be given. The standard bicarbonate solution (B.P.) is 1·4% and contains 167 mmol/l (mEq/l) of bicarbonate and sodium. The 8·4% bicarbonate used in cardiac arrest and forced alkaline diuresis of salicylate and barbiturate overdose contains 1 mmol/ml (1 mEq/ml) of bicarbonate and is hypertonic. Sodium salts, and especially saline, may be dangerous in renal failure since the kidney may not be able to excrete the sodium (or chloride) and dialysis may be needed.

Alkalosis
Alkalosis is the tendency towards a rise in the pH of the extracellular fluid.

Causes may be respiratory or metabolic:

    A. *Respiratory alkalosis* is due to loss of carbon dioxide ($\equiv$ carbonic acid) via the lungs by hyperventilation (over-breathing). This occurs in hysteria, anxiety, brain damage, salicylate poisoning.

    B. *Metabolic alkalosis.*
      1 Loss of acid is due to repeated vomiting or gastric aspirations.
      2 Gain of bicarbonate is due to excessive intake of sodium bicarbonate (in peptic ulcer) or to hypokalaemia, as in Cushing's syndrome, aldosteronism, and intestinal fistulae (because of the hypokalaemia potassium leaves the cell to enter the e.c.f. and is replaced by hydrogen ions. The hydrogen ions come from carbonic acid and therefore leave excess bicarbonate in the e.c.f.).

Clinically: There is drowsiness, paraesthesiae (numbness, pins and needles) and tetany (due to a low ionised calcium in the plasma) and fits may occur. In metabolic alkalosis respiration is decreased because the body tries to compensate for the alkalosis by retaining carbon dioxide.

Treatment is of the cause; e.g. hysterics should be made to breathe in and out of a paper bag (rebreathing increases the carbon dioxide in the blood). Correction of fluid and electrolyte imbalance. 10 ml 10% calcium chloride i.v. for tetany.

4 BODY TEMPERATURE, INFLAMMATION, IMMUNITY, AND INFECTION

BODY TEMPERATURE

The enzyme systems of the body can only function within a narrow range of temperature, so the normal temperature is regulated at 36·8°C ± 0·6°C (98·1°F) being highest at 6 p.m. and lowest at 3 a.m. The temperature is higher in the rectum than in the mouth and lowest in the axilla, the maximum normal being 37·4°C in the rectum, 36·9°C in the mouth, and 36·7°C in the axilla. A clinical thermometer is often marked '½-minute'; i.e. it will reach its highest reading in half a minute in a water-bath, but in the body heat transfer is slower and takes 2–5 minutes, thus half a minute gives a false low reading. The thermometer should be replaced until a constant reading is obtained. A false high reading occurs after a hot bath or exercise. Muscular exercise may raise the rectal temperature to 38°C or even 40°C. The oral temperature gives false readings for 30 minutes after smoking, mouth breathing or the ingestion of warm or cold food and drink.

Subcutaneous fat acts as an insulator. If the air surrounding the body is cold, the skin temperature may fall to, e.g., 17°C, but the temperature of the body core remains normal. But the *sensation* of heat and cold depends on skin temperature and therefore on skin blood flow; thus dilated vessels in the skin give a feeling of warmth and constricted vessels a feeling of cold, whatever the body temperature is. The optimum skin temperature for comfort is 33°C.

In order to maintain a constant body temperature the heat produced by the body must balance the heat lost.

Heat is Produced by muscular exercise, including shivering, the contractions of muscles of vital organs (diaphragm, heart, gastro-intestinal peristalsis) and by the metabolic processes in all the tissues, especially the liver. The source of heat is the 'burning' of carbohydrate, fat and excess protein for energy.

Heat Loss from the body depends upon the difference between body and environmental temperature, the amount of body surface exposed to the air, and the type of clothing. Air is a poor conductor of heat and air trapped in layers of clothing acts as an insulator. Heat is lost from the body mostly via the skin by radiation, conduction, convection and evaporation, but a little is lost from the lungs in water vapour and warm air expired, and in urine and faeces.

Radiation is the loss of heat by infra-red waves and occurs without the warm body being in contact with anything. The sun's rays reach earth by radiation. White shiny surfaces reflect infra-red waves, therefore less heat is lost or gained. Rough and dark surfaces absorb infra-red waves, therefore more heat is lost or gained.

The skin is rough and acts as a dark object. White clothing is more suitable than black both in the tropics, where less heat will be gained, and in the arctic where less heat will be lost from the body.

Conduction is the transfer of heat to a cooler object in contact with the warmer one.

Convection is the movement of molecules in a gas or liquid, the warmer molecules rising; e.g. hot air rising from a radiator. Similarly, warm air rises from the body. Movement of air (wind, draughts) increases heat loss by convection and evaporation. Clothing traps air and prevents convection.

Evaporation is the change of a liquid into a gas (vapour) and this absorbs a large amount of heat. It occurs easily in a dry atmosphere, but with difficulty in a humid one no matter how much sweat is produced.

Very hot humid climates may cause heatstroke and death.

Temperature Regulation. The body temperature is controlled by the nervous system via the skin. The loss of heat from the skin depends on the amount of blood flowing through it. The greater the blood flow the greater is the heat loss. Blood flow is increased by vasodilatation. Reducing the blood flow, which is by vasoconstriction, reduces heat loss.

Blood flow through the skin is controlled by the temperature-regulating centre ('thermostat') in the hypothalamus which is part of the brain. Temperature-sensitive cells there can detect a difference of $0.1°C$ in the temperature of the blood which it receives from the carotid artery. If the blood is cooler than normal the hypothalamus sends impulses to the vasomotor centre in the medulla oblongata. The vasomotor centre is part of the autonomic nervous system and sends impulses via sympathetic nerves to cause vasoconstriction of the arterioles in the skin, thus reducing the blood flow in the skin and reducing heat losses. If necessary, the temperature-regulating centre also increases heat production by shivering via the motor nerves to the muscles. If the body temperature rises the hypothalamus sends impulses, again by the vasomotor centre, to cause vasodilatation of arterioles in the skin, which increases heat loss from the skin by radiation, conduction and convection. Autonomic impulses also causes sweating which causes further heat loss by evaporation.

Recording the Temperature

Oral Recording. Thermometers are kept dry in individual holders marked with the patient's name. They are changed and cleaned in soap and water on discharge of the patient.

1   The thermometer is taken from the holder and wiped with a swab damped in water from a gallipot.
2   The used swab is placed in a waste receiver.
3   The thermometer is shaken using a wrist action until the mercury is at its lowest level.
4   The patient is asked to hold the thermometer under the tongue, but not to bite on the thermometer.

5 The thermometer is read after two to five minutes by holding it horizontally and rotating it until the mercury column is visible.

6 It is wiped before replacing it in the holder.

7 The reading is recorded on the patient's temperature chart.

Rectal Recording. In children up to three years of age or in adults who are unconscious or restless the rectal temperature is recorded, using a special rectal thermometer. The patient is placed in the lateral position, the thermometer lubricated with a damp swab and gently inserted into the rectum until the bulb of the thermometer is covered. In children the legs are held firmly together. After 2 minutes or longer the thermometer is removed, wiped and read as above.

Axillary Recording is used in children aged three to ten years and where the oral method is impracticable, as in unco-operative patients. The thermometer is placed in the axilla and the patient's arm placed to hold it firmly in position. It is read after five minutes, or when the rise in the mercury column ceases.

Pyrexia

Pyrexia is an increase in temperature above the normal.

Causes:

1 Failure of heat loss due to a high environmental temperature (the body gains more heat than it can lose); excess of clothing (diminished heat loss); dehydration, especially in infants (inability to sweat, also the low blood pressure causes skin vasoconstriction, preventing heat loss); and pontine haemorrhage (damaged nerve fibres descending from the hypothalamic temperature-regulating centre).

2 Excessive heat production: severe exercise, emotional tension (increased muscle tension), thyrotoxic crisis (increased metabolic rate).

3 Reset thermostat due to pyrogens (heat-producers) released from bacteria, damaged body cells (as in infarction) and some tumours. Pyrogens enter the circulation to reach the temperature-regulating centre and 'reset' it to a higher temperature than normal. *Note:* antipyretics, e.g. aspirin, act on the heat-regulating centre to reset it at a lower level.

4 Uncertain causes: severe anaemia, deep venous thrombosis, collagen diseases, some drugs.

P.U.O. (pyrexia of unknown origin) is pyrexia without sufficient symptoms and signs to be able readily to diagnose the cause.

Causes:

1 Infection (the commonest cause), particularly tuberculosis, bacterial endocarditis, brucellosis, typhoid, infectious mononucleosis and other viral infections, pyelonephritis, subclinical viral hepatitis, and malaria. Corticosteroids may mask the signs of infection.

2 Auto-immune diseases, e.g. systemic lupus erythematosus.

3 Malignancy, e.g. Hodgkin's disease, leukaemia and renal carcinoma.

Investigations: a thorough history and examination, blood count (a polymorph leucocytosis is usual in bacterial infection, and a lymphocytosis in viral infection), culture, E.S.R. (erythrocyte sedimentation rate, which is increased in most diseases, thus a high E.S.R. indicates organic disease), serology (agglutination and other tests on serum). Urine for albumin, leucocytes, blood and organisms. Sputum for pus and T.B. Faeces for salmonellae and shigellae. Chest X-ray.

Hyperpyrexia

Hyperpyrexia is a temperature above 41·2°C (106°F). It causes weakness, headache, confusion and finally coma.

Treatment is by sponging with tepid water at about 26°C for 20-minute periods, without drying, so that evaporation cools the body, and by giving abundant fluid.

Hypothermia

This is a subnormal temperature, usually below 35°C. Compensatory shivering and vasoconstriction fail if the body temperature falls below 32°C (90°F), death occurs at 26°C (77°F). A special low-reading thermometer must be used.

Causes:

1   Immersion in water (e.g. shipwreck) causes rapid heat loss.
2   Exposure to cold, wind and rain.
3   Old age. Subcutaneous fat and bodily activity diminish with age, reducing insulation and heat production. Hypothermia occurs if the elderly are in a cold environment, especially if they also have cerebrovascular disease damaging the brain's heat-regulating centre, motor centres (paralysis preventing mobility), or intellectual centres (inadequately clothed because of self-neglect).
4   Hypothyroidism (myxoedema) reduces the metabolic rate, hence less heat is produced.
5   Drugs such as phenothiazines, sedatives and alcohol. These cause vasodilatation, reduce bodily activity and abolish shivering. Anaesthetics or poisons causing coma.
6   Diseases of the nervous system. Mental impairment (failure of subjects to protect themselves from cold), damaged hypothalamus.
7   Shock: trauma, haemorrhage, or surgical operation. In shock there is depression of bodily activity.

Treatment: slowly rewarm, covered with blankets, in a room at 25°C, or in water at 43°C. Oxygen, hydrocortisone, antibiotic. Tri-iodothyronine for myxoedema.

Artificial Hypothermia

This is used in cases of head injury to reduce cerebral metabolism and hence the brain's need for blood, and in surgical operations on the heart and large blood vessels, which allows interruption of the circulation for 15 minutes. The patient is surrounded by ice and covered with a wet sheet cooled by a fan.

INFLAMMATION

Inflammation is the local reaction in the tissues in response to injury. It helps to fight against further injury and aid healing by improving the blood supply to the inflamed area. Sterile inflammation follows injury by mechanical causes (pressure e.g. fractured bone, friction), chemicals (acids, alkalis), thermal causes (burns, frostbite), radiation (X-rays, radium), or hypersensitivity (allergy, e.g. allergy to grass pollen causes hay fever or asthma). Inflammation also follows infection by bacteria, fungi and viruses. It may be pyogenic (pus-forming) in acute infection, e.g. a boil, or granulomatous (forming granulation tissue) in chronic infection, e.g. tuberculosis. Granulation tissue also forms in sterile wound healing, in a thrombus and in infarcted (dead) tissue.

Mechanisms of Acute Inflammation. Damaged cells release histamine and kinins which dilate arterioles, capillaries and venules, thus increasing the blood flow in the area which causes the part to be red, hot and pulsating. The increased blood flow brings more oxygen, glucose and other nutrients to the inflamed part as well as antibodies and leucocytes (leuco = white, cyte = cell) to combat infection. Histamine and kinins also increase the permeability of the capillaries so that fluid (plasma) escapes from the blood into the tissues, providing the tissues with extra nutrients and antibodies; but this also causes swelling (oedema) and pain. Thus the signs of inflammation are redness, heat, swelling and pain. There is also loss of function of the part due to the mechanical effects of swelling and to reflex inhibition of muscles by pain, and this helps to rest the part, thus aiding healing.

Leucocytes can migrate from the blood, passing between the capillary endothelial cells into the inflamed tissue (*Fig. 4.1*). Large numbers of neutrophil polymorphs do this in bacterial infection and ingest (phagocytose) the bacteria. This may kill the polymorphs as well as the bacteria, and dead polymorphs which have given up their lives for the sake of the body, bacteria and dead tissue cells and particles, form

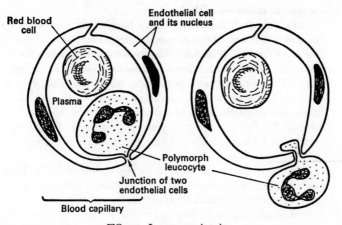

FIG. 4.1   Leucocyte migration

pus. An abscess is a collection of pus. Eosinophil polymorphs (eosinophils) enter the tissues from the blood in allergic inflammation where there is either insoluble foreign protein, e.g. pollen, or an antigen–antibody reaction is occurring. Eosinophils are attracted towards histamine and inactivate it; they are found in the sputum in asthma. Lymphocytes enter the tissue in chronic infection, e.g. tuberculosis.

Where there has been destruction of tissue, healing occurs by the formation of vascular young connective (granulation) tissue which finally becomes a fibrous tissue scar. Granulation and fibrous tissue formation in chronic inflammation, e.g. chronic peptic ulcer, is an attempt at healing.

The body 'cavities' are lined by membranes—the pleura, pericardium, peritoneum and synovial membranes of joints—and exudation of plasma may occur through inflamed membranes to produce effusions, e.g. pleural effusion.

IMMUNITY

Immunity is resistance to disease, particularly infectious disease.

Factors Influencing Immunity to Micro-Organisms

A.   The Organism

1   The number of organisms; and

2   Their virulence (ability to cause disease). The larger the infecting dose and the more virulent the organism the more likely it is to cause disease.

3   The portal of entry; e.g. many organisms enter the stomach only to be killed by gastric acid; the same organisms if entering the lung may cause pneumonia.

4   Products of the organism; e.g. hyaluronidase is an enzyme produced by haemolytic streptococci and allows the organism to spread by dissolving connective tissue.

B.   Non-specific resistance of the Host

1   Genetic (inherited) factors; e.g. many Negroes are resistant to malaria because their red blood cells contain an unusual haemoglobin (HbS) which the malarial parasite (*Plasmodium falciparum*) is unable to metabolise.

2   General health. Correct nutrition: adequate protein, fat, carbohydrate, minerals and vitamins, without an excess. Adequate sunlight, exercise and fresh air. Sunlight kills bacteria, including those on the skin, and also causes advantageous metabolic changes in substances in the skin, e.g. it makes vitamin D. Polluted air predisposes to respiratory disease, especially bronchitis. Resistance is lowered by cold and damp, by diabetes mellitus, chronic renal failure and Addison's disease.

3   Skin and mucous membranes act as barriers to infection, aided by mucus and cilia on respiratory mucosal cells. Cilia are fine hairs which mechanically remove particles; mucus is sticky and traps particles (*Fig. 4.2*).

4   Microbicidal (microbe-killing) substances in the body secretions and plasma; e.g. gastric hydrochloric acid kills many organisms, fatty acids on

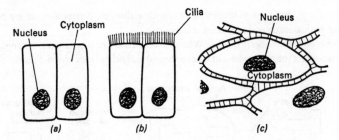

FIG. 4.2   Epithelium: (*a*) columnar; (*b*) ciliated columnar; (*c*) squamous

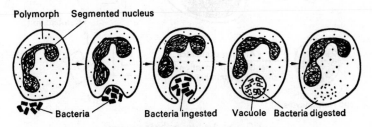

FIG. 4.3   Phagocytosis

the skin destroy some (e.g. streptococci). Lysozyme is an enzyme which kills cocci and is present in saliva, nasal mucus, and tears.

5   Microbicidal substances liberated from damaged tissues, e.g. lysozyme, phagocytins, and blood lysins (e.g. complement).

6   The normal flora (the bacteria normally present in a given site) has antibiotic activity which prevents the growth of certain pathogens, thus if the organisms normally present in the mouth are killed by antibiotic drugs then monilia (Candida, 'thrush') can grow.

7   Phagocytosis. Polymorphs and monocytes ingest ('eat', phagocytose) bacteria and digest them (*Fig. 4.3*). A low white cell count in the blood (leucopenia) predisposes to infection.

8   Interferon is secreted by cells and acts against viruses.

C.   Specific Resistance. Foreign protein (antigen), such as bacteria, causes two main types of response in the body:

1   Humoral immunity (antibody formation).
2   Cellular immunity.

1 Humoral Immunity. Antibodies and *antitoxins* are immunoglobulins (gamma-globulins) which circulate in the blood plasma. Antibodies act against particles, e.g. bacteria, whereas antitoxins act against dissolved toxins. Each antibody acts against a specific antigen; e.g. diphtheria antibody acts only against diphtheria bacilli, diphtheria antitoxin acts only against diphtheria toxin.

Antibodies act not only against bacteria but also against other foreign proteins as in allergy, or against transplanted organs, e.g. renal transplant, and sometimes against the body's own tissues (= auto-immune disease). Antibodies act by combining with antigen and rendering it harmless.

Formation of antibodies (Fig. 4.4). When bacteria enter the tissues some are engulfed by phagocytes (polymorphs and macrophages) and others are carried directly along

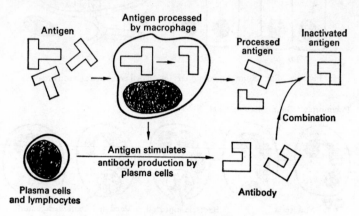

FIG. 4.4   Antigen–antibody response

the lymphatics to the lymph nodes. In the lymph nodes toxins or bacteria and their phagocytosed breakdown products, cause the multiplication of B-lymphocytes (these are lymphocytes which make serum antibodies) and the formation of plasma cells. Lymphocytes and plasma cells then make antibodies which are released into the plasma to circulate as gamma-globulin (γ-globulin) and to act against the specific bacteria causing the infection. This is natural active immunity, i.e. the body has produced *its own* antibodies because of natural infection. *Active immunity* can also be produced artificially by vaccination. A vaccine of dead organisms, of living organisms which have been attenuated (rendered harmless), or of toxin (also first rendered harmless) can be injected. The injected organisms or toxins pass along the lymphatic vessels to the lymph nodes and, just as in natural infection, antibodies and antitoxins are made by the lymphocytes and plasma cells. This is artificial active immunity (it is active immunity because the body itself has produced antibodies).

Passive immunity is quite different and is provided by the injection of antibody (serum or γ-globulin) obtained from animals or from other humans. The patient is receiving antibody, not making it himself; therefore this is passive immunity and it is artificial (injected). Infants under three to six months of age do not produce antibody but rely on passive immunity provided by γ-globulin received from the mother across the placenta during fetal life. Specific immunity therefore may be (1) *active*; or (2) *passive*, and active immunity may either (*a*) be due to natural infection or (*b*) be produced artificially by vaccination (*Fig. 4.5*).

Vaccination (Table 4.1) is used in the prevention of smallpox, diphtheria, whooping cough, tetanus, measles, rubella, poliomyelitis, typhoid, cholera and yellow fever. Passive immunity is used in rubella, measles, virus hepatitis, diphtheria and

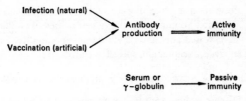

FIG. 4.5   Immunogenesis

TABLE 4.1   *Active immunisation schedule*

Age	Vaccine
6 months	Triple vaccine* 0·5 ml i.m. or s.c., plus poliomyelitis (Sabin vaccine) 3 drops on a lump of sugar orally.
8 months	Triple vaccine 0·5 ml. Poliomyelitis.
12–20 months	Triple vaccine 0·5 ml. Poliomyelitis.
15 months	Measles 0·5 ml i.m. or s.c.
2 and 5 years	Smallpox (in endemic areas only).
5 years	Diphtheria/tetanus 0·5 ml, poliomyelitis.
12 years	Rubella 0·5 ml s.c. to girls only.
13 years	B.C.G.† 0·1 ml i.d., if tuberculin negative.
15–19 years	Tetanus 0·5 ml i.m. or s.c. plus poliomyelitis.

* Triple vaccine = Diphtheria, pertussis and tetanus (D.P.T.).
† B.C.G. = Bacille Calmette Guérin; an attenuated bovine tubercle bacillus.

tetanus. Its action lasts only a short time—up to one month, whereas active immunity lasts for months or years.

2   *Cellular Immunity* is provided by small lymphocytes (T-lymphocytes). These fight fungal and viral infections and are also the cause of the rejection of kidney and heart transplants and of delayed allergic reactions.

Disorders of Immunity

Allergy (hypersensitivity) means an abnormal reaction. Persons with an allergy develop symptoms and signs to substances which do not affect normal people. An allergic reaction may occur in almost any tissue in the body, including skin (eczema, urticaria, contact dermatitis), joints (serum sickness) and respiratory system (hay fever, asthma). Allergens (the substances causing the allergy) include food (eggs, shellfish, strawberries), pollens (especially grass), dust (dandruff from the skins of dogs and cats), drugs (penicillin, streptomycin), chemicals (washing powders, industrial chemicals), and cement.

Treatment: ephedrine, antihistamines (e.g. Phenergan), corticosteroids, desensitisation—a series of small doses of allergen are injected as a 'vaccine'.

Anaphylaxis (anaphylactic shock) is sudden collapse, shock, and spasm of bronchi which may be fatal. It follows the second injection of foreign protein, e.g. anti-tetanus serum, insect stings; the first dose having sensitised the patient, in 10 days, to the protein. Prevention is by giving a small test dose (0·1 ml) of serum s.c. (subcutaneously) and after 10 minutes noting whether there is swelling around the injection site or an increased pulse rate. If symptoms appear allergy is present, and serum must not be given, except under special circumstances.

Treatment: adrenaline s.c., corticosteroid (e.g. prednisolone), antihistamine.

Autoimmune Disease is due to antibodies acting against the body's own tissues. These autoantibodies are made by lymphocytes 'by mistake' and occur in acute nephritis, rheumatoid arthritis, some haemolytic anaemias, systemic lupus erythematosus, hypothyroidism, and pernicious anaemia.

Reduced Immunity may be due to certain drugs, e.g. corticosteroids and anti-mitotic drugs such as azathioprine and methotrexate; these suppress specific immunity and are therefore used to prevent the rejection of tissue transplants. Immunity is reduced by splenectomy (since the spleen makes lymphocytes), irradiation of lymphoid tissue, or by giving antilymphocytic serum (serum containing antibodies to lymphocytes). Agammaglobulinaemia (no γ-globulin in the blood) is a rare disease in which there is congenitally defective development of B-lymphocytes (antibody-forming lymphocytes). All these conditions cause suscepti-bility to bacterial infection.

Immune Serum

Serum is the liquid part of the blood after removal of the clot. It is plasma which has lost its fibrinogen. Immune serum is serum containing an unusually high concentration of antibody.

Horse serum is used to provide temporary passive immunity in diphtheria, tetanus and gas gangrene. Horses are injected with antigen, e.g. diphtheria toxin, and respond by making antitoxin. Blood is taken from the horses and the serum, containing antitoxin, is separated. Unfortunately horse serum differs from that of humans and when injected into man it acts as a foreign protein and may cause a reaction. The reaction may be acute (anaphylactic shock) and severe enough to kill the patient. Thus to test for sensitivity a small test dose must be given first. If any reaction then occurs no serum should be given, except under special circumstances.

Antilymphocytic serum (A.L.S.) is made by immunising horses with human lymphocytes. The serum is used to counter the rejection of organ transplants, but has its own complications.

Human γ-globulin is extracted from human serum and contains concentrated antibodies. It is less likely to cause reactions than is horse serum, and is given to provide passive immunity in measles, rubella, poliomyelitis and infectious hepatitis, if the contact has not previously had the disease (in which case he would already have circulating antibodies). It is given to children in whom measles would be dangerous (those with chronic heart or lung diseases), to women during the first three months of pregnancy, since rubella may cause congenital malformations in the fetus, and to hepatitis and unvaccinated poliomyelitis contacts. Concentrated human anti-D globulin is given to prevent haemolytic disease of the newborn ('rhesus babies').

INFECTION

Infection is the entry of pathogenic micro-organisms into the body, but infection does not necessarily cause disease since the host may immediately overcome it.

Micro-organisms are present in soil, town air, bowel, on the skin, the ground and furnishings. Some are completely harmless, others are harmless only while in their normal habitat but cause infection if they enter certain tissues. Staphylococci are normally present on the skin and in the nose without harm, but if they enter a wound may cause an abscess. *E. coli* are normally present in the bowel, but may cause cystitis and pyelonephritis on entering the bladder or kidney. Organisms capable of causing disease are called pathogens. Any disease due to micro-organisms is infec*tive*, i.e. capable of being spread, but only those which are easily spread are called infec*tious* diseases.

Infection may be *sporadic*, i.e. a few scattered and unrelated cases occur, *endemic* when a few cases repeatedly occur in the same area, *epidemic* when many cases occur together, and *pandemic* when large areas of the world are affected.

Types of Pathogenic Microbes (*Fig. 4.6*)

A   Protozoa, e.g. Amoeba, Malaria, Giardia, Trichomonas.

B   Bacteria.
1. Cocci. Spheres 1 um (micrometre) in diameter, e.g. staphylococci, which grow in bunches; streptococci, which form chains; diplococci, in pairs (pneumococci, gonococci, meningococci).
2. Bacilli. Rods 3 μm long by 0·5 μm wide, e.g. tubercle bacilli, typhoid, *E. coli*, and the rickettsiae, which are smaller. Some bacilli form spores which resist drying and survive a long time, e.g. anthrax, tetanus.
3. Spirochaetes. Spirals, e.g. treponema (syphilis, leptospira).
4. Vibrio. Comma-shaped, e.g. cholera.

C   Fungi. Fungi have hyphae (filaments) and spores, e.g. Candida (monilia), Tinea (ringworm).

D   Viruses. These are very tiny organisms which cannot be seen through the ordinary microscope but can be seen by using an electron microscope.

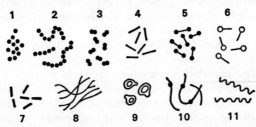

FIG. 4.6   Types of bacteria: (1) Staphylococci; (2) Streptococci; (3) Diplococci; (4) Bacilli; (5) Diphtheria; (6) Tetanus; (7) Anthrax; (8) Actinomyces; (9 and 10) Candida; (11) Spirochaete

Source, Mode of Spread and Entrance of Infection

1 Inhalation into the respiratory tract of droplets sprayed into the air by sneezing, coughing, talking or spitting. Dried droplets, i.e. dust, may remain suspended in the air for days. Brushing floors with a dry brush or dusting with a dry duster disperses dust into the atmosphere and these methods should not be used.

'Wet' methods avoid this; for example mop and bucket, damp dusting. Droplets and dust spread measles, influenza, colds, smallpox, diphtheria, whooping cough, human tuberculosis.

2 Ingestion of food, milk and water contaminated with faecal and other organisms such as typhoid, dysentery, cholera and poliomyelitis. Faecal contamination may occur through cracked drains leaking into a water supply, unwashed hands of food-handlers, shellfish from contaminated rivers. Bovine tuberculosis spreads via milk which has not been properly pasteurised.

3 Implantation of dirt or dust into wounds, or direct contact, e.g. staphylococci, streptococci, E. coli, Proteus vulgaris, tetanus, gas gangrene.

4 Direct contact, e.g. infectious mononucleosis transferred by kissing; syphilis, gonorrhoea and trichomonas by venereal contact; scabies by skin contact. Spread from maternal blood across the placenta to the fetus, e.g. syphilis, rubella.

5 Fomites—inanimate articles, e.g. clothing, furniture, tableware, drinking-glasses, catheter.

6 Injection—by insects, e.g. malaria and yellow fever by mosquitoes; plague by fleas; serum hepatitis by blood transfusion.

Clinical Effects of Infection

The incubation period is the time between infection and the appearance of symptoms and signs. Microbes may cause only local signs of inflammation, as in a boil; or both local and general signs as in streptococcal sore throat. In this condition the infection is localised to the throat but general symptoms such as pyrexia, headache and skin rash (= scarlet fever) occur, and acute nephritis may follow two weeks later.

Pyrexia is caused by a resetting of the thermostat of the temperature-regulating centre in the hypothalamus. This causes vasoconstriction of the skin which conserves heat. In addition rigors (shivering) may occur and increase heat production. Pyrexia, within reasonable limits, increases the body's metabolism, thus increasing antibody production.

The skin is hot, flushed and dry at first, but sweating occurs later, and the temperature falls.

There is tachycardia which is partly due to toxaemia and partly to the pyrexia which increases the body's metabolic rate and blood flow. Increased respirations are partly due to the increased metabolic rate causing production of carbon dioxide and an increased need for oxygen. A dry furred tongue and concentrated urine are common, and are signs of dehydration due to increased loss of fluid from the skin and from the lungs and to decreased fluid intake due to illness.

Consequence of Infection

1 Healing (resolution).

2 Suppuration, i.e. the formation of pus.

3 Secondary infection of inflamed tissue by another pathogen.

4 Spread of infection, e.g. an infection in the nose may spread to the sinuses (sinusitis), larynx (laryngitis), or pharynx (pharyngitis). These are upper respiratory tract infections (U.R.T.I.). Spread from the pharynx along the Eustachian tube may cause otitis media. Spread into the lymphatics to the glands in the neck causes cervical adenitis. U.R.T.I. may descend to the trachea (tracheitis), bronchi (bronchitis) and lungs (pneumonia, pneumonitis). Pneumonia is especially liable to occur if there is pain or weakness which prevents the coughing-up of secretions from the trachea and bronchi, or if there is shallow respiration, since this causes alveolar atelectasis and pulmonary congestion which predispose to infection.

5 Fibrosis, i.e. healing by the replacement of destroyed tissue with fibrous tissue which contracts to form a scar.

6 Organisms may spread to other tissues if they enter the bloodstream (septicaemia).

Prevention of Infection

General:

1 At ports and frontiers: prohibit importation of parrots (psittacosis), dogs (rabies), and monkeys (yellow fever). Report illness on ship or aircraft. Landing permission by the community medical officer of environmental health. Contacts are either isolated for the incubation period of the disease (= period of quarantine) by which time the disease (if present) will show itself, or are vaccinated and kept under observation.

2 Notification of certain infectious diseases to the community medical officer, i.e. acute encephalitis, acute meningitis, acute poliomyelitis, cholera, dysentery, typhoid, paratyphoid, typhus, anthrax, diphtheria, infective jaundice, leprosy, leptospirosis, malaria, measles, ophthalmia neonatorum, plague, relapsing fever, scarlet fever, smallpox, tetanus, tuberculosis, whooping cough, rabies, Lassa fever and yellow fever.

3 Strict isolation in an isolation ward is required for diphtheria, measles, tuberculous meningitis, mumps, smallpox, 'open' pulmonary tuberculosis, whooping cough, herpes zoster, typhoid, paratyphoid, and cholera. Barrier nursing in a side room is satisfactory in infectious hepatitis, leprosy, and haemolytic streptococcal infection (scarlet fever, erysipelas). The isolation period for some commoner diseases is given in *Table 4.2*.

4 Carriers are treated and prohibited from handling food. Chronic carriers are individuals who have a pathogenic (disease-causing) organism in their body but are not themselves suffering from disease because of natural resistance or acquired immunity due to previous infection. They transmit typhoid, paratyphoid, diphtheria, meningococci and staphylococci. Patients who are recovering from an infection are 'convalescent' carriers.

TABLE 4.2   *Incubation, quarantine and isolation periods*

Disease	Incubation period (days)	Quarantine period (days)	Isolation period
Diphtheria	2–4	7	Until bacilli are absent from nose and throat, usually 4–5 weeks
Scarlet fever	2–4	7	2–4 weeks
Whooping cough	7–14	15	3–4 weeks
Measles	10–14	16	7 days from the appearance of the rash.
Rubella	14–21	21	5 days.
Smallpox	10–14	14	Until all scars have healed.
Chickenpox	14–21	16	Until all scars have healed.
Mumps	16–21	25	9 days from onset of swelling.
Typhoid	10–14	—	Until bacilli are absent from 6 consecutive daily faeces, usually 6 weeks.

5 Control of food, milk, and water by regional health authorities. Healthy cattle (tuberculous cattle are slaughtered), pasteurised milk, cows milked by machine (sterilised) not by hand. Food cooked. General cleanliness. Water supply filtered through sand and chlorinated.

6 Adequate sanitation and sewage disposal.

7 Control of insects with insecticides, e.g. malathion for mosquitoes and flies.

8 Avoidance of overcrowding which facilitates the spread of disease.

9 Education of the public in hygiene and the benefits of vaccination.

Specific: by immunisation using vaccines. A vaccine may consist of attenuated live organisms (B.C.G., vaccinia, poliomyelitis) or dead organisms, e.g. typhoid and paratyphoid A and B (T.A.B.). A timetable for active immunisation of children is shown in *Table 4.1*, p. 37.

General Treatment of Infection
The origin and cause of infection must be found and contacts vaccinated in order to prevent spread to others (prophylaxis). The disease itself and its complications are treated (specific therapy), and unpleasant symptoms alleviated (symptomatic treatment).

Precautions Taken to Prevent Spread of Infection in the Isolation Unit
Good ventilation of each room, preferably with an extractor fan, prevents contaminated air from entering the rest of the ward and reduces the risk of airborne infection of the other patients and staff. All staff and visitors are taught isolation technique. The thermometer is kept in the cubicle. Gowns are kept in the cubicle. On taking them off only the outside should be handled, and the inside is considered clean and hung folded inward. Masks must be worn to protect the attendant. Paper masks are burnt. After each visit to the patient, the hands and arms must be scrubbed with soap and water, having removed the gown and dealth with crockery, linen, excreta, etc. The washbasin is outside the room. Feeding utensils—crockery and cutlery—are marked and are boiled after each use. Bedpans and urinals should be sterilised with steam or placed in disinfectant such as cresol 1·25% or lysol 5%.

Excreta—stools, urine, vomit, sputum, and discharges are mixed with 5% lysol or cresol and left for two hours. Linen is placed in a mobile tank containing formalin, 5% phenol or 1·25% sudol for two hours, or in plastic bags, sealed and marked 'infectious', and sent to the laundry for disinfection and boiling or autoclaving. Blankets are autoclaved. Autoclaving is the use of steam under pressure for 30 minutes, e.g. steam at 2·3 kg pressure has a temperature of 106°C. Handkerchiefs should be of paper, placed in a paper bag and burnt. Newspapers, books and toys must be burnt or capable of being disinfected. Mattresses should be in a complete plastic cover and wiped with hypochlorite, 5% lysol or formalin and left for two hours. Other mattresses and pillows are autoclaved. Furniture, such as the table and bed, is wiped with 5% phenol or lysol then scrubbed with soap and water. Floors are disinfected by regular mopping with lysol or white cyllin (crude cresols). Gaseous ethylene oxide is used for materials and instruments which do not tolerate heat. When the patient is discharged, thermometers, B.L.B. oxygen masks and stethoscopes are wiped with disinfectant then washed with soap and water, and the room fumigated with formaldehyde and left for 24 hours.

Prevention of spread of infection both in isolation and in general wards also includes the avoidance of creating dust—'wet' methods are used for cleaning floors and furnishings. Dirty and clean work should not be done at the same time, and dressings should be done before bedmaking, which causes dust. Staff with infections should not do the dressings. Use of clean operation on wounds using sterile instruments and techniques. Sterilisation using ultraviolet light, dry heat, moist heat (boiling, steaming, or autoclaving), filtration for liquids, chemicals—formalin, phenol, lysol, iodine, alcohol, chlorhexidine ('Hibitane'—this is inactive against tubercle bacilli, viruses, and spores). Instruments must be dismantled before sterilisation. Beds a minimum of 1·2 m (4 ft) apart.

Patient Care. Rest in bed helps the body to combat disease, but predisposes to stiff joints, weak muscles, bedsores, constipation and venous thrombosis, especially in the elderly. Therefore ambulation should be as early as possible.

Well ventilated, warm (60°F, 16°C) room.

Care of the mouth, skin and bowels.

Sedation provides rest and helps to keep the temperature down. Tepid sponging for hyperpyrexia.

Fluid intake should be high to prevent dehydration due to sweating and apathy (the patient is too ill to be bothered to drink).

Electrolyte balance (sodium, potassium) must be maintained. Diet should be suitable for the particular disease, e.g. low residue in typhoid (to reduce the possibility of bowel haemorrhage), high calorie if there is weight loss or pyrexia (pyrexia increases the metabolic rate and therefore the need for calories and fluid), and adequate protein to reduce muscle-wasting and allow healing of tissues. Vitamins A, B, and C, for healthy metabolism and repair of tissues.

Local treatment of an infected area: rest (immobilise) in the position of function (e.g. arm in a sling) to relieve pain and swelling. Local heat for comfort. Prevention of further (secondary) infection by covering with dressings, using sterile precautions, including masks worn by the staff and patients.

Antitoxin when applicable. Chemotherapy—sulphonamide or antibiotic. Rehabilitation to return the patient to the maximum degree of fitness as soon as possible.

ANTIBIOTICS

Antibiotics are drugs which kill bacteria, or prevent their growth. Sulphonamides are antibiotics although they are usually spoken of as a separate group, i.e. chemotherapy.

Bacteria may have a *natural resistance* to an antibiotic, e.g. pseudomonas to penicillin, or may *acquire resistance*, e.g. some staphylococci to penicillin; therefore the organisms should be tested for sensitivity to antibiotics so that the correct one can be given.

Antibiotics which are poorly absorbed will remain in the gut and thus kill certain of the organisms normally present in the gut (= the normal flora) causing an imbalance which allows other organisms to take over, and these may cause disease (e.g. Candida, staphylococcal enteritis).

Table 4.3 shows the most suitable choice of antibiotic for given infections.

The most important antibiotics are benzylpenicillin, ampicillin, erythromycin, streptomycin, and tetracycline. The most important sulphonamides are sulphadimidine and co-trimoxazole.

1   Penicillins

These are active against cocci (streptococci, pneumococci, gonococci, meningococci and some staphylococci). Their action is prolonged by giving probenecid (Benemid) which reduces the urinary excretion of penicillins.

Side-effects: penicillins are the least toxic of all the antibiotics but may cause allergy—urticarial rash, arthralgia, and anaphylactic shock (rare).

Benzylpenicillin (Penicillin G) is mostly destroyed by gastric acid and is therefore given intramuscularly. It is the first choice for infection with β-haemolytic streptococci, pneumococci, *Streptococcus viridans*, syphilis, sensitive staphylococci, anthrax, actinomyces, diphtheria, and *Clostridium welchii*. Some staphylococci are insensitive to penicillin since they produce penicillinase, an enzyme which destroys penicillin.

Dose: 300 mg (0·5 mega units, Mu) eight-hourly intramuscularly. Up to 6 g (10 Mu) daily may be used for certain infections, e.g. bacterial endocarditis.

Procaine Penicillin is slowly absorbed after i.m. injection, thus giving a more prolonged action (24 hours) than benzylpenicillin.

Dose: 900 mg daily i.m.

Benzathine Penicillin has a very long action—up to four weeks, according to dose.

Dose: 900 mg (1·2 Mu) i.m. two to four times weekly.

TABLE 4.3   *Choice of antibiotics*

Organisms	First choice	Antibiotics Second choice(s)	Others
GRAM-POSITIVE COCCI			
Pneumococcus	Penicillin	Erythromycin,	Streptomycin
Streptococcus viridans		Sulphadimidine,	Tetracycline
Haemolytic streptococcus		Co-trimoxazole	Cephalosporins
Staphylococcus-Penicillinase neg.			
Staphylococcus-producing Penicillinase	Methicillin Flucloxacillin	Erythromycin Gentamicin	Lincomycin, Fucidin
Streptococcus faecalis	Penicillin+ Streptomycin Ampicillin	Penicillin+ Kanamycin Carbenicillin	Sulphonamides Co-trimoxazole Vancomycin
GRAM-NEGATIVE COCCI			
Gonococcus	Penicillin	Erythromycin,	Ampicillin,
Meningococcus		Sulphadimidine	Tetracycline
GRAM-NEGATIVE BACILLI			
Bacteroides	Tetracycline	Mezlocillin	Erythromycin
Brucella	Tetracycline	Streptomycin+ Sulphadimidine	Co-trimoxazole
E. coli (a) Sepsis	Ampicillin	Kanamycin	Gentamicin
(b) Urinary	Sulphadimidine, Co-trimoxazole	Nalidixic acid, Streptomycin	Nitrofurantoin, Ampicillin
Haemophilus influenzae	Ampicillin Sulphadimidine	Co-trimoxazole Tetracycline	Streptomycin Chloramphenicol
Klebsiella	Cephalosporin+ Ampicillin	Tetracycline+ Streptomycin	Gentamicin Co-trimoxazole
Proteus mirabilis (a) Sepsis	Penicillin	Ampicillin	Kanamycin
(b) Urinary	Sulphadimidine	Nalidixic acid	Streptomycin
Proteus vulgaris and others	Kanamycin	Gentamicin	Co-trimoxazole
Pseudomonas	Carbenicillin Mezlocillin	Gentamicin Tobramycin	Streptomycin Polymyxin
Salmonella	Ampicillin	Chloramphenicol Tetracycline	Streptomycin Sulphonamides
Shigella	Ampicillin	Tetracycline	Streptomycin
GRAM-POSITIVE BACILLI			
Actinomyces	Penicillin	Tetracycline	Sulphadimidine
Anthrax	Penicillin	Erythromycin	Tetracycline
Clostridia (tetanus, gas gangrene)	Penicillin	Erythromycin Carbenicillin	Ampicillin Tetracycline
Diphtheria	Penicillin	Erythromycin	Ampicillin
RICKETTSIAE	Tetracycline	—	Chloramphenicol
SYPHILIS	Penicillin	Erythromycin	Tetracycline
TUBERCLE BACILLUS	Streptomycin+ I.N.H.+P.A.S.	Ethambutol Rifampicin	Pyrazinamide
FUNGI			
Tinea	Griseofulvin	Econazole	
Candida	Nystatin	Amphotericin B	
VIRUSES			
Herpetic keratitis	Iododeoxyuridine		
Smallpox prophylaxis	Methisazone		

Phenoxymethyl Penicillin (penicillin V), **Phenethicillin** (Broxil), **Phenbenicillin** (Penspek), **Propicillin** (Ultrapen, Brocillin) all resist gastric acid and are given orally, but do not provide as high a concentration in the blood as does injected penicillin; they are better used only in mild infections.

Dose: 250–500 mg six-hourly.

Methicillin (Celbenin), **Cloxacillin** (Orbenin), and **Flucloxacillin** (Floxapen) are not inactivated by penicillinase and are used in place of other penicillins when there is penicillinase-producing staphylococcal infection (sometimes called 'resistant' staphylococci).

Dose: Methicillin: 1 g four-hourly i.m. or i.v. (destroyed by gastric acid). Cloxacillin: 500 mg six-hourly orally or 250–500 mg six-hourly i.m. Flucloxacillin: 250 mg six-hourly orally or i.m.

Ampicillin (Penbritin), **Amoxycillin** (Amoxil) and **Mezlocillin** have a broad spectrum and are active against bacilli—shigella, salmonella, *H. influenzae*, some *E. coli* and proteus—as well as cocci, but are destroyed by penicillinase.

Dose: Ampicillin: 0·5–1·5 g eight-hourly orally or 250–500 mg six-hourly i.m. In penicillinase-producing staphylococcal mixed infection it is combined with cloxacillin (Ampiclox). Amoxycillin: 250 mg eight-hourly.

Carbenicillin (Pyopen) and **Ticarcillin** also have a broad spectrum and are active against cocci and bacilli including *Pseudomonas aeruginosa* and proteus.

Dose: Carbenicillin: 2 g six-hourly i.m., or 12 to 30 g by i.v. infusion daily.

Carfecillin (uticillin) 500–1000 mg t.d.s. orally for urinary infection.

Mecillinam (Selexid) is effective against Gram-negative bacteria.

Cephalosporins

These have a similar action to ampicillin but resist penicillinase.

Use: penicillinase-producing staphylococcal infection and in patients allergic to penicillin.

Side-effects: rash, pain on i.m. injection, thrombophlebitis, nephrotoxicity at doses above 6 g daily.

Dose: Cefuroxime (Zinacef) 750 to 1500 mg t.d.s. i.m. Cephalothin (Keflin) 1–2 g six-hourly i.m. or i.v. Cephalexin (Ceporex, Keflex) 1 g six-hourly orally. Cefazolin (Kefzol) 500 mg six- to twelve-hourly i.m.

2   Aminoglycosides

Active against cocci and bacilli, including tubercle bacilli, but are not absorbed orally.

Side-effects: rash (nurses who regularly handle streptomycin may get dermatitis), eighth nerve damage—vestibular disturbance first, then deafness, especially if there is renal insufficiency since these drugs are largely eliminated in the urine.

Streptomycin (Soluvone, Strepolin) is used with penicillin in respiratory tract infections—bronchitis, and pneumonia. Tubercle bacilli rapidly become resistant to streptomycin alone, but not if it is given with other drugs (P.A.S., I.N.H.). Dihydrostreptomycin is obsolete owing to ototoxicity.

Dose: 0·5 g b.d., i.m. Oral streptomycin is used in gut infections.

Kanamycin (Kannasyn, Kantrex) is toxic. It is used in serious Gram-negative infections except pseudomonas.

Dose: 0·5–1 g i.m. twelve-hourly.

Gentamicin (Genticin, Cidomycin), 80 mg i.m. eight-hourly, is used in serious Gram-negative infections, e.g. *Pseudomonas aeruginosa*, but is toxic to the kidney and vestibular nerve. A cream is used for topical infections.

Tobramycin (Obracin), 4 mg per kg daily i.m. or by i.v. infusion, is similar.

Neomycin (Neomin) is too toxic for injection, but is used orally in hepatic failure and *E. coli* enteritis, since it is poorly absorbed from the gut, and topically in skin infection.

Dose: 0·5–2 g six-hourly orally.

Paromomycin is similar to neomycin.

3 Tetracyclines

These have a very wide spectrum. They are active against cocci (but penicillin is more active), bacilli, rickettsiae, mycoplasmas, psittacosis and lymphogranuloma venereum, but not against pseudomonas and some proteus. They are used in low dosage over months in acne vulgaris.

Side-effects: nausea, vomiting, loose stools due to a laxative action, diarrhoea due to staphylococcal or pseudomonas enterocolitis; this does not occur until after several days of oral treatment and is due to alteration in the bowel flora with only resistant organisms remaining. Loss of the normal flora may also cause superinfection of the mouth and anus with candida, and vitamin B deficiency. Tetracyclines cause staining of the teeth and bones in young children. Outdated tetracycline may cause renal damage.

Dose: tetracycline (Achromycin) 250 mg six-hourly orally, or i.v. in 0·9% saline or 5% dextrose. Chlortetracycline (Aureomycin) and oxytetracyline (Terramycin) 250–500 mg six-hourly. Methacycline (Rondomycin) 150–300 mg six-hourly orally. Demethylchlortetracycline (Ledermycin) 300 mg b.d. orally. Doxycycline (Vibramycin) 200 mg stat. then 100 mg daily.

4 Macrolides

Macrolides are active against Gram-positive organisms including penicillinase-producing staphylococci, but are less effective than penicillin. They are used in place of penicillin in penicillin allergy. Resistance to erythromycin rapidly develops.

Side-effects: fever, diarrhoea (especially with lincomycin), cholestatic jaundice (with erythromycin estolate but not plain erythromycin). They have to be given 30 minutes before meals since they are slowly destroyed by gastric acid.

Dose: erythromycin 250–500 mg six-hourly orally. Lincomycin (Lincocin, Mycivin) 500 mg eight-hourly orally a.c. or i.m. Clindamycin (Dalacin-C) 150–450 mg six-hourly orally a.c. Spiramycin and oleandomycin are less effective.

5   Others

Chloramphenicol (Chloromycetin) has a wide spectrum and is used in typhoid and paratyphoid fevers, *H. influenzae* meningitis, and locally in eye infections.
Side-effects are serious and may be fatal: granulocytopenia, thrombocytopenia, aplastic anaemia (rare), grey syndrome in infants (circulatory collapse).
Dose: 250–750 mg six-hourly orally.

Vancomycin (Vancocin) is used against 'resistant' staphylococci.
Side-effects: very toxic. Causes deafness, renal damage, rash.
Dose: 0·5 g eight-hourly i.v.

Fusidic Acid (Fucidin) has a moderate spectrum, penetrates bone and is used in staphylococcal osteomyelitis. It is active against penicillinase-producing staphylococci but these rapidly become resistant so it is best combined with erythromycin.
Side-effects: gastro-intestinal upset, rash.
Dose: 500 mg six- to eight-hourly orally.

Colistin (Colomycin, Polymyxin E) *Dose:* 300 mg i.m. daily. **Sulphomyxin** (Thiosporin) *Dose:* 0·5 Mu six-hourly i.m. **Polymyxin B.** *Dose:* 150 mg daily i.v. Not absorbed orally.
These have a similar action and are active against Gram-negative organisms, e.g. *Pseudomonas.*
Side-effects: toxic to the nervous system and kidney, local pain if given i.m.

Nitrofurantoin (Furadantin) has a broad spectrum and is used in *E. coli* and *Proteus* urinary infection. It produces low blood levels but is concentrated in the urine.
Side-effects: nausea, rash, diarrhoea, peripheral neuropathy, pulmonary infiltration, haemolytic anaemia.
Dose: 50–150 mg orally p.c. six-hourly.

Nalidixic Acid (Negram) is active against Gram-negative organisms but they rapidly become resistant. Used in urinary infection, e.g. *Proteus.*
Side-effects: gastro-intestinal upset, rash, toxic to the nervous system. Causes a positive Clinitest and Benedict's test.

Hexamine (Methenamine) Mandelate (Mandelamine) is broken down to formaldehyde and mandelic acid in an acid urine but is useless in an alkaline urine.
Side-effects: nausea, overdose causes chemical cystitis.
Dose: 1–1·5 g six-hourly orally.

Metronidazole (Flagyl) 800 mg t.d.s. orally is active against anaerobic infection and amoebiasis.

6   Antifungal Agents

Griseofulvin (Fulcin, Grisovin) is deposited in keratin and used in ringworm.
Side-effects: rash, headache, leucopenia, alcohol intolerance. Toxic by injection.
Dose: 125–250 mg q.i.d. orally for several months.

Nystatin (Nystan, Nitacin) is active against candida. Little is absorbed orally.

Side-effects: toxic by injection.

Dose: applied topically—lozenges or mouthwashes (1 ml, = 100,000 u, q.i.d.) for oral candida, pessaries for vaginal, tablets 0·5–1 Mu t.d.s. for gastro-intestinal infection.

Amphotericin B (Fungilin, Fungizone) and **Flucytosine** are active against candida, aspergillus and cryptococcal infection. Amphotericin B is poorly absorbed from the gut. Flucytosine is excreted in the urine.

Side-effects: Amphotericin B: fever, headache, nausea, vomiting, uraemia, local thrombophlebitis at the site of the injection. Flucytosine: pancytopenia.

Dose: Amphotericin B: 0·25–1 mg/kg daily i.v. (freshly prepared), often for two months. Flucytosine: 100 mg/kg daily orally or as 1% i.v. solution.

Natamycin (Primaricin) is active against aspergillosis, cryptococcus, histoplasmosis, trichomonas and candida.

Side-effects: anorexia, nausea, diarrhoea.

Topical use: 1 ml 1% suspension under the tongue for oral thrush (candida) in infants; pessary.

Tolnaftate and **Pecilocin** are used topically in dermatophyte infection.

Imidazoles are active against dermatophytes, yeasts, and filamentous fungi. They include Clotrimazole (Canesten), Miconazole (Daktarin) and Econazole (Ecostatin).

7 Sulphonamides

Sulphonamides have a wide spectrum. The 'old' sulphonamides, e.g. sulphathiazole, are poorly soluble in acid and form crystals in the urine which damage the kidneys; large amounts of fluid have to be given to prevent this, but this dilutes their action. The new sulphonamides used in urinary infection are soluble, but those used to sterilise the bowel are insoluble and therefore are not absorbed. Urinary infection should be treated for three to six weeks to avoid recurrence.

Side-effects: vomiting, rash, agranulocytosis, fever, haemolytic anaemia, purpura.

Sulphadimidine or **Sulphadiazine** are soluble and are used for systemic or urinary infection. Either is given with penicillin in meningitis.

Dose: 3 g stat. then 1 g six-hourly orally.

Sulphafurazole (Gantrisin) is used in urinary infection.

Dose: 4 g stat. then 1 g six-hourly orally.

Co-trimoxazole (Bactrim, Septrin) consists of sulphomethoxazole 400 mg plus trimethoprim 80 mg. It is used in urinary and respiratory Gram-nagative infection.

Dose: 2–3 tabs. b.d. for five days.

Phthalylsulphathiazole and **Succinylsulphathiazole** are poorly soluble and are used to 'sterilise' the bowel prior to bowel surgery.

Dose: phthalylsulphathiazole 1–1·5 g four- to six-hourly. Succinylsulphathiazole 2–3·5 g four- to six-hourly.

Sulphasalazine (Salazopyrin) is used in ulcerative colitis.
  Dose: 0·5 – 2 g six-hourly.

SPECIFIC INFECTIONS

A Boil is a localised staphylococcal infection of a hair follicle or sebaceous gland which begins as a white spot with a hair in the centre and later becomes red, hot, swollen and tender. Prevention is by cleanliness, antisepsis and the treatment of predisposing conditions, e.g. diabetes mellitus.
  Treatment: removal of the hair to drain pus, absorbent dressing. Incision or antibiotic is needed occasionally. Auto-vaccination for recurrent boils, i.e. pus is taken from a boil and a vaccine made from the staphylococcus cultured from it.

Cellulitis is a spreading infection due to organisms such as β-haemolytic streptococci which release hyaluronidase, an enzyme which destroys connective tissue, and fibrinolysin which dissolves (lyses) fibrin. The area is red, tender and oedematous.
  Treatment: penicillin G 300 mg i.m. eight-hourly.

Erysipelas is cellulitis due to the entry of the β-haemolytic streptococcus through a wound in the skin or mucous membrane.

β-HAEMOLYTIC STREPTOCOCCAL INFECTIONS

β-haemolytic streptococci cause several diseases:
  1 Tonsillitis with or without a rash. If a rash is present the disease is called scarlet fever.
  2 Erysipelas, in patients with a low resistance.
  3 Streptococcal puerperal fever, due to infection of the genital tract after childbirth.
  4 Rheumatic fever, which is an allergic response to streptococcal toxins.
  5 Acute nephritis, which is also an allergic response to toxins.

SCARLET FEVER (SCARLATINA)

This is due to β-haemolytic streptococcal tonsillitis. The organism produces an exotoxin which causes a skin rash. In subsequent infections of acute streptococcal tonsillitis the rash does not occur because circulating antitoxin has been produced by the previous infection and neutralises the toxin. The disease is then no longer called scarlet fever. The rash pales around an injection of antitoxin into the skin (Schultz–Charlton reaction).
  Spread is by droplets, direct contact, or infected milk from a cow with streptococcal mastitis. It is notifiable.

Clinically: it is commonest in children aged two to ten years. The incubation period is two to four days. It has a sudden onset with sore throat, headache, shivering (rigors), pyrexia 39°±0·7°C, tachycardia (often 120 a minute), nausea, vomiting due to toxaemia, and constipation due to anorexia and dehydration. The tonsils are enlarged and covered with follicular exudate which is yellow (pus) and easily wiped off (unlike diphtheritic membrane which adheres), and the throat is inflamed. The tongue is furred with prominent red papillae ('strawberry tongue'). The punctate erythematous rash (tiny red spots on a flushed skin) appears in 24 hours. The area around the mouth is pale (circumoral pallor) and contrasts with the flushed face. The rash fades in one week, and the skin desquamates (peels) over one month. There is cervical adenitis, i.e. the glands of the neck, draining the inflamed throat, are enlarged and tender.

Complications:
1   Acute otitis media, due to spread of infection along the Eustachian tube (*Fig. 4.7*).

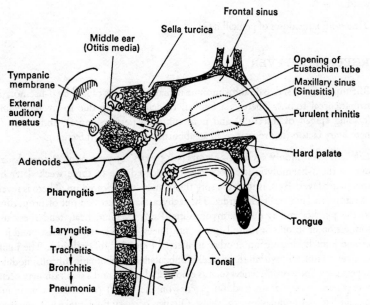

FIG. 4.7   Complications of upper respiratory infection

2   Quinsy (peritonsillar abscess), which requires incision and drainage.
3   Rarely, rheumatic fever or acute nephritis due to hypersensitivity to the streptococcal toxins.

Diagnosis: throat swab cultured for haemolytic streptococcus. Serum shows a high level (above 125 units) of antibody to streptolysin i.e. antistreptolysin (A.S.O.). Streptolysin is a toxin produced by the streptococcus which causes haemolysis (haemo = blood, lysis = destruction).

Treatment: isolation. General treatment for infectious diseases. Rest in bed for one to four weeks (until apyrexial). Regular mouthwashes, four-hourly temperature, pulse and respirations in order to detect complications. Diet: fluid or semi-solid while swallowing is painful, iced drinks. Earache (otitis media), joint pains (rheumatic fever), puffy eyelids or albuminuria after the second week (acute nephritis) must be reported. The urine is examined for albumin and blood in the second and third weeks.

Drugs: Penicillin V 250 mg orally six-hourly for six days, or sulphadimidine 3 g then 1 g six-hourly orally. Aspirin 0·6 g four-hourly to relieve sore throat.

PUERPERAL FEVER

Puerperal fever is infection following childbirth. Streptococci cause 40% of cases. Droplet infection or the use of an infected instrument during delivery allows infection of the uterus (endometritis). This is followed by septicaemia and sometimes a rash.

Treatment: large doses of penicillin G i.m.

RHEUMATIC FEVER

Rheumatic fever is due to auto-immune damage to tissues caused by β-haemolytic streptococcal toxins. There is a familial tendency, partly due to overcrowding (causing spread of infection) and poor nutrition (less resistance), and partly to hereditary factors (less resistance, or an abnormal response, to infection).

Clinically: commonly aged 10–25 years (5–15 years, 25 years ago). A sore throat, due to the β-haemolytic streptococcus, is followed one to three weeks later by rheumatic fever. By this time the sore throat may have cleared up. There is fever, sweating, malaise and tachycardia. The tachycardia is increased out of proportion to the pyrexia and is due to myocarditis. Pain, swelling, heat, tenderness and stiffness occur in one or more larger joints (knees, elbows, ankles, wrists) and just as one joint is clearing up another is affected ('flitting' polyarthritis). The joints recover completely within three weeks. Subcutaneous rheumatic (fibrous) nodules appear over bony prominences such as elbows and wrists, and a skin rash may occur —erythema marginatum (reddish patches on the trunk) or erythema nodosum (purplish tender nodules over the shins). Oliguria occurs if fluid intake is inadequate.

Investigations: throat swab to demonstrate the streptococcus. Blood: polymorph leucocytosis up to 20×10^9/l (20,000 per mm³), anaemia, raised E.S.R. (erythrocyte sedimentation rate) and raised A.S.O. level (anti-streptolysin O, i.e. antibody to streptolysin, a toxin produced by the streptococcus).

Complications:
1   *Endocarditis* (inflammation of the endocardium, the inner lining of the heart) causes damage to the heart valves. This may be mild and improve, but if there are recurrent attacks of rheumatic fever over years the valves eventually thicken and become distorted by fibrosis, causing stenosis or incompetence, especially of the mitral and aortic valves.

2   *Chorea.* This is due to damage to the basal ganglia in the brain, and consists of irregular involuntary restless (fidgety) movements causing weight loss and 'clumsiness'. The movements are absent during sleep. Ketosis occurs if carbohydrate intake is not increased and is due to the metabolism of fat for energy.

   Treatment: Quiet room, padded bed with sides to prevent injury. Aspirin. Sedation with phenobarbitone. Warm clothes rather than bed-clothes, which are soon tangled due to the restlessness.

Treatment: complete rest in bed, to prevent cardiac failure, for a mimimum of six weeks and until symptoms have been absent for one week and the E.S.R. is normal. Bed cradle to take the pressure of the bedclothes off inflamed joints. Joints supported in a position of comfort. Absorbent sheet or clothing (flannelette) to absorb sweat, and damp clothing is changed several times daily. Abundant fluids to compensate for sweating. Fluid intake and output record. Temperature, pulse rate and respirations four-hourly, and any change should be reported. A rising pulse indicates cardiac involvement or pericarditis. The sleeping pulse rate is raised (the sleeping pulse is not increased by anxiety or excitement).

   Adequate sleep. Encourage appetite. Care of the skin, mouth, and hair. Occupational therapy. Education.

   Drugs: penicillin V 250 mg orally six-hourly for the infected throat. Soluble (calcium) aspirin 300–900 mg (tab. = 300 mg) two-hourly, i.e. up to 80 mg/kg body-weight daily, omitting two night doses, or sodium salicylate 120 mg/kg daily. Continue until one week after symptoms have subsided. *Side-effects:* nausea, headache, dizziness, tinnitus, deafness; larger doses produce vomiting, hyperventilation due to acidosis, and mental symptoms. Sodium bicarbonate should not be given with salicylates since it increases their excretion in the urine and reduces their effectiveness. Prednisolone also relieves symptoms but has no long-term advantage and does not prevent mitral stenosis.

   Convalescence: gradual resumption of normal activity. For maximum recovery a long convalescence is advisable before return to school or work if cardiac complications were present and the general condition of the patient is poor. Parents should be told to report further attacks immediately so that treatment can be given, and to avoid exposure of the child to infection.

Prevention: improved nutrition and living conditions. It is not the nurse's duty to preach to the child's parents that it would be better to spend more of their wages on better nutrition for their children than on cigarettes, beer and bingo for themselves!

   Penicillin V orally daily continued until age 20 years, for recurrent attacks.

TETANUS ('Lockjaw')

Tetanus is due to *Clostridium tetani*, a drumstick-shaped anaerobic spore present in soil and in the intestines of animals, including horse and man.

Clinically: after an incubation period of two to thirty (average ten) days it germinates into vegetative bacilli, but only in anoxic injured tissues. The organisms remain localised to the site of injury but make a neurotoxin which enters the blood and results in muscle spasm by stimulating motor nerves. Spasm of the jaw muscles (trismus, 'lockjaw') occurs first and is followed by generalised rigidity and tonic spasms. Any stimulus, e.g. a noise or bump, may precipitate a painful convulsion.

Prevention: active immunisation with tetanus toxoid. A second dose is given six weeks after the first, a third three to six months later, and a fourth ('booster') dose after another 1 year, then every 10 years. Children are immunised before the age of 1 year, using 'triple' vaccine (diphtheria, pertussis, tetanus). Wounds contaminated with soil should be properly cleaned and necrotic tissue removed.

Treatment: passive immunisation with 250–500 units i.m. of human antitoxin protects for four weeks. Horse antitoxin (1500–20,000 units) may be used but contains foreign (horse) serum which may cause a sensitivity reaction. Toxoid is also given, at a different site, to initiate active immunity. Antibiotic—benzyl-penicillin 300 mg i.m. (0·5 Mu) b.d., or erythromycin 500 mg six-hourly. The patient should be in a quiet dark room and stimuli should be avoided. Sedation with phenobarbitone 30–120 mg t.d.s. or chlorpromazine 25–100 mg six-hourly to inhibit spasms; thiopentone 1 g in 500 ml of i.v. fluid, or curare in severe spasms. Control fluid and electrolyte balance by mouth if possible, but i.v. if necessary. Prevention of bronchopneumonia—the patient lies on his side, and oropharyngeal secretions are aspirated. Death is from asphyxia, aspiration pneumonia, or hypotension and pulmonary oedema.

GAS GANGRENE

Gas gangrene is a serious infection due to anaerobic putrefying bacteria such as *Clostridium (Cl.) perfringens (welchii)*, *Cl. septicum*, and *Cl. novyi*. These live only on dead tissue where there is no oxygen, e.g. lacerated muscle or crush injury. Clostridial spores enter a wound in soil or faecal matter and grow anaerobically (without oxygen) to produce several toxins, such as lecithinase (an enzyme which hydrolyses the lecithin of cell walls and thus kills the cells), collagenase which destroys collagen (connective tissue), and fibrinolysin which dissolves fibrin. These toxins allow the infection to spread. The organisms also ferment carbohydrate to produce gas. Gas and oedema distend the tissues and reduce their blood supply, thus providing anaerobic conditions for growth.

Clinically: the infection begins as an anaerobic cellulitis or myositis, with a foul-smelling thin brownish discharge, gas in the tissues (causing crepitations), pain (myositis), oedema and discoloured skin. The foul odour is due to hydrogen sulphide ('bad eggs') formed from destroyed haemoglobin. Lack of bleeding indicates dead tissue, later the tissue becomes green or black due to putrefaction. General signs are tachycardia, fever (which may be very high), tachypnoea, toxaemia, shock with fall in blood pressure, stupor, delirium, coma and death.

Complications: shock and haemolysis cause acute oliguric renal failure.

Diagnosis: the type of injury indicating tissue death, the presence of dirt. Pus or tissue from the wound contain Gram-positive rods ± spores, which show haemolysis on anaerobically incubated blood agar plates.

Treatment: excision of devitalised tissue; amputation if necessary. Multiple incisions and fasciotomy to allow the escape of exudate and reduce tissue tension in order to maintain a blood supply to the tissues. Hysterectomy or curettage of the uterus in puerperal gas gangrene. Anti-gas-gangrene serum (polyvalent antitoxin) 40,000 units i.v. six-hourly. Penicillin 600 mg (1 Mu) i.m. three-hourly. Hyperbaric oxygen. Fluids and electrolytes i.v., plasma.

Prevention: prompt excision of devitalized (dead and dying) tissues, antibiotic (penicillin), anti-gas-gangrene serum.

INFLUENZA

Influenza is due to influenza A or B viruses, which are myxoviruses, spread by droplets. It occurs in epidemics, and occasionally in pandemics as in 1918 and 1957. Illnesses caused by other viruses, or the common cold, are often wrongly called 'flu' by the layman.

Clinically: the incubation period is one to three days and the infection lasts about a week. There is malaise, headache, aching in the limbs, anorexia, flushed face, tachycardia, shivering and a pyrexia of up to 39°C. The fauces are red and there may be mild conjunctivitis and a dry cough.

Complications:

1 Tracheitis, bronchitis, or bronchopneumonia due to the influenza virus or to secondary bacterial infection with staphylococci, streptococci or *H. influenzae* bacilli.
2 Acute toxic myocarditis which may cause sudden death.
3 Encephalitis, rare.
4 Post-influenzal weakness and depression which may last a few weeks.

Treatment: isolation at home in bed until apyrexial.

Symptomatic: soluble aspirin or codeine Co. tab. 1 to 2 t.d.s. for aches, linctus codeine 5 ml for dry cough. Antibiotic for bacterial bronchopneumonia.

Prevention: annual vaccination each November for patients with chronic respiratory disease, e.g. chronic bronchitis, or chronic cardiac disease, e.g. congestive cardiac failure.

THE COMMON COLD (ACUTE CORYZA)

A cold is due to one of many viruses, spread by droplets and direct contact. There are three main types of coryza:

1   Apyrexial Acute Catarrhal Rhinitis

Inflammation of the nose without pyrexia. This is due to Rhinoviruses, the commonest cause of a cold.

Clinically: the incubation period is two to four days. Inflammation of the upper respiratory tract (U.R.T.) causes irritation with sneezing, watery nasal discharge and mild cough. There is malaise and headache, but pyrexia is mild or absent. Temporary deafness may occur due to obstruction of the Eustachian tubes by inflammation.

Complications:
1   Secondary bacterial infection of the nose (purulent rhinitis), which may spread to the sinuses (sinusitis).
2   Acute otitis media, due to spread of infection along the Eustachian tube to the middle ear.

2   Apyrexial Acute Rhinitis with Sore Throat

This is due to coronaviruses. The symptoms are the same as above, but there is also a sore throat.

3   Rhinitis with Pyrexia and Other Symptoms

This is due to adenoviruses, of which there are over thirty types.

Clinically: there is pyrexia, malaise, nasal catarrh, pharyngitis with cough, headache and conjunctivitis. The cervical lymph nodes may be swollen and tender.

Complications: (Fig. 4.7)
1   Purulent rhinitis.
2   Sinusitis.
3   Acute otitis media.
4   Laryngitis, causing a hoarse voice.
5   Tracheo-bronchitis.
6   Pneumonitis.

Treatment: there is no specific cure. Bed in a warm room. 1% ephedrine nasal drops or spray to relieve congestion. Steam inhalations may be soothing. Soluble aspirin 300 mg four-hourly for headache. Antibiotic for secondary infection.

Prevention: isolation of the patient for three days.

GLANDULAR FEVER

Glandular fever is fever with lymph gland enlargement which is not due to pyogenic infection. It has several causes, including viruses, rickettsiae and drugs.

Infectious Mononucleosis

This is the commonest cause of glandular fever. It is due to the Epstein–Barr (E.B.) virus, which is spread by droplets and direct contact (kissing).

Clinically: the incubation period is 5–10 days. It most commonly affects those aged 10–25 years. There is malaise, tiredness, general aching, headache, pyrexia, petechial haemorrhage on the palate, sore throat and enlargement of lymph nodes and spleen. Mesenteric adenitis (inflammation of mesenteric lymph nodes) causes pain in the right iliac fossa. A maculopapular rash occurs in 5% of patients.

Complications are rare, but include:
1 Mental depression.
2 Jaundice due to hepatitis.
3 Rupture of the spleen, which is enlarged and soft.
4 Lymphocytic meningitis.
5 Thrombocytopenia.
6 Autoimmune haemolytic anaemia, i.e. the body makes antibodies against its own red cells and these cause haemolysis.
7 Respiratory obstruction due to oedema of the pharynx and larynx.

Diagnosis: the white cell count is raised from the end of the first week, e.g. to $15 \times 10^9/l$ (15,000 per mm³), due to an increase in mononuclear cells and lymphocytes. The Paul-Bunnell test for antibodies in the serum is positive after 6–10 days.

Treatment: rest in bed until apyrexial. No specific treatment is available or required, and recovery is complete. Symptomatic treatment: aspirin for headache.

WHOOPING COUGH (PERTUSSIS)

Whooping cough is due to the bacillus, *Bordetella* ('*Haemophilus*') *pertussis*, which is spread by droplets. A similar infection is caused by adenoviruses.

Clinically: pertussis usually occurs in children under five years of age. The incubation period is 7–14 days. The first week (catarrhal stage) resembles a cold and there is rhinitis, conjunctivitis and cough. The second stage (paroxysmal stage) is due to bronchitis and lasts 2–4 weeks. There are several bouts of coughing, each bout consisting of a series of about 20 short sharp coughs which may bring up thick sputum, and end in a deep inspiration through partly closed vocal cords causing a 'whoop', followed by vomiting. Facial congestion and cyanosis are marked, the tongue protrudes and may ulcerate beneath from trauma by the lower teeth.

Complications:
1 Bronchopneumonia due to invasion of the lungs by other organisms.
2 Atelectasis (collapse of lung tissue) due to mucus obstructing the bronchi.
3 Bronchiectasis (dilatation of bronchi) may follow atelectasis.
4 Convulsions due to cerebral hypoxia during a bout of coughing.
5 Epistaxis or subconjunctival haemorrhage, due to venous congestion in the head.
6 Umbilical hernia or prolapsed rectum, due to increased intra-abdominal pressure due to coughing.

Diagnosis:

1 Pernasal swab from the posterior nasopharynx, or cough plates, cultured for *B. pertussis*.
2 Fluorescent antibody test.
3 The white blood cell count is increased by a lymphocytosis often to $20 \times 10^9/l$ (20,000 per mm^3).
4 Chest radiograph to show atelectasis.

Treatment: isolation for four weeks. The milder cases are better isolated out of doors if kept warm. Rest in bed. Feeds are given immediately after vomiting at the end of a coughing bout, since this allows the most time for digestion before the next bout. Dry foods (biscuits) irritate the pharynx, causing coughing and should be avoided. Steam inhalations loosen thick sputum. Maintain hydration.

Drugs: cough suppressant, e.g. linctus codeine. Sedation with diazepam or chloral. Sulphonamide, erythromycin or tetracycline syrup 100 mg in 1 ml b.d., given early, prevents bronchopneumonia.

Prevention: notifiable. Contacts are examined for catarrhal symptoms and a swab cultured. Immunisation with D.P.T. vaccine.

MUMPS (EPIDEMIC PAROTITIS)

Mumps is a paramyxovirus infection of the salivary glands spread by droplets or direct contact.

Clinically: the incubation period is 18 days. It affects schoolchildren and young adults. There is anorexia, nausea, malaise and fever of 38·5°C followed on the second day by tender swelling of one or both parotid glands which makes eating painful and pushes the lobe of the ear outwards. The submandibular salivary glands may also be involved.

Complications: other glands may be affected.

1 Orchitis (inflammation of the gonads—testis or ovary). Usually only one testis is affected and is swollen, tender and painful and may later atrophy. If both testes are affected the patient may be sterile and cease to produce androgen (male hormone).
2 Pancreatitis (inflammation of the pancreas) causes nausea, vomiting, epigastric pain and tenderness.
3 Acute lymphocytic meningitis, causing headache.
4 Encephalomyelitis, rarely. This causes headache, fever, photophobia, and drowsiness.

Treatment: isolation until the swelling has subsided (14 days) plus a further week. In bed for 10 days. Oral hygiene is important, since the mouth is dry due to lack of saliva. Chewing is painful, therefore the patient may need semisolid or minced food or feeding through a straw.   *Drugs:* analgesics for pain, e.g. aspirin.

For orchitis the testes should be supported with a sling. Morphine 15 mg is given s.c. or i.m. Prednisolone may reduce the testicular inflammation, and 15 mg is given six-hourly for three days then rapidly reduced over four days.

MEASLES (MORBILLI)

Measles is due to a virus (paramyxovirus) spread by droplets which enter the respiratory tract or conjunctiva. Epidemics occur every two to three years.

Clinically: it usually affects children aged three to five years. The incubation period is 10 days. The first stage (catarrhal stage) is highly infectious and resembles a cold, with fever up to 39·5°C, watery nasal discharge (catarrh), sneezing and conjunctivitis. A loud brassy cough and hoarse voice due to laryngitis, photophobia (dislike of light), and Koplik's spots, occur on the second day. Koplik's spots are diagnostic and are tiny white spots, like grains of salt, surrounded by a red zone of inflammation, on the mucous membrane of the mouth.

The second (exanthematous) stage occurs on the fourth day, a macular rash appearing behind the ears and on the forehead, spreading to the face and in a few hours affecting the trunk and limbs. The macules tend to fuse causing the rash to appear blotchy, and the child is irritable and crying. The rash then fades and the skin shows a faint brown-staining and a powdery fine desquamation (scaling).

Complications:

1 Stomatitis.
2 Croup, i.e. severe laryngitis and bronchitis.
3 Febrile convulsions (fits due to fever) in young children.
4 Acute suppurative otitis media due to secondary infection of the middle ear by bacteria. The child rolls the head, screams and puts a hand over the ear, and these signs should be reported.
5 Corneal ulceration due to severe conjunctivitis.
6 Bronchiolitis (inflammation of small bronchi), which may cause:
7 Bronchiectasis (dilatation of bronchi).
8 Bronchopneumonia, which may be fatal.
9 Rarely, acute encephalitis or subacute sclerosing panencephalitis.

Treatment: notifiable. The child is kept off school for 14 days from the onset of the rash, isolated in bed in a well-ventilated room or outdoors, if kept warm, to reduce the possibility of bronchopneumonia. The room should be darkened to relieve photophobia, the mouth kept moist, the eyes bathed frequently with weak boracic lotion, and steam inhaled, using a humidifier or steam kettle, for laryngitis.

Drugs: analgesic, e.g. soluble aspirin tab. 1 or 2 t.d.s. for headache. Linctus codeine 5 ml b.d. (or linctus codeine paediatric 10 ml if under age five years). Antibiotic e.g. penicillin, for bronchopneumonia.

Prevention: examination of contacts for catarrh and Koplik's spots. Active immunisation with live attenuated (weakened) virus vaccine s.c. Passive immunisation with human immunoglobulin within five days of exposure will prevent measles and is given to contacts under 18 months of age and to debilitated children. Dose: 250 mg i.m. if under one year, 500 mg for those over one year.

RUBELLA (GERMAN MEASLES)

Rubella is due to a virus spread by droplet infection. Epidemics occur every six to nine years. Not notifiable.

Clinically: the incubation period is 14–21 (average 18) days. It is a mild disease affecting children over six years, adolescents, and young adults. There is malaise, slight fever, sore throat, mild conjunctivitis and vague aches in the joints. The rash of pink macules begins on the first day, behind the ears and on the forehead, and spreads to the face then the trunk and limbs and disappears on the third day. The lymph nodes in the posterior cervical region (the back of the neck) become enlarged and tender and this may cause neck 'stiffness'.

Complications:

1 Polyarthralgia (pain in many joints) in adults.
2 Thrombocytopenic purpura—small pinpoint haemorrhages in the skin (purpura) due to a low blood platelet count. This recovers completely.
3 Encephalomyelitis, seven to 10 days after onset of rash.
4 Rubella occurring in women during the first three months of pregnancy may cause congenital malformations in the unborn child, e.g. cardiac defect, mental defect, cataract, deafness.

Treatment: isolation is not necessary but pregnant women should avoid contact with the patient. If a woman in the first three months of pregnancy has not previously had rubella, her serum will not contain antibodies (these can be tested for). If she does come in contact with rubella then 1·5 g of human immunoglobulin should be given in order to provide passive immunity. If immunoglobulin is not given immediately abortion is permitted. Girls should try to contract the disease before childbearing age. If they have not had rubella before the age of 14 years they may be given a vaccination of live attenuated virus.

SMALLPOX (VARIOLA)

Smallpox is due to poxviruses and is spread by droplets, direct contact or fomites, e.g. clothing. The virus can survive at room temperature for months. Infection is by inhalation of virus into the upper respiratory tract. The virus passes through the mucosa, multiplies in the reticuloendothelial system, then enters the circulation to reach all the organs.

Clinically: the incubation period is 12–14 days. On the first day of illness there may be a prodromal scarlatiniform rash. There is malaise, frontal headache, backache, rigor(s), sore throat, cough and fever. The fever is 39·8°C for the first three days then falls, but rises again (= secondary fever) on the eighth day when the rash becomes pustular. On the second day the typical rash appears as macules (flat red spots), becoming papules (raised spots) on the third day, and vesicles (small blisters) on the sixth day. The vesicles are depressed centrally ('umbilicated') and vesicles on the nasal and oral mucosa become ulcers. On the eighth day the clear fluid in the vesicles becomes cloudy, forming pustules. These dry to form scabs on the tenth day and the scabs separate after several days leaving 'pocks' (pitted scars). The rash is more dense on the limbs and forehead than on the trunk, and is worse where the skin is chafed by clothing. The cervical lymph nodes, liver and spleen may enlarge. There are two smallpox viruses: (1) *Variola major*, and (2) *Variola minor* (Alastrim), a mild form. In variola major the disease shows one of three degrees of severity: (1) discrete spots, the usual form; (2) confluent rash in which the pocks merge together; (3) haemorrhagic smallpox, the most severe form, usually fatal. Smallpox causes mild disease if it occurs in vaccinated individuals (modified smallpox).

Complications:
1 Bronchopneumonia.
2 Secondary bacterial infection of the skin causing boils and impetigo, or of the middle ear causing otitis media.
3 Corneal ulcer (danger of blindness) due to conjunctivitis.
4 Occasionally encephalitis.

Diagnosis: laboratory examination for 'elementary bodies' in fluid from vesicles, electronmicroscopic demonstration of virus, tissue or egg culture of virus.

Treatment: notifiable. Isolation of patient and staff. Staff and contacts must have been recently vaccinated. Contacts are then kept under observation, or may be quarantined for 16 days. General treatment of infectious disease. Light bedclothes and cradle to avoid chafing against pustules. Hair cut short. Skin, eyes and mouth require special care to prevent secondary infection. The mouth is cleansed frequently with weak phenol solution. Frequent bathing reduces the offensive odour and helps to relieve itching. The patient is infectious until all scabs have separated. For conjunctivitis the eyes are bathed with weak boracic lotion. Diet: high fluid and high calorie intake. Antibiotic for secondary infection.

Prevention: vaccination before travelling to an epidemic area and for contacts, except in patients with active skin disease, e.g. infantile eczema, since these patients may develop generalised vaccinia which may be fatal.

Vaccination: the skin is inoculated with 'lymph' which is fluid from a vesicle containing the vaccinia (cowpox) virus taken from calves. Vaccination should be performed in contacts, ambulance drivers, and hospital staff every 7 years. Routine vaccination is avoided in infantile dermatitis, intercurrent illness, and during corticosteroid therapy since a severe vaccinial rash may occur in these conditions, and in pregnancy owing to the danger of damage to the fetus. Methisazone 200 mg/kg followed by 50 mg/kg six-hourly for eight doses may prevent the disease in close contacts but does not affect established disease.

CHICKENPOX (VARICELLA)

Chickenpox is due to the varicella-zoster virus. The same virus causes shingles in adults. Spread is respiratory in chickenpox and via ruptured skin lesions in herpes zoster. It is a highly infectious but mild disease. Not notifiable.

Clinically: it usually affects children under 10 years old. The incubation period is 14–18 days. There is malaise and fever, then a rash on the skin and mucous membranes of the mouth. The rash consists of successive crops of macules becoming papules then vesicles containing clear fluid, which within 48 hours become pustules. They itch and are ruptured by scratching, then dry to form crusts. Suboccipital and posterior cervical lymph nodes enlarge.

Complications are unusual but include:

1   Secondary infection of skin lesions by staphylococci and streptococci.
2   Encephalomyelitis, rare.
3   Spread to adults causing herpes zoster (shingles) is very rare.
4   Haemorrhagic chickenpox, with haemorrhage into skin, melaena (blood in the faeces) and haematuria (blood in the urine). It may be fatal and occurs in patients with a low resistance, leukaemia, or on corticosteroid therapy.
5   Varicella pneumonia.
6   Glomerulonephritis (inflammation of the glomeruli of the kidney).

Diagnosis: chickenpox resembles modified smallpox and must be distinguished from it (*Table 4.4* and *Fig. 4.8*). The lesions in chickenpox are more dense on the trunk and the illness is mild. In smallpox the lesions are more dense on the limbs than on the trunk.

TABLE 4.4   *Distinction between chickenpox and smallpox*

	Chickenpox	Smallpox
General symptoms	mild	severe
Rash		
appearance	first day	second or third day
greatest density	on trunk	on limbs and face
evolution of lesions	all stages present	all at same stage
in axilla	present	rare
vesicles	unilocular, superficial	multilocular, deep

Treatment: mild disease is treated at home. Local care of lesions by a daily bath, with added antiseptic e.g. chlorhexidine. Isolation is needed until the dry scab stage, usually for three weeks. Dry scabs are not infectious. Fingernails are cut short to reduce scratching. Antihistamine, e.g. Phenergan 10 mg t.d.s. orally to relieve itching, and provide sedation. Antibiotic for bacterial superinfection.

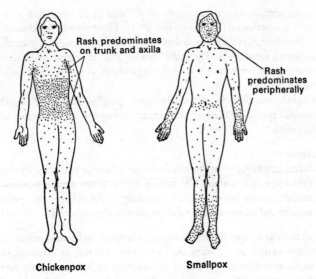

Rash predominates
on trunk and axilla

Rash
predominates
peripherally

Chickenpox

Smallpox

FIG. 4.8 Distribution of pocks in chickenpox and smallpox

HERPES ZOSTER (SHINGLES)

Herpes zoster is due to infection of posterior root sensory ganglia of the spinal cord or sensory ganglia of the cranial nerves by the varicella-zoster virus, by the reactivation of dormant virus from previous chickenpox infection, or rarely by contact with chickenpox.

Clinically (Fig. 4.9): shingles begins with severe continuous burning pain in the distribution of the affected nerve roots, usually on the trunk, and usually affecting

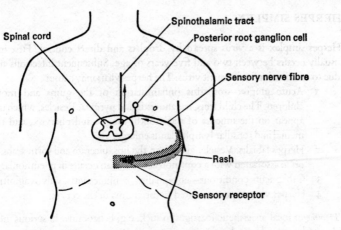

Spinal cord

Spinothalamic tract

Posterior root ganglion cell

Sensory nerve fibre

Rash

Sensory receptor

FIG. 4.9 Distribution of the rash of shingles

two or three dermatomes (a dermatome is the area of skin supplied by a single nerve root). It is unilateral (affects one side only). There may be mild pyrexia and malaise. After three days the affected skin becomes red and vesicles appear, then dry over six days to form scabs. The scabs then separate and leave small scars. The dermatome may be permanently anaesthetic (without sensation) due to the death of sensory nerve cells.

If the ophthalmic division of the trigeminal ganglion is infected (ophthalmic herpes) vesicles appear on the cornea and may lead to corneal ulceration, scarring and visual defect.

Complications:

1 Secondary infection of the rash due to scratching or to chafing by clothes.
2 Post-herpetic neuralgia. The pain of herpes zoster usually subsides as the rash disappears but sometimes, especially in the elderly, pain persists for months and may cause mental depression leading to suicide.

Treatment: there is no specific treatment, and corticosteroids, amantadine, vitamin B_{12}, pituitary extract and X-rays are ineffective. Talcum or calamine powder applied to the area dries the vesicles. A dry dressing excludes secondary infection. An ointment containing local anaesthetic (Ung. cinchocain co. B.P.C.) applied to the rash relieves pain. Clothing should be loose. Simple analgesics, e.g. codeine co. may be given, but drugs of addiction such as morphine should be avoided. An antibiotic is given for secondary infection of the rash. In ophthalmic herpes, chloramphenicol and 2% homatropine and corticosteroid eye drops are used six-hourly to prevent secondary infection and scarring.

For post-herpetic neuralgia analgesic, e.g. codeine co., is given, if necessary with a tranquilliser, e.g. chlorpromazine 50–100 mg t.d.s. In intractable pain section of the spinothalamic tract may benefit but section of a nerve or a posterior nerve root is ineffective.

HERPES SIMPLEX

Herpes simplex is a virus spread by droplets and direct contact. First infection usually occurs between two and five years of age. Subsequent infections are often due to reactivation of dormant virus. The herpes virus may cause:

1 Acute gingivo-stomatitis (inflammation of the gums and mouth) in children. The child frets, has anorexia and pyrexia. Vesicles, which ulcerate, appear on the mucosa of the mouth, tongue and pharynx, and the sub-mental and tonsillar lymph glands enlarge.
2 Herpes labialis. Vesicles appear on the lips, ulcerate and form scabs. This is often associated with a common cold but also occurs in pneumonia.
3 Other acute conditions—encephalitis, conjunctivitis, vulvovaginitis.
4 Herpes virus type 2 is related to carcinoma of the cervix.

Treatment: local anaesthetic lozenges to suck, e.g. benzocaine. In serious infections idoxuridine may be used.

TUBERCULOSIS

Tuberculosis is due to mycobacterium tuberculosis, of which there are several different types, including human, bovine (in cattle), avian (in birds), and piscine (in fish). There are also atypical (anonymous) mycobacteria.

Many people are infected with tuberculosis in childhood but only a small proportion (those with low resistance or receiving a massive infection) develop disease. Most people overcome the infection and acquire a specific immunity to it. The immunity is shown by a positive tuberculin skin (Mantoux, Heaf, or Tine) test, and this becomes positive within six weeks of infection whether the infection has been overcome or not. The incidence in the population of a positive tuberculin test due to natural infection fell from 56% in 1952 to 9% in 1978, due to improved nutrition, better housing (less overcrowding, hence a reduced chance of spread of infection), mass radiography (detection and treatment), and B.C.G. vaccination (which provides acquired active immunity).

Most infections in man are due to human tubercle bacilli inhaled in infected droplets and dust, causing pulmonary tuberculosis, but about 1% of cases are due to bovine T.B. ingested in infected milk and causing lymph gland infection in the neck (via the tonsil) and mesentery (via the ileum). Pasteurisation of milk kills tubercle bacilli and other pathogens.

Pathology: Tubercle bacilli enter the body and multiply in the lung or lymph nodes. The body defences act and cause inflammation. Macrophages (histiocytes) surround the area, phagocytose the bacilli and either change into epithelioid cells or fuse together to form multinucleated giant cells. Many lymphocytes, but only a few polymorphs, also surround the area. Toxins from the bacilli kill the tissue at the centre of the area which becomes whitish, like cheese, and this is called caseous necrosis (caseation). This rounded area of central caseation surrounded by epithelioid cells, giant cells and lymphocytes is called a tubercle follicle (*Fig. 4.10*). Tubercle follicles enlarge and may coalesce. Healing of the area is by the formation of granulation tissue (young connective tissue) followed by fibrosis. Calcium may be deposited (calcification) in the caseous part. The calcium is seen on X-ray of the lungs and abdomen for many years after the lesion has healed.

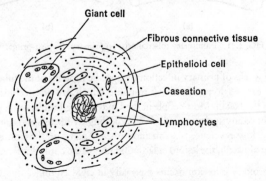

FIG. 4.10   A tuberculous follicle (tubercle)

Tubercle bacilli may spread via the lymphatics to the draining lymph nodes, causing tuberculous lymphadenitis, and may enter the bloodstream and spread to other organs, especially to bone and kidney, causing osteomyelitis or renal tuberculosis. If numerous bacilli enter the bloodstream and overwhelm the body, they cause miliary tuberculosis, i.e. infection scattered throughout the liver, spleen, lungs, kidneys, meninges and other organs, which is often fatal.

Pulmonary Tuberculosis (Phthisis)

Predisposing conditions are:

1   Poor socioeconomic conditions—overcrowding, poor health.
2   Occupation. Miners with pneumoconiosis are prone to tuberculosis, as are tuberculin-negative nurses if receiving massive infection, and laboratory workers handling T.B. cultures.
3   Disease, e.g. diabetes mellitus, congenital heart disease.
4   Drugs, e.g. corticosteroids.

The body's response to first (primary) infection with tubercle bacilli differs from that in subsequent (post-primary) infection.

Primary Pulmonary Tuberculosis. Inhaled bacilli enter the lung and tubercle follicles form. From this focus of infection (Ghon focus) tubercle bacilli pass along the lymphatics to infect and cause tubercle formation and caseation in the interpulmonary and mediastinal (hilar) lymph nodes, which enlarge (*Fig. 4.11*). During

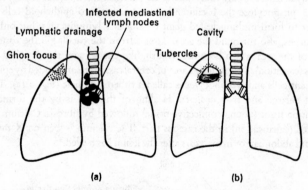

FIG. 4.11   Pulmonary tuberculosis: (*a*) primary; (*b*) post-primary

the first few weeks of primary infection the specific proteins of the tubercle bacillus (tuberculin) cause a hypersensitivity response which provides cellular immunity and destroys the bacilli. Most people in the United Kingdom have a high resistance and do not have any symptoms, the lesions healing by fibrosis and calcification. In those with a low resistance, e.g. malnourished Asians, or those infected with a massive dose of bacilli, the lesions enlarge and may cause complications.

Clinically: primary infection occurs especially in children under five years of age, but also in some adults. Most cases are symptomless. In others there may be mild fever, anorexia, malaise, fatigue and rash (erythema nodosum). Compression of the trachea and bronchi by the enlarged lymph nodes causes dry cough, stridor and dyspnoea.

Complications:

1 Pressure by enlarged lymph nodes may obstruct a bronchus and cause collapse of a segment of lung as air is absorbed from the alveoli supplied by the obstructed bronchus.
2 Lung abscess, due to necrosis of a volume of lung tissue.
3 Pleurisy and serous (clear) pleural effusion, due to spread of inflammation to the pleura.
4 Tuberculous bronchopneumonia due to aspiration of caseous material into bronchi from ulcerated lymph nodes.
5 Ulceration of a caseous focus into a vein allows spread of tubercle bacilli via the blood stream and causes (*a*) miliary tuberculosis; (*b*) tuberculous meningitis; (*c*) renal tuberculosis; (*d*) bone tuberculosis. Renal and bone tuberculosis may remain dormant for many years.
6 Bronchiectasis of the upper lobes of the lungs.
7 Emphysema due to bronchostenosis.
8 Progression to post-primary tuberculosis.
9 A cold abscess may follow cervical lymphadenitis and is due to pus tracking from the cervical lymph glands to the subcutaneous tissue.

Post-primary Pulmonary Tuberculosis. This occurs only if there is a low general bodily resistance. It is due either to a second infection with tubercle bacilli or (usually) to reactivation of the primary lesion (e.g. by giving corticosteroids). Tubercles form and caseation occurs but the presence of hypersensitivity from the start localises the infection at the site of entry, thus lymph-node involvement is less likely than in primary tuberculosis. There may be rapidly caseating bronchopneumonia and cavitation or a chronic fibrosing cavity.

Clinically: it affects the middle-aged and elderly. The onset is insidious, with fever in the evening, tachycardia, sweating especially at night, malaise, anorexia (loss of morning appetite is due to gastritis), loss of weight, dyspepsia (due to gastritis from swallowed sputum), persistent cough, sputum (mucoid or purulent), haemoptysis —usually slight streaking of the sputum but sometimes sudden and fatally large due to the erosion of an artery in a cavity—amenorrhoea, pleuritic pain, and later dyspnoea on exertion. Immigrants from Asia, Africa, and the West Indies often have bone and joint tuberculosis.

Complications:

1 Pleural. Dry pleurisy, causing pleuritic pain. Pleural effusion. Tuberculous empyema (pus in the pleural 'cavity').
2 Pulmonary. Haemoptysis, tuberculous bronchopneumonia, airways obstruction, spontaneous pneumothorax due to ruptured pleura, fungus infection in a cavity, emphysema, and pulmonary fibrosis. Either emphysema or pulmonary fibrosis may cause respiratory failure and cor pulmonale.
3 Tuberculous spread to the trachea, larynx (causing hoarseness), gut

(swallowed bacilli) causing enteritis, fistula-in-ano (tubercle bacilli enter through an abrasion in the rectal mucosa), and ischio-rectal abscess. Secondary infection of the last two with pyogenic bacteria is common.

Diagnosis of Pulmonary Tuberculosis. History of contact. Sputum, gastric aspiration of fasting juice, and laryngeal swabs for Ziehl–Neelsen stain and fluorescent microscopic examination for T.B., also for culture and sensitivity to antibiotics. A positive sputum indicates 'open' tuberculosis. Radiology of the chest shows the shadows of inflammation or translucencies of cavities, and there may be calcification in the upper lobes of the lungs. The erythrocyte sedimentation rate is raised. A four-hourly temperature chart may detect an occasional rise.

Tuberculin skin test: Mantoux test; 0·1 ml of 1:10,000(= 1 unit) of old tuberculin (O.T.) is injected intradermally. Induration (thickening) 10 mm in diameter at the second to third day is positive. If this is negative it is repeated after one week using 1:1000 (= 10 u) and if this is negative 1:100 (= 100 u) is used. Purified protein derivative (P.P.D.), which is purified protein from O.T., may be used. The Heaf test uses a multiple-puncture gun. A ring of small papules is positive. These tests become positive within six weeks after infection or B.C.G. vaccination, but may be negative in overwhelming infection, Hodgkin's disease, measles or during immunosuppressive drug therapy. B.C.G. (Bacille Calmette-Guérin) is a living attenuated bovine tubercle bacillus.

Treatment.

A General: patients may be treated in hospital or at home. Those admitted to hospital are the very ill, infectious ('open') cases if there are susceptible (tuberculin-negative) family contacts, unco-operative patients, alcoholics, and the mentally disturbed (the last three are likely to be unreliable in taking their drug therapy). 'Open' cases (sputum positive for T.B.) must have full isolation precautions with maximum ventilation of their room, or be nursed outdoors if possible. Staff must be tuberculin-positive and have regular chest X-rays. Sputum should be examined by smear and culture, monthly while positive, then three-monthly. A patient is considered 'closed' (non-infective, even though he still may be suffering from infection) when several successive sputa are negative for T.B.

Mild cases are treated at home and for economic reasons they may be allowed to work if 'closed'.

The diagnosis is a shock to the patient and the disease and the good prognosis must be explained to him to relieve anxiety.

Rest in bed until apyrexial. With antituberculous drugs the patient should cease to be infectious within a few weeks; isolation precautions may then be discontinued.

Good nutrition—high protein, milk, vitamins and iron. The patient should be weighed weekly to determine calorie requirements. Calories are increased if there is weight loss. Sedation with phenobarbitone 60 mg b.d. Gradually increasing exercise; e.g. walking. Occupational therapy to relieve boredom while in hospital and, if necessary, to provide a job after the patient is discharged. Provision of financial help for dependents.

B *Chemotherapy* with anti-tuberculous drugs is required for six to 24 months. Combined treatment with three drugs is given for the first two months. This is because the drugs are given without knowing whether or not the tubercle bacilli are sensitive to them, and the organisms may be resistant to at least one. Once the results of sensitivity tests, which take four to eight weeks, are known two appropriate drugs are given together. If only one drug is given, resistant bacilli may rapidly emerge. Failure of therapy is usually due to patients failing to take their drugs, therefore the urine should be monitored (e.g. Phenistix detects P.A.S.).

Streptomycin 1 g i.m. daily for two months then twice weekly for patients under 40 years old, to a total dose of 70 g. The dose is 0·75 g for patients over the age of 40 years because streptomycin is excreted via the urine and renal function diminishes after the age of 40. A plasma level of up to 1 μg per 1 ml (1·5 μmol/l) is required. *Side-effects:* rash, fever, nausea, giddiness then deafness due to damage to the vestibular and auditory branches of the eighth nerve.

Isoniazid (I.N.H.) 100 mg t.d.s. then b.d. *Side-effects:* anorexia, nausea, rash, peripheral neuritis. Pyridoxin 10 mg orally is given with each dose of isoniazid to prevent peripheral neuritis.

Para-aminosalicylic Acid (P.A.S.) 6 g orally b.d. *Side-effects:* nausea, vomiting, diarrhoea, rash.

Ethambutol (Myambutol) 25 mg/kg orally daily for two months, then 15 mg/kg daily. Used in place of streptomycin or P.A.S. *Side-effects:* retrobulbar neuritis, causing reduced visual acuity and scotomata, which is often reversible on withdrawal of the drug. Tuberculosis tends to be cured in 9–12 months.

Thiacetazone 150 mg orally daily. *Side-effects:* nausea, vomiting, headache, jaundice, agranulocytosis, exfoliative dermatitis.

Rifampicin (Rimactane) 450–600 mg orally a.c. daily. Expensive, used in place of streptomycin or P.A.S. *Side-effects:* nausea, jaundice, thrombocytopenic purpura.

Prothionamide 500 mg b.d. orally. *Side-effects:* anorexia, nausea, vomiting.

Ethionamide 500 mg b.d. orally. *Side-effects:* anorexia, nausea, vomiting, metallic taste, stomatitis, hepatotoxicity, neuropathy.

Pyrazinamide up to 40 mg/kg daily. *Side-effects:* anorexia, nausea, vomiting, fever, hepatotoxicity, hyperuricaemia.

Viomycin 0·5–1 Mu (0·4–0·8 g) i.m. daily or twice weekly. Used in place of streptomycin. *Side-effects:* as for streptomycin.

Cycloserine 0·25–1 g orally daily. *Side-effects:* neurotoxic—confusion, drowsiness, epilepsy.

Common combinations of three drugs are: Streptomycin and I.N.H., with either P.A.S., thiacetazone, ethambutol or rifampicin, for two months, then two drugs, e.g. I.N.H. plus one of these.

Symptomatic Linctus codeine, pholcodine or methadone 5 ml to suppress unproductive (dry) cough. Cough with sputum should not be suppressed. Pleuritic pain is relieved by warmth to the chest and an analgesic, e.g. soluble aspirin; sometimes pethidine 50–100 mg orally or i.m.

C *Local Treatment of the Lung:* postural drainage to drain sputum from a cavity. Prior to the advent of chemotherapy the treatment was to rest the lung by collapsing it using artificial pneumothorax (introduction of air into the pleural cavity) or by thoracoplasty (resection of ribs allowing collapse of the chest wall). Crushing the phrenic nerve is now obsolete.

Lobectomy or segmental resection of lung is occasionally required in patients with localised severe disease which is not responding to drugs. Effusion may be aspirated for diagnostic investigation, e.g. the detection of tubercle bacilli, or for the relief of dyspnoea, but small effusions do not need treatment.

Prevention. Notification to the area community medical officer, and the tracing of contacts. Better housing with less overcrowding; improved standard of living providing better diet and open-air recreation; early treatment; pasteurisation of milk and tuberculosis-free herds (slaughter of tuberculous cows); better ventilation and avoidance of dusts in industries which cause predisposing disease, e.g. coal mines (pneumoconiosis); vaccination with B.C.G.—an attenuated living bovine tubercle bacillus—if Mantoux negative. Protection by B.C.G. lasts 15 years. Mass radiography was used to detect early cases but is no longer used in the U.K. owing to the low incidence of tuberculosis.

DIPHTHERIA

Diphtheria is due to the bacillus *Corynebacterium diphtheriae*, which is spread by carriers, usually in droplets, but sometimes by direct contact or fomites. The incidence in England and Wales has fallen from 50,000 cases a year to less than 20, due to immunisation.

Pathology: diphtheria bacteria multiply on mucous membranes or in skin abrasions causing inflammation and exudation. Surface cells die and exudate clots to form a membrane. The bacteria remain localised in the upper respiratory tract, but produce a toxin which enters the tissues and bloodstream and damages the heart muscle and nervous system.

Clinically: the incubation period is two to four days. The throat is sore and on it is a cream or pearl-grey, raised, and closely adherent membrane surrounded by inflammation. Removal of the membrane with a swab leaves a bleeding surface. The lymph nodes in the neck are tender and swollen ('bull-neck' if swelling is marked). Infection may occur in the larynx causing a husky voice and cough due to laryngitis, and stridor (noisy inspiration) due to narrowing of the larynx by thick membrane. The breath is foul-smelling. Toxaemia causes apathy, headache, mild fever up to 38·5°C, albuminuria and, if severe, a haemorrhagic rash. Toxic myocarditis produces a rapid pulse of small volume, low blood pressure and pallor. Infection occasionally occurs in the anterior part of the nose causing a bloodstained discharge and a milder disease since less toxin is present.

Complications:
1 Acute toxic myocarditis may cause heart failure or arrhythmia which may be fatal.
2 Respiratory. Respiratory obstruction by the membrane in laryngeal

diphtheria causes dyspnoea and cyanosis, and requires tracheostomy. Inhalation of detached membrane causes pulmonary collapse, and broncho-pneumonia may follow.

3 Neurological. Neuritis begins with paralysis of the soft palate on the tenth to the fourteenth day, thus the posterior part of the nose cannot be shut off from the pharynx, the voice becomes nasal and fluids regurgitate through the nose on swallowing. In the fourth week paralysis of accommodation causes difficulty in reading and paralysis of the external muscles of the eye causes squint. After the seventh week paralysis of the diaphragm (causing respiratory failure) and polyneuritis ('inflammation' of the peripheral nerves) occur. Recovery from cardiac complications and paralysis is complete.

Diagnosis: appearance of the throat. Throat swab for direct microscopy and culture for diphtheria on media containing serum.

Treatment: general treatment for infectious disease. Notifiable. Since there is the danger of heart failure due to myocarditis the patient is kept in bed at complete rest, lying down for three to six weeks. He is not allowed to do anything for himself and is fed, lifted onto a bedpan. and rolled on his side for bedmaking. On recovery, activity is gradually increased. Care of the mouth with moist tissues which are put in a bag to be burnt. Enema if unduly constipated.

Diet: semi-solid or solid to minimise nasal regurgitation, or a pernasal intragastric tube may be used. Glucose is given orally or i.v. Fluid intake should be high to dilute the exotoxin. In palatal paralysis the patient is unable to swallow saliva; the foot of the bed is therefore raised to keep the airway clear of secretions, which are removed from the mouth by swabbing or suction. Heart failure is treated with a diuretic, and salt restriction. Intubation of the larynx or tracheostomy may be necessary in laryngeal diphtheria if laryngoscopic suction fails to remove the membrane from the larynx.

Drugs: antitoxin is given 10,000 units i.m. in mild cases, to 100,000 units i.v. in severe cases, but a small s.c. test dose must be given first since there is the danger of anaphylactic shock or serum sickness due to the presence of horse serum. Benzyl-penicillin 300 mg (0·5 Mu) six-hourly i.m. or erythromycin 250 mg six-hourly orally.

Prevention: throats are examined and swabs taken from all contacts. Carriers are treated with penicillin and unhealthy tonsils removed. A Schick test determines whether or not the patient is immune to diphtheria toxin. 0·2 ml of toxin is injected intradermally into one forearm and a control of 0·2 ml of destroyed toxin into the other arm. In the absence of immunity redness and swelling appear in 48–72 hours (= positive test), and the subject needs immunising. If the subject has circulating antitoxin, toxin is neutralised, the test is negative and the patient immune.

Immunisation: formol toxoid (F.T.) three doses of 0·5–1 ml s.c. or i.m. at four- to eight-week intervals, begun at age three to nine months; 1 ml at age five years; 0·5 ml at 10 years and 15 years. Triple vaccine is an alternative in children.

TYPHUS

Typhus is due to Rickettsiae, small bacteria living in cells. It must not be confused with typhoid. It is spread by fleas, lice, ticks and mites which live on small animals, e.g. rodents. Spread is by insect-bites, by insect faeces getting into a skin abrasion or dried faeces being inhaled.

Treatment: tetracycline or chloramphenicol.

ENTERIC FEVERS

These are typhoid, paratyphoid and other salmonella infections.
Spread: bacilli spread via swallowed faecally contaminated water, food and milk, and by flies, fomites and carriers. Spread by water is due to drinking from contaminated streams or rivers, or leakage from cracked sewage pipes into fresh water supplies. Spread by food includes shellfish caught in sewage-contaminated rivers, imported tinned meat cooled in infected water, dried eggs and coconut, and via carriers handling food. Unpasteurised milk, ice-cream, and cheese may contain salmonellae. Epidemics occur where there is poor sanitation.

TYPHOID

Typhoid is due to *Salmonella typhi*. It must not be confused with typhus.

Pathology: from the small intestine *S. typhi* enters the intestinal lymphatics and mesenteric lymph nodes and travels via the thoracic duct into the blood, causing bacteraemia. The bacilli are taken up from the blood by phagocytes (monocytes) in the reticulo-endothelial system (liver, spleen, bone marrow) where the bacilli multiply. By the tenth day the organisms flood into the blood and cause illness (septicaemia), spreading to many organs including kidneys, bronchi and intestines, hence urine, sputum and faeces are infectious. In the small instestine the lymphoid tissues (Peyer's patches) swell, ulcerate and bleed and may perforate and cause peritonitis. The ulcers heal in the fourth week by the formation of granulation tissue. The spleen and mesenteric lymph nodes enlarge.

Clinically: the incubation period is 10–14 days.
  First week: the temperature rises stepwise to 39·4°C over four to five days and there is anorexia, malaise, insomnia, severe frontal headache, aching, epistaxis, drowsiness and usually constipation. The pulse rate is increased but is not as fast as expected from the height of the temperature.
  Second week: a scanty rash of rose-red spots occurs on the abdomen and chest and lasts three days. It is due to bacterial emboli. Diarrhoea occurs, the stools being yellow ('pea soup' stools) and offensive. There is splenomegaly (enlargement of the spleen), furred tongue, abdominal distension, tenderness in the abdomen, especially in the right iliac fossa, cough (bronchitis), and there may be delirium.

Third week: lethargy, rapid soft pulse, muscular weakness, tremors and toxaemia. Coma and death may occur. There may be haemorrhage or perforation of ulcerated Peyer's patches.

Fourth week onwards: gradual recovery, but there may be relapses.

Complications:

1 Haemorrhage from the ileum is of sudden onset, with shock (faintness, increased pulse rate, fall in temperature) but bright red or tarry stools may not be passed for some hours.
2 Perforation of the ileum allows bowel contents to enter the peritoneal cavity, causing peritonitis.
3 Bronchopneumonia due to low resistance to secondary infection.
4 Others—cholecystitis, osteomyelitis, meningitis, arthritis, parotitis, venous thrombosis.

Diagnosis: in the first week there are few diagnostic signs, but typhoid must be distinguished from other causes of P.U.O. (pyrexia of unknown origin). In typhoid the pulse rate is slow compared with the height of the temperature. Blood or bone marrow culture for organisms is positive in the first week, faeces culture from the second, and urine culture in the third week. Culture is made in selenite broth or on McConkey's bile agar plates, which favour the growth of salmonellae. Suspicious colonies will agglutinate if mixed with known antibody on a slide. Blood for serology (Widal agglutination test) after the tenth day shows a rising level (titre) of typhoid antibodies, and 1:100 or more is positive. The white cell count is slightly low (leucopenia) due to granulocytopenia (reduced numbers of granulocytes, i.e. polymorphs); thus there is a relative lymphocytosis (apparent increase in lymphocytes).

Treatment: as for infectious disease in general. Rest in bed in a warm (16°C) well-ventilated room, preferably having an extractor fan. Plastic-covered mattress. Care of the mouth and pressure areas, and the patient is turned four-hourly. Abundant fluids according to the urinary and faecal losses (fluid balance chart), with allowance for increased fluid loss from the skin by sweating due to an increased metabolic rate caused by fever.

Diet: must be semifluid at first (*see* diet 1, Appendix) with three pints of milk daily to supply protein and calories, followed by a low roughage diet (*see* diet 2, Appendix); food should be digested and liquid by the time it reaches the terminal ileum since gas and roughage predispose to perforation and haemorrhage. Fish or minced meat is given at the end of the fourth week, and a normal diet after six weeks. If antibiotic is given from the start of the illness it will prevent damage to the ileum and therefore a normal diet can be given after a few days. Pulse, blood pressure, respiratory rate and four-hourly temperature must be recorded in order to detect the onset of complications.

A pyrexia above 39·5°C requires tepid sponging for 15 minutes every four hours. Stools for culture. The patient is infective until six consecutive stools are salmonella-negative.

Drugs: analgesic for headache e.g. Sod. salicylate B.P.C. 10 ml t.d.s. Sedative for insomnia, e.g. amylobarbitone 60 mg at night. Ampicillin or chloramphenicol 0·5 g six-hourly. For diarrhoea: fluid and electrolytes, drugs which constipate, e.g. codeine phosphate 15–30 mg t.d.s. Enema for constipation, NOT an aperient since this may precipitate perforation by increasing peristalsis.

Treat Complications. Haemorrhage: the patient should be horizontal, or, in severe shock, the foot-end of the bed elevated, and ice sucked. Morphia 15 mg s.c. or i.m., phenobarbitone. Blood grouping and haemoglobin should be done and a blood transfusion given if necessary.

Perforation: gastric suction via a pernasal Ryle's tube, intravenous fluids, antibiotic. Surgery with repair of the perforation may be considered, but has a high mortality.

Venous Thrombosis: anticoagulants may be used if blood is absent from the faeces, but there is danger of haemorrhage from the bowel. They cannot be given if blood is present in the faeces.

Carriers: 3% of cases become carriers and carry the bacilli in the gall bladder and bile ducts. A three-month course of co-trimoxazole or ampicillin with probenecid may cure, but often cholecystectomy is also required.

Prevention: notification to the area community medical officer, who will trace the source of infection and remedy it, and warn and immunise contacts. Immunisation is by the injection of killed *S. typhi* and *S. paratyphi* A and B (= T.A.B. vaccine) 0·5 ml s.c. (or 0·2 ml intradermally), then four weeks and six months later 1 ml s.c. (or 0·2 ml i.d.) is given, this dose being repeated every three years. For children under 12 years the dose is halved. Prevention of direct spread is by isolation of the patient and barrier nursing. The stools, urine and sputum are treated by covering with 5% phenol (carbolic) or 5% lysol for two hours. Linen is put into plastic bags marked 'infectious' and treated with formalin, 5% phenol or 1·25% (1 in 80) sudol for 2 hours, then laundered by boiling. Marked feeding utensils, boiled after each use. The nurse should scrub her hands and arms with soap and water after each visit to the patient. The patient's case notes and X-rays should be kept outside the cubicle.

PARATYPHOID

Paratyphoid is commonly due to *S. paratyphi* B, sometimes to *S. paratyphi* A. It is a milder disease than typhoid, but otherwise symptoms, diagnosis and treatment are similar.

OTHER SALMONELLAE

These cause food poisoning if ingested in large numbers. There is acute onset of headache, nausea, vomiting, abdominal pain and diarrhoea, lasting three days. Diagnosis is by faecal culture and agglutination tests.

Treatment: rehydration and mist. kaolin 10 ml (= 2 g kaolin) for diarrhoea.

Antibiotics should not be given in simple enteritis since they do not shorten the illness but paradoxically may prolong the carrier state!

DYSENTERY

Types: (1) Bacillary (Shigellae); (2) Amoebic; (3) Flagellate ('Ciliate').

Bacillary Dysentery
This is due to infection of the wall of the large bowel with bacilli called Shigellae, of which there are several types. *Shigella (Sh.) sonne* is mild and common in the U.K. *Sh. shiga* is severe and common in the tropics. *Sh. flexneri* and *Sh. boydi* are moderately severe. Spread is by the ingestion of food or drink contaminated through poor hygiene and flies.

Clinically: the incubation period is one to seven days. There is acute inflammation of the colon causing fever, nausea, abdominal colicky pain, tenderness over the large bowel, tenesmus (severe straining at stool), and diarrhoea. The faeces contain blood, mucus ('red-currant jelly') and pus.

In severe cases loss of fluid and electrolytes causes dehydration, especially in children. A person may continue to excrete bacteria after symptoms have subsided (= carrier).

Complications:
1   Severe dehydration causes fall in the blood pressure and renal failure.
2   Haemorrhage.
3   Anaemia.
4   Peritonitis.

Investigations: faeces or rectal swab cultured for shigellae.

Treatment: bed. Isolation. General treatment of infectious disease. The nurse looking after the patient must not prepare food. Adequate fluid by mouth to prevent dehydration; i.v. fluid if necessary. Fluid balance chart. Low residue diet.

Drugs: chemotherapy (usually not required). One of the following may be given according to sensitivity:
1   Phthalylsulphathiazole 30 mg/kg body-weight four-hourly until less than four stools are passed in a day, then eight-hourly for three days.
2   Sulphadiazine 3 g stat. then 1 g six-hourly with abundant fluids to prevent dehydration; the urine should be made alkaline by giving sodium bicarbonate 1 to 3 g two-hourly. Resistance is common.
3   Tetracycline 0·5 g orally six-hourly.
4   Streptomycin 500 mg orally b.d. for one week.
5   Neomycin 0·5 g orally six-hourly.
        Also codeine phosphate for pain. Kaolin for diarrhoea.

Amoebic Dysentery
This is due to *Entamoeba histolytica*, the cysts of which are passed in the faeces. After the ingestion of food contaminated with non-motile cysts the cysts transform into

active motile amoebae (vegetative form) which invade the mucosa of the large intestine, producing ulcers.

Clinically: amoebic dysentery is usually a mild afebrile chronic disease with grumbling abdominal pain, tender colon, and two or three loose stools daily, often alternating with periods of constipation. The stools are offensive and contain mucus.

Complications: (1) perforation of the large bowel; (2) spread of the parasite in the portal bloodstream causing an amoebic abscess in the liver which causes pyrexia, sweating, an enlarged tender liver and a raised diaphragm.

Diagnosis: mucus from several freshly passed motions is examined for motile vegetative amoebae (which soon die outside the body) and for cysts (which live for months). Sigmoidoscopy demonstrates ulcers, and allows a biopsy to be taken and examined for amoebae. Isotope or ultrasonic liver scan for hepatic abscess.

Treatment: low residue diet. Iron for anaemia.

Drugs: metronidazole (Flagyl) 400–800 mg t.d.s. for five days is the drug of choice. Emetine hydrochloride 60 mg s.c. daily for three to five days, the patient being kept in bed since emetine has a toxic action on the heart, followed by emetine bismuth iodide (E.B.I.) 200 mg for each of eight evenings (with water) four hours after the last meal and no further food or fluid is taken for 12 hours. E.B.I. causes vomiting; to prevent this the patient is given an hypnotic, e.g. amylobarbitone 0·2 g, one hour before. An alternative to E.B.I. is diloxanide furoate (Furamide) 0·5 g t.d.s. orally for ten days.

After six weeks six or more stools are re-examined for amoebae and cysts and sigmoidoscopy is performed. This is repeated monthly for six months to be sure of a cure.

For hepatic amoebiasis metronidazole is given for 5 days, emetine for 10 days or chloroquine 600 mg (base) daily for two days then 300 mg daily for 21 days. A liver abscess may need draining.

Flagellate (Ciliate) Dysentery
Giardiasis is due to *Giardia lamblia*, a parasite having four pairs of flagellae. Spread is by the ingestion of cysts in contaminated food or drink.

Clinically: it causes acute or chronic diarrhoea in children by causing inflammation of the small intestine. Cysts are excreted in the stools.

Treatment: metronidazole 50–200 mg t.d.s. for five to seven days has outdated mepacrine (Quinacrine) 50–100 mg t.d.s. for five days.

LEPTOSPIROSIS

Leptospirosis is due to one of many spirochaetes, e.g. *Leptospira canicola*, spread by dogs, or *Leptospira icterohaemorrhagica*, spread by rats, mice and other animals.

Leptospira Icterohaemorrhagica (Weil's Disease)

The animals excrete the organisms in the urine and man is infected, via the skin and mucous membranes, by bathing or working in infected water (coal miners, sewermen, ditchers, canal bathers) or by taking food or drink contaminated by a rat.

Clinically: the incubation period is seven to fourteen days. The disease begins as a septicaemia, with pyrexia, headache, anorexia, nausea, vomiting, conjunctivitis, enlarged spleen and skin rash, often petechial. The temperature then falls and the patient recovers, or the disease continues with jaundice and a tender liver due to hepatitis, albuminuria due to renal damage, haemoptysis due to haemorrhagic pneumonia, myocarditis and meningitis. There is a general bleeding tendency—epistaxis, skin bruising, haematuria. A polymorph leucocytosis is present.

Diagnosis: (1) blood and urine culture or guinea-pig inoculation; (2) the presence of leptospiral antibodies in the serum from the second week.

Treatment: isolation is unnecessary. Rest in bed, general treatment (p. 42). Fluid balance chart to detect early renal or cardiac failure (these cause fluid retention). Benzylpenicillin 600 mg six-hourly i.m. for one week, then b.d. for one week.

PSITTACOSIS (ORNITHOSIS)

Psittacosis is an infection with a small bacterium (once thought to be a virus) spread by birds (parrots, pigeons, canaries). The incubation period is 10 days. It causes sore throat and pneumonia.

Treatment: isolation, tetracycline.

CHOLERA

Cholera is due to *Vibrio cholerae*, a curved bacillus shaped like a comma, spread by the ingestion of faecally contaminated food and water, and by flies. The organism is confined to the gastro-intestinal tract.

Clinically: the incubation period is two to five days. There is nausea, vomiting, abdominal cramp and severe watery diarrhoea ('rice-water' stools), causing dehydration, oliguria and fall in blood pressure. Death is from circulatory failure.
Treatment: i.v. glucose–saline in abundance. Oral tetracycline may be given but antibiotic is not essential providing enough saline fluid is given.

RABIES ('HYDROPHOBIA')

Rabies is due to a virus which invades the nervous system. It is spread by the bite of a rabid animal, e.g. dog, wolf, vampire bat.

Clinically: the incubation period is two to sixteen weeks or longer. There is restlessness, delirium, convulsions, painful spasm of the pharynx on swallowing (saliva therefore drools from the mouth), paralysis and death.

Prevention: strict quarantine of imported animals for six to twelve months.

Treatment: attenuated rabies vaccine may help if given soon after the patient has been bitten, but is useless once symptoms are present.

LEPROSY

Leprosy is due to *Mycobacterium leprae*, which is spread by close contact or droplets and enters through mucous membranes; possibly also through the skin by biting-insects. It was described in Egypt in 1350 B.C. and affects 15 million people in the tropics and subtropics. It is notifiable.

Clinically: the incubation period is one to five years. There are two extremes and various intermediate forms of disease depending on the patient's resistance.
1 Tuberculoid leprosy occurs if the patient has a high cell-mediated immunity, hence there are few leprosy bacilli in the body. The skin rash (tuberculides) consists of scanty red macules, then papules. There is polyneuritis (inflammation of peripheral nerves) which causes thickening of the nerves. Damage to sensory nerves causes burning, tingling, then anaesthesia (loss of sensation) of the skin which allows injury to occur. Damage to motor nerve fibres causes muscle-wasting which is followed by fibrosis and contractures of muscles leading to deformities. Autonomic nerve damage produces a dry skin due to lack of sweating.
2 Lepromatous leprosy. The patient has a low cell-mediated immunity, and the tissues contain numerous bacilli. The skin rash consists of macules, papules or red tender nodules (erythema nodosum) lasting a few days, and the skin thickens. Although the nerves are invaded by bacilli there is little cellular response and little neurological damage. Rhinitis and iritis occur.

Diagnosis: the Lepromin skin test is positive in tuberculoid leprosy owing to the patient's response to infection, but is negative in lepromatous leprosy since the patient does not produce a reaction to the lepromatous antigen. Scrapings from the skin or nasal mucosa show numerous organisms.

Treatment: isolation of patients with the lepromatous form in a colony until they are free from bacteria, or removal of young children from infected families. The tuberculoid form is relatively non-infectious and is treated at home.
Diet should be adequate in protein, vitamins and calories.
Drugs: dapsone, beginning with 25 mg orally twice weekly, gradually increasing to 50 to 100 mg daily for six days a week, and continuing for two years or longer. Tetracycline or rifampicin 600 mg daily a.c. for two weeks may be used, followed by dapsone. Surgical correction of deformities.

BRUCELLOSIS

Brucellosis is due to the bacilli *Brucella* (*Br.*) *abortus* (in cattle), *Br. melitensis* (in goats) or *Br. suis* (in pigs). Spread is by the ingestion of infected unpasteurised milk, droplets entering the respiratory tract or conjunctiva, or by direct contact through the skin. It is an occupational hazard in veterinary surgeons, slaughter-house, laboratory and farm-workers, and hide-handlers. *Brucella abortus* causes undulant fever in man and abortion in cows.

Clinically the incubation period of *Br. abortus* is usually three weeks but may be months. There is sweating and pyrexia alternating with apyrexial periods; weakness, headache, anorexia, depression, constipation, rigors, pains in the limbs and back and an enlarged spleen. There is neutropenia (a low polymorph count).

Complications: (1) arthritis; (2) spondylitis (inflammation of the spine); (3) anaemia.

Diagnosis: (1) blood culture daily for one week; (2) serum agglutination and complement-fixation tests show rising antibody levels.

Treatment: rest in bed. Oral or i.v. fluids if dehydrated. Tetracycline 500 mg six-hourly orally for three to six weeks for acute disease. Tetracycline 1 g daily and sulphadimidine 4 g daily for three to six weeks in chronic disease (streptomycin 1 g daily is sometimes given in addition). Prevention is by boiling or pasteurising milk, slaughter of diseased animals, and vaccination of young female calves.

VENEREAL DISEASE

Venereal disease is disease contracted during coitus (sexual intercourse) with an infected person. Venereal diseases are: gonorrhoea, syphilis, non-specific urethritis, trichomonas, Reiter's disease, candida vaginitis and balanitis.

Note: In 1864 and 1866 the contagious diseases acts were passed whereby a person with syphilis could be locked up until cured! They were repealed 10 years later.

Gonorrhoea

This is due to infection of the mucous membrane of the genito-urinary tract with the diplococcus *Neisseria gonorrhoeae* (gonococcus). There are 16 million cases a year in the world.

Clinically: the incubation period is three to ten days. In the male the infection begins in the anterior part of the urethra and spreads to the posterior part of the urethra, and from there to the bladder (cystitis), prostate (prostatitis), and seminal vesicles (vesiculitis) (*Fig. 4.12*). There is dysuria (painful micturition), increased frequency of micturition, and a yellowish discharge from the urethra. In the female the infection is in the urethra (urethritis), cervix of the uterus (cervicitis), and Bartholin's glands (glands in the vulva; Bartholinitis), causing dysuria, frequency of micturition, and vaginal discharge, but the symptoms are often so mild as to be

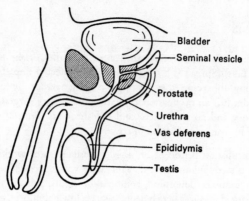

FIG. 4.12   Spread of gonorrhoea

unnoticed. The anal canal may be affected in homosexual males. Infants born of infected mothers have gonorrhoeal conjunctivitis (ophthalmia neonatorum), which must be notified; it may cause corneal scarring and blindness.

Complications:

1 Local spread to the epididymis (epididymitis) in males which may cause sterility due to obstruction of the vas deferens by scar tissue.
2 Spread to the Fallopian tubes causes acute salpingitis in females, and may cause sterility.
3 Septicaemia causing spread via the blood to joints (gonococcal arthritis), iris of the eye (iritis), heart valves (endocarditis) especially of the aortic valve, skin (septic dermatitis—a rash of papules and pustules).

Diagnosis: a swab of the pus shows the presence of gonococci in polymorphs (*Fig. 4.13*) and on culture. Gonococci soon die outside the body and if cultures cannot be made immediately the swab should be put in Stuart's transport medium which keeps the organisms alive for 48 hours. A serum gonococcal fixation test (G.C.F.T.) is positive in chronic cases.

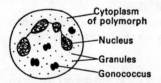

FIG. 4.13 Gonococci in a polymorph

Treatment: sexual intercourse is prohibited until cured. Contacts should be traced and treated. The patient must be told that he is infectious to others, must have his own towel and must wash his hands after micturition.

Drugs: benzylpenicillin 300 mg i.m. plus procaine penicillin 600 mg (0·6 Mu) i.m., repeated in 24 hours, or ampicillin 2 g plus probenecid 1 g orally.

Tetracycline or erythromycin may be used if the patient is allergic to penicillin or if the gonococci are penicillin-resistant. Unfortunately these short courses of penicillin, erythromycin or tetracycline may mask the presence of syphilis, although curing the gonorrhoea; so sometimes drugs which do not affect syphilis are given, e.g. Co-trimoxazole 1 tablet six-hourly for five days, kanamycin or streptomycin.

For gonococcal conjunctivitis penicillin is given both i.m. and intensively as eye-drops. Prevention: at childbirth the baby's eyes are wiped with sterile swabs before they are opened.

Non-specific Urethritis

This is urethritis due to organisms other than gonococci, e.g. mycoplasma, chlamydia (small intracellular bacteria).

Treatment: oxytetracycline 250 mg q.i.d.

Reiter's Disease

Reiter's disease is probably due to chlamydia, usually spread by sexual intercourse.

Clinically: there is acute urethritis (or sometimes diarrhoea in non-urethral infection), followed by purulent conjunctivitis, uveitis (inflammation of the uvea, the pigmented vascular layer of the eye, including the iris), polyarthritis, balanitis, shallow painful ulcers on the penis and in the mouth. A rash may occur over the palms and soles, and rarely there is pericarditis and myocarditis. The condition lasts for three months; sometimes longer.

Complications: (1) deformities of the feet; (2) spondylitis.

Treatment: tetracycline 500 mg q.i.d. for 10 days, or sulphadimidine plus strepto-mycin. Analgesic, rest in bed, then physiotherapy for arthritis. Local corticosteroids for conjunctivitis.

Lymphogranuloma Venereum (Lymphogranuloma Inguinale)

This is due to a bacterium (chlamydia) spread by venereal contact.

Clinically: the incubation period is three to twenty days. It begins on the genital mucous membrane as a papule which becomes a vesicle and ulcerates. The lymph nodes draining the ulcer enlarge and these and the surrounding tissues become hard and swollen and suppurate, forming sinuses. There is pyrexia and often a rash.

Complications:

1   Elephantiasis (marked oedema) of the genitals.
2   Arthritis.
3   Iritis.
4   Urethral stricture if the ulcer was in the anterior urethra, rectal stricture due to proctitis in male homosexuals.

Diagnosis: (1) Frei skin test; (2) blood for complement-fixation test.

Treatment: sulphonamides. Tetracycline.

Granuloma inguinale is a chronic infection of the genital and perianal areas due to an intracellular organism which forms 'Donovan bodies'. Treatment: tetracycline 2 g daily.

Syphilis

Syphilis (Σ) was known in 3000 B.C. It is a chronic disease due to the spirochaete (spiro = coil, chaete = bristle), *Treponema pallidum*, spread by sexual intercourse, or occasionally by kissing, or through the placenta. There is a rising incidence in the world due to promiscuity. About 50% of cases in Britain are due to homo-sexuality.

Clinically: the incubation period is 10 days to 12 weeks; average 25 days. The organisms enter directly through a mucous membrane or through a tiny abrasion in the skin, enter the lymphatics and pass into the blood to be dispersed throughout the body within 24 hours. There are three stages.

The primary stage: the primary lesion (chancre) develops at the original site of infection, usually the genitals (glans penis, vulva, cervix), but occasionally the lip, anus, or finger. It is a painless, red, indurated (hard), small nodule (papule) which ulcerates. The regional lymph nodes enlarge and are discrete, rubbery and painless. The chancre heals in two to six weeks.

The secondary stage begins between the sixth and twelfth weeks and is due to the generalised infection. The patient feels ill, has malaise, anorexia, mild pyrexia, headache from meningeal inflammation, sore throat due to ulcers in the fauces, anaemia, patchy ('moth-eaten') alopecia (baldness), hoarse voice (laryngitis), mucous patches (silver-grey—'snail-track'—ulcers on mucous membranes) in the mouth and pharynx, macular, papular or scaly coppery-red skin rash which does not itch, bone pain due to periostitis (inflammation of the periosteum), iritis and retinitis (inflammation of the iris and retina of the eye), and generalised painless lymphadenopathy (enlargement of the lymph nodes). Condylomata lata appear in moist areas on the skin, especially around the genitals and anus, and are due to the coalescence (running together) of papules to resemble flat warts. Mucous ulcers and condylomata are highly infectious. These changes disappear in about one year to be followed by a latent period of two to thirty years before the third stage.

Tertiary stage: local necrotic swellings (gummata) appear anywhere, especially in the skin where they ulcerate, and also in testis, liver, bone, and meninges. In the brain they cause symptoms of a cerebral tumour. Inflammation of the aorta weakens the wall and causes it to bulge, forming an aneurysm, which may rupture (*Fig. 4.14*). Involvement of the nervous system (neuro-syphilis) causes general paralysis of the insane (G.P.I.), tabes dorsalis, and Argyll Robertson pupils—small, irregular, unequal pupils which do not react to light.

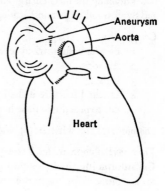

FIG. 4.14   Aortic aneurysm

Diagnosis:

1   Exudate (serum) from the chancre, condylomas or mucous ulcers, is ex-amined for spirochaetes.

2   Blood Wassermann (W.R.), Kahn, venereal disease research laboratory (V.D.R.L.) tests become positive from the fourth week but may give a temporary false positive in glandular fever, infective hepatitis, systemic lupus erythematosus and chickenpox. The Reiter protein complement-

fixation test (R.C.F.T.) is more specific. Specific tests on blood serum are the fluorescent treponemal antibody (F.T.A.) and treponemal immobilisation (T.P.I.) tests.

Treatment: procaine penicillin 0·6–1·2 g i.m. daily for 10–20 days. Tetracycline or erythromycin 500 mg q.d.s. for one month is used if the patient is allergic to penicillin. Patients are seen monthly for six months then three-monthly for two years, in case further courses are needed. Benzathine penicillin 2·4 g i.m. single injection lasts two weeks but is not as reliable as procaine penicillin and is only used in patients unable, or unlikely, to attend for daily injections. Prednisolone is given with the first injection of penicillin to prevent the Jarisch–Herxheimer reaction (fever and fall in blood pressure lasting a few hours, due to endotoxin released as the spirochaetes die). Prednisolone+1% atropine eye-drops for keratitis. Contacts must be traced and treated.

Congenital Syphilis. This is due to infection of the fetus via the placenta in a syphilitic mother. The fetus may die in the uterus and abort or be still-born; or may be born alive and infected. The child may be born wasted; fail to thrive; have 'snuffles' (nasal discharge) and a skin rash, e.g. pemphigus (bullae) on the soles, palms and buttocks; or appear normal at birth but within a few months develop changes similar to acquired syphilis—skin rashes (papules, blisters); mucous patches; enlarged liver and spleen; rhagades (scars due to healed lesions at the angles of the mouth); Hutchinson's teeth (peg-shaped, notched separated incisors); saddle-shaped nose (flattened bridge); periostitis; 'sabre' tibia; eighth nerve damage causing deafness; eye disease (keratitis, optic atrophy); condylomas; gummas. Tabes and G.P.I. may occur in adolescence, but are rare.

PARASITES

Parasites obtain their nourishment from others and are common where there is a lack of hygiene. They cause itching, scratching and secondary bacterial infection.

Fleas
Fleas are insects living on animals which they bite to obtain blood. They can survive three months without a meal. The bite causes an itching papule. Eggs are laid in cracks in furniture and floors. Development is from eggs to larva to pupa (chrysalis) to flea. Fleas spread plague, typhus and anthrax. They are destroyed with insecticides e.g. Dicophane or malathion.

Lice
Lice are also insects living on blood. Prevention is by simple hygiene. There are three types, all killed by insecticides; e.g. 0·5% carbaryl (Carylderm), 0·1% gamma-benzene hexachloride (Lorexane), or 0·5% malathion (Prioderm).

The Head Louse (*Pediculus capitis*) lays pale grey eggs (nits) attached to the base of the hair. These lice are spread by direct contact or fomites (pillows, hats).

Treatment: insecticide is applied to the entire scalp and the head is covered for 24 hours. The hair is not washed and insecticide is again applied to the scalp one week later to kill any new lice that hatch. The hair is left unwashed for a further week, then the hair is shampooed and nits removed by careful combing with a special fine-toothed metal nit-comb. The operator should wear overalls, and a waterproof cover is placed around the patient's neck. Hats are sterilised by heat; hair brushes and combs by hot 2% lysol. All infected members of the family should be treated at the same time.

The Body Louse (*Pediculus corporis*) lays its eggs on clothing, including bed clothing. It transmits typhus. Lorexane cream is applied over the whole body below the chin. Underclothing and bedclothing are treated with formalin or are boiled.

The Pubic Louse (*Phthirus pubis*) lives in the pubic and axillary hair and is spread by direct contact, usually sexual. The pubic hair is cut short and insecticide applied to pubic and axillary regions.

Bedbugs

These live in cracks in rooms in slums and feed on blood at night. They are killed with insecticide.

Scabies

Scabies is due to the mite *Sarcoptes* (*Acarus*) *scabiei* which burrows in the skin to lay eggs. The burrow is a thin grey line 1 cm long, with a small vesicle at one end containing a tiny speck which is the mite. Infection is by close contact or fomites. It infects the clefts of the fingers, fronts of the wrists, axillae and genital skin and causes irritation, especially at night when the patient is warm in bed. Scratching causes secondary infection and impetigo, which is contagious and the patient should be segregated until cured.

Treatment: 25% benzyl benzoate, 1% gamma-benzene hexachloride (Lorexane) cream, or monosulphiram (Tetmosol) diluted to 25% before use. The patient has a bath, scrubs the affected areas with a nail-brush to open the burrows and is painted completely from chin to toe with the solution, and allowed to dry. He is repainted on the second day and has a bath and a complete change of clothing on the third day. Underwear and bed linen are steam-ironed. All other members of the family are treated at the same time to prevent re-infection.

HELMINTHIC (WORM) INFECTIONS

Nematodes (Roundworms) (*Fig. 4.15*)

Threadworm (*Enterobius vermicularis*). The male is 3 mm, the female 10 mm, long. The female lays eggs (ova) around the anus, causing itching. Eggs are transferred from the anus, via clothing and unwashed hands, to the mouth and are swallowed to develop into worms in the ileum. Most adult worms live in the colon. Ova are detected by pressing sticky Sellotape to the anus in the morning and examining it microscopically.

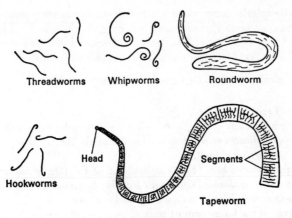

FIG. 4.15   Helminths

Treatment: piperazine phosphate (4 g) with senna (Pripsen 10 g) orally in a single dose at night, repeated after two weeks. Viprynium embonate (Vanquin) is used similarly but stains the faeces red. Check weekly for eggs. Mercury ointment around the anus o.n., secure pyjamas, forbid scratching and nail-biting (or gloves worn at night), nails kept short, hands washed. The whole family should be treated simultaneously since most are likely to be infected. Pyjamas, underclothing and bed linen should be boiled, and lavatory seats kept clean.

Roundworm (*Ascaris lumbricoides*) is 20 cm long and resembles an earthworm, but it is pale yellow. Eggs from food or drink develop into larvae and migrate through the wall of the small intestine to reach the lungs. They ascend the trachea and are swallowed to develop into adults. Ova are found in the faeces.
Treatment: piperazine as for threadworms.

Roundworm of Dogs and Cats (*Toxocara canis* and *T. cati*) are common in these animals (which should be de-wormed at an early age) and ova from faeces may be ingested by children in close contact with their pet. Ova develop in the stomach into larvae which migrate into the bloodstream and may cause asthma with eosinophilia. The toxocara skin test is positive.

Treatment: diethylcarbamazine (Banocide) 9–12 mg/kg body weight daily for three weeks kills larvae, plus piperazine to expel the adult worms.

Filaria of various types are spread by mosquitoes and flies.

Treatment: diethylcarbamazine 2 mg/kg body weight t.d.s. for three weeks.

Whipworm (*Trichuris trichiura*) is 4 cm long. Infection is via soil-contaminated food.

Treatment: thiabendazole 50 mg/kg body weight over two days, difetarsone 0·5 g b.d. with food, for one week, or mebendazole 100 mg b.d. for 3 days.

Trichinella spiralis causes trichinosis. It is spread by ingesting partially cooked pork sausages or ham. There is nausea, vomiting, diarrhoea and abdominal pain followed by pyrexia, tachycardia, muscle stiffness and allergic oedema of the face, eyelids and conjunctivae. The blood shows an eosinophilia.

Treatment: thiabendazole 50 mg/kg body weight over two days.

Cestodes (Tapeworms, *Fig. 4.15*)
These have a life cycle in two 'hosts'. They are ribbon-shaped worms consisting of numerous segments attached to the head (scolex). The larvae (cysticerci) are ingested in undercooked meat.

The **tapeworm of beef** (*Taenia saginata*) and **of fish** (*Diphyllobothrium latum*) are treated with niclosamide (Yomesan) 1 g orally; the tablets are taken fasting and chewed before swallowing. The dose is repeated in 1 hour.

The larvae of the **tapeworm of pork** (*Taenia solium*) migrate throughout the body and in the brain may cause epilepsy.

Treatment: Felix mas, niclosamide or mepacrine (Quinacrine) for the worm. Anticonvulsants for the epilepsy.

Taenia echinococcus is the canine tapeworm. The dog excretes ova in its faeces. Man may swallow ova after handling a dog. Sheep, cattle, pigs and camels ingest the eggs while grazing. The embryo hatches from the ovum in the duodenum and penetrates the intestinal wall to be carried, in the portal bloodstream and lymphatics, to the organs of the host, commonly the liver and lungs, sometimes the spleen, brain, kidney or muscle. In the organ the embryo develops into the larval stage, the hydatid cyst. The cyst slowly enlarges and may be symptomless or may cause pressure symptoms. Numerous scolices are produced in a cyst. Each scolex (worm's head) can develop into a tapeworm in the dog and its relatives. Cysts may calcify, degenerate or become infected to form an abscess. Cysts may be removed surgically. The Casoni skin test (intradermal injection of cyst fluid) is positive.

Hookworms (*Ancylostoma duodenale* and *Necator americanus*)
These larvae penetrate the skin of those who walk barefoot and the worms in the intestine cause anaemia. They may cause pneumonia. Eggs are found in the faeces.

Treatment: tetrachloroethylene 4 ml (fasting) followed two hours later by a saline purge, or bephenium hydroxynaphthoate 2·5–5 g daily for three days for *A. duodenale*, thiabendazole for *N. americanus*. Iron for anaemia.

Trematodes (blood flukes)
Schistosomiasis (bilharziasis), which affects about 150 million people in the world, including 400,000 in the U.S.A., is due to *Schistosoma*, flukes which live in the circulatory system. The adult worms mature in the branches of the portal vein in the liver, then migrate, against the portal blood flow, to the intestinal wall (*S. masoni* and *S. japonicum*) or to the bladder wall (*S. haematobium*) where eggs are deposited. Eggs rupture into the lumen of the gut or bladder to be excreted in faeces or urine. In fresh water, eggs hatch into miracidia which penetrate snails and transform into thousands of cercariae (infective larvae), which penetrate

human skin, enter the bloodstream, and develop into schistosoma. *S. mansoni* and *S. japonicum* lead to allergic itching, urticaria, fever and headache, and to diarrhoea. There may be an enlarged, tender liver and anaemia. Ova are found in the stools. Treatment is with niridazole 25 mg/kg orally daily for 7 days, oxamniquine (Vansil) 30 to 60 mg/kg total dose, hycanthone, stibocaptate (Astiban), or tartar emetic.

S. haematobium causes dysuria, frequency of micturition, haematuria and anaemia. Ova are present in urine. Treatment is with the drugs used for *S. mansoni* or with metrifonate.

MALARIA

Malaria is due to one of the five *Plasmodia* (malarial parasites), transmitted by mosquito bites or infected blood transfusion in the tropics.

Types

1 *Plasmodium* (*P.*) *falciparum* causes malignant tertian malaria, the most dangerous form. It is the commonest type in tropical Africa.
2 *P. vivax* causes benign tertian malaria. It is common in India and South-East Asia.
3 *P. malariae* causes quartan malaria.
4 *P. ovale* causes benign tertian malaria.
5 *P. knowlesi*, in Malaya.

The Life Cycle of the Malarial Parasite

The female Anopheles mosquito sucks infected blood containing the sexual forms (gametocytes) of the parasite which form eggs. These develop, in about two weeks, into asexual forms (sporozoites) which reach the mosquito's salivary glands to be injected into the next person bitten. In man the sporozoites develop in the liver cells which rupture to release merozoites into the blood, and these enter red blood cells where asexual multiplication occurs. The invaded cells rupture to release merozoites into the plasma and cause a rigor. Merozoites enter new red cells and the cycle is repeated causing rigors every 48 hours in tertian malaria, and every 72 hours in quartan malaria. Some sexual forms (gametocytes) develop in the erythrocytes, but these must be ingested by the Anopheles mosquito for the completion of the sexual cycle. Sporozoites persist in the liver, if untreated, for several years, except for *P. falciparum* infection which terminates spontaneously within two years.

Clinically: the incubation period is 10–30 days. An acute attack is due to rupture of red cells which causes haemolytic anaemia and releases parasites into the plasma, the patient feels cold and has rigors (violent shivering) which cause fever. There is severe headache, nausea and vomiting, then the patient feels hot. Sweating then reduces the temperature and the patient feels better until the next rigor in two days (tertian malaria) or three days (quartan malaria), and rigors continue for about six weeks. The spleen is enlarged and tender and may rupture from minor injury, and herpes labialis is common. Blood films reveal malarial parasites.

Parasites may persist in the liver and enter the bloodstream at intervals, producing relapsing malaria.

Complications: abortion. Falciparum malaria may cause cerebral symptoms (cerebral malaria), e.g. fits, hemiplegia, drowsiness, coma; acute renal failure; and blackwater fever (severe haemolysis) which is usually precipitated by quinine.

Prevention: insecticide spray for houses and mosquito-breeding sites. Eliminate stagnant water by drainage or filling-in with earth. Wire mesh over windows at night, mosquito nets over beds.

Drugs: proguanil (Paludrine) 100–200 mg daily, pyrimethamine (Daraprim) 25–50 mg once weekly, or chloroquine 300 mg (base) weekly, for one week before entering, and one month after leaving, the malarial zone. This suppresses acute attacks of haemolysis but does not prevent infection, and should be followed by primaquine to destroy the exoerythrocytic parasite.

Treatment: rest in bed, abundant fluids, i.v. for severe vomiting and dehydration. Aspirin or paracetamol for headache. Bathing and change of clothes after sweating. Treat anaemia.

Drugs: Acute malaria—chloroquine or amodiaquine 600 mg (base) orally, or 300 mg i.m., stat., 300 mg after six hours, then 150 mg b.d. for three to six days. Quinine or sulphadoxine with pyrimethamine is given for parasites resistant to these. These drugs destroy the parasites in red blood cells, but do not destroy those in the liver.

Relapsing malaria—as for acute malaria, followed by primaquine, 7·5 mg b.d. for three weeks to destroy the parasites in the liver.

5 BLOOD, RETICULOENDOTHELIAL AND LYMPHATIC SYSTEMS, AND THYMUS

THE BLOOD

The blood consists of plasma, the faintly yellow fluid portion, and cells. Serum is the liquid remaining after clotting has removed the fibrinogen from the plasma. The volume of blood in a 70 kg man is 5·6 l. Of this, 55% (3 l) is plasma, and 45% (2·5 l) is cells. The blood volume of the 3·2 kg (7 lb) baby is 270 ml.

THE PLASMA

The plasma contains numerous ions and molecules; the important ones are shown in *Table 5.1*. The function of the plasma is the transportation of nutrients from the sites of absorption (intestine, skin) or of manufacture (liver) to all the tissues, of hormones from the endocrine glands to their target tissues, of wastes to the lungs and kidneys, and of antibodies from the lymphoid tissues to sites of infection. The plasma proteins provide the osmotic function required for the reabsorption of fluid from the interstitial tissues, a protein reserve, a buffer to neutralise acids and bases, and haemostasis due to its clotting factors. The plasma proteins albumin, fibrinogen and prothrombin are made in the liver, γ-globulins are derived from lymphocytes and plasma cells and are antibodies and antitoxins; α-globulins transport bilirubin, cortisol, and thyroxin; β-globulins transport cholesterol, fats and iron.

Plasma Transfusion. Whole plasma is given for shock due to burns or pancreatitis. Fresh frozen plasma or concentrated antihaemophilic globulin purified from plasma is used in haemophilia. Other purified fractions of the plasma are also prepared:
1. γ-globulin, used in the prevention of measles, rubella and poliomyelitis, and in agammaglobulinaemia, a rare inherited deficiency of γ-globulin from which children die at an early age due to infection.
2. Fibrinogen.

Blood Clotting (Coagulation) is required for haemostasis—a sealing-off of damaged blood vessels to stop bleeding. There are twelve plasma clotting factors including fibrinogen (factor I), prothrombin (factor II), thromboplastin (thrombokinase, factor III), calcium (factor IV), and antihaemophilic globulin (A.H.G., factor VIII).

Mechanism. Vasoconstriction temporarily reduces the bleeding. Factors released from damaged tissue cause platelets to adhere and form plugs in capillaries: they also activate prothrombin to form thrombin which changes soluble fibrinogen into

TABLE 5.1 *Normal values of plasma constituents*

	SI units	Old Units
Water	91%	
Proteins, total	73±7 g/l	
albumin	48±7 g/l	
globulins, total	25±7 g/l	
α-globulin	8 g/l	
β-globulin	6 g/l	
γ-globulin	11±3 g/l	
Clotting factors		
fibrinogen	2 to 4 g/l	
prothrombin	200 mg/l	
Mineral salts, mmol/l		
sodium	141±5	141±5 mEq/l
chloride	102±5	102±5 mEq/l
bicarbonate	27±3	27±3 mEq/l
potassium	4·5±0·7	4·5±0·7 mEq/l
magnesium	0·9±0·02	2·1±0·3 mEq/l, 3 to 4 mg%
calcium	2·4±0·2	5±0·4 mEq/l, 10±0·8 mg%
phosphate (as P)	1·2±0·4	2·5 to 4·5 mg%
Other minerals, μmol/l		
iron	23±9	70–180 μg%
iron-binding capacity	56±20	250–410 μg%
iodide (protein-bound, PBI)	0·3 to 0·6	3·8–7·5 μg%
Nutrients, mmol/l		
amino acids (as nitrogen)		5–8 mg%
glucose, fasting	3·4–5·6	60–100 mg%
sugar, fasting	4·4–6·7	80–120 mg%
fatty acids, total	2–4·5	200–450 mg%
cholesterol	4·7–6·5	180–250 mg%
triglycerides	0·28–2	25–180 mg%
Vitamins and hormones, nmol/l		
folic acid	14–41	6–18 ng/ml = μg/l
cobalamin	110–660	150–900 pg/ml = ng/l
thyroxine	55–155	
Enzymes, i.u./l		
amylase (diastase)	70–300	
transaminases		
S.G.O.T.	4–17	4–40 u/ml
S.G.P.T.	4–17	1–45 u/ml
lactic dehydrogenase	60–250	200–500 u%
phosphatase, acid	4–20	1–4 KAu%*
phosphatase, alkaline	20–90	3–13 KAu%*
Wastes		
urea	3·3–6·7 mmol/l	20–40 mg%
uric acid (urate)	0·12–0·36 mmol/l	2–6 mg%
creatinine	60–120 μmol/l	0·7–1·4 mg%
bilirubin	5–14 μmol/l	0·3–0·8 mg%

*KAu = King Armstrong units.

strands of fibrin (*Fig. 5.1*). The fibrin threads enmesh red and white cells to form a clot. After a time the clot shrinks and becomes firm (clot retraction).

Blood is prevented from clotting inside vessels by the smooth endothelial lining, by the removal of any activated clotting factors by the liver, and by the presence

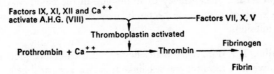

FIG. 5.1   The blood clotting mechanism

of heparin in the basophils in the blood and mast cells in the tissues. Heparin prevents the conversion of prothrombin into thrombin but does not affect any clot already present. Any unwanted clot that does form is broken down by plasmin in the plasma, which breaks down small amounts of fibrin, but there is not sufficient to break down the large amounts of clot formed at the site of an injury.

Haemorrhagic Disorders (also see purpura, p. 111)

Causes:

1   Deficiency of clotting factors in the plasma—prothrombin, fibrinogen, antihaemophilic globulin. There is a normal bleeding time since the platelets are normal, but a prolonged clotting time.

2   Capillary defects—scurvy; congenital defects; chemicals, e.g. corticosteroids; infections, e.g. septicaemia, smallpox, typhus; allergic disorders e.g. Henoch-Schonlein purpura. These have a normal clotting time but a prolonged bleeding time and increased capillary fragility.

3   Platelet deficiency (thrombocytopenia) The clotting time is normal, but the bleeding time is prolonged.

Investigations:

1   The bleeding time is normally 2–7 minutes. It does not test blood clotting since the lesion produced by the needle prick is of the capillaries and requires only platelet plugging. It is prolonged in thrombocytopenia or capillary damage.

2   The clotting time is normally 3–9 minutes at 37°C. It is prolonged by deficiency of any plasma clotting factor and is usually normal in thrombocytopenia.

3   Capillary fragility (Hess's) test, using a pressure cuff inflated to midway between systolic and diastolic blood pressures, increases capillary pressure and produces a large number of petechiae if the capillaries are fragile.

4   The prothrombin time is normally 12–15 seconds. It may be expressed as a percentage of normal, normal being 100%, or as an index (test time/normal time).

5   Platelet count.

Hypoprothrombinaemia. A low prothrombin concentration in the blood is due to vitamin K deficiency, as in obstructive jaundice, impaired synthesis of prothrombin from vitamin K in liver disease, or to patients receiving oral anticoagulants (phenindione, warfarin) which interferes with the use of vitamin K by the liver.

Afibrinogenaemia. A deficiency of fibrinogen in the blood may be acquired during toxaemia of pregnancy, or rarely may be congenital. Treatment is by fibrinogen infusion.

Haemophilia. This is inherited deficiency of antihaemophilic globulin (A.H.G., factor VIII) which is recessive and sex-linked; i.e. the abnormal gene is carried on the X-chromosome, therefore it is transmitted by the female but affects only males (*Fig. 1.6*). All the daughters of an affected male are carriers but his sons are normal. Queen Victoria was a carrier.

Clinically: prolonged haemorrhage occurs following minor injury or operation, e.g. tooth extraction, in childhood. Haemorrhage into a joint (haemarthrosis) causes pain and swelling of the joint and fever. The blood clot may become fibrous tissue and cause ankylosis and deformity. The blood clotting time is prolonged; the bleeding time, prothrombin time and platelet count are normal.

Treatment: rest in bed. Fresh blood for shock due to haemorrhage. To stop the bleeding fresh frozen plasma or concentrated A.H.G. ('cryoprecipitate') is given i.v., and local dressings soaked in a haemostatic substance, e.g. Russell's viper venom 1:10,000, or thrombin, is applied to bleeding wounds. A bleeding nose or tooth socket may need packing. Affected joints are splinted and lightly bandaged and cold packs or icebags are applied to relieve pain. Pethidine, morphine (addiction), aspirin (haematemesis) and i.m. injections (haematoma) are avoided.

Prevention: fresh frozen plasma or A.H.G. is given before and after operations. Trauma is avoided. A card should be carried stating that the patient is a haemophiliac. Haemophiliacs, their sisters and daughters (= carriers) are advised not to have children, and to consider sterilisation.

Christmas Disease. This is a rare form of haemophilia and is due to factor IX deficiency.

THE CELLS

The cells in the blood are red blood cells (erythrocytes), white blood cells (leucocytes) and platelets (thrombocytes). The white cells are of three main types: polymorphs, lymphocytes and monocytes.

Haemopoiesis (blood formation, *Fig. 5.2*). Red cells, polymorphs and platelets are made in the bone marrow. In the fetus red cells are also made in the spleen and liver. Lymphocytes and monocytes are made in the lymphoid tissues, especially the lymph nodes and spleen.

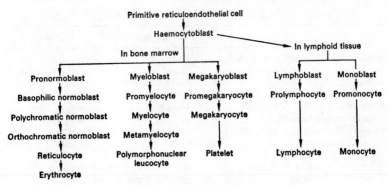

FIG. 5.2   Blood cell development

RED BLOOD CELLS (ERYTHROCYTES)

Anatomy and Function: each red cell is a biconcave disc, i.e. a disc which is slightly hollowed on each side (*Fig. 5.3*) and is therefore thinner in the centre than around the edge. Like any cell it consists of a membrane on the outside, and contains protein, but unlike other cells the major protein is haemoglobin and the human red cell does not have a nucleus. There are normally $5 \times 10^{12}/l$, i.e. 5 million per mm³ of blood (a mm³, cubic millimetre, is about the size of a pinhead). Normal values of the red cells are shown in *Table 5.2*. The haemoglobin in the cells carries oxygen from the lungs to the tissues and assist in the buffering of the blood.

Formation: the red cell precursors in the bone marrow contain nuclei. The haemocytoblast divides and can form any of the early precursor cells in the blood. In red cell production the precursor cell is the pronormoblast which divides to form normoblasts. Normoblasts mature and take in iron to form haemoglobin. They

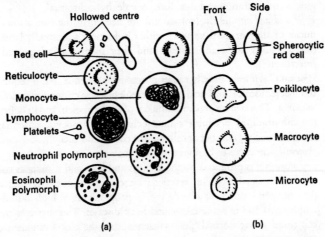

FIG. 5.3   The cells of the blood; (*a*) normal cells; (*b*) abnormal red cells

TABLE 5.2   *Normal haematological values*

	Normal range	Average
Haemoglobin (Hb) 100% = 14·8 g/dl	13·5–17 g/dl	14·8 g/dl
Red cells (R.B.C.s), millions (M) per mm³	4·2–6M	5M(= 5 × 10¹²/l)
Colour index (C.I.)	0·9–1·1	1·0
Packed cell volume (P.C.V.)	38–52%	45%
Mean cell volume (M.C.V.) μm³ (fl)	80–94 fl	90 fl
Mean cell haemoglobin (M.C.H.)	27–32 pg	30 pg/cell
Mean cell Hb concentration (M.C.H.C.)	32–35 g/dl	34 g/dl
Mean cell diameter (M.C.D.)	6·7–7·7 μm	7·2 μm
Reticulocytes	0·2–2%	
White cells (W.B.C.s), total count	5 to 10 × 10⁹/l(= 5000–10,000 per mm³)	
Neutrophil polymorphs	50–75% (3000–7000 per mm³)	
Eosinophil polymorphs	1–4% (50–400 per mm³)	
Basophil polymorphs	0–1% (0–100 per mm³)	
Lymphocytes	25–35% (1250–3500 per mm³)	
Monocytes	2–8% (200–800 per mm³)	
Platelets	150–400× 10⁹/l (150,000–400,000 per mm³)	
Serum iron	23 ±9 μmol/l (70–180μg%)	
Folic acid, serum	14–41 nmol/l (6–18 ng/ml)	
Folic acid, red cell	340–1450 nmol/l (150–640 ng/ml)	
Serum vitamin B₁₂	110–660 nmol/l (150–900 pg/ml)	
Bleeding time	2–7 minutes	
Coagulation time	3–9 minutes	

lose their nuclei to become reticulocytes which contain fragments of reticular material. Reticulocytes leave the marrow and enter the blood to become erythrocytes. The main substances necessary for the production of red cells are iron, folic acid, vitamin B_{12}, vitamin C, thyroxin, protein and erythropoietin.

1 *Iron:* 2·5 g of the 4 g of iron in the body is in the haemoglobin. Iron deficiency produces small cells (microcytes) which have a low haemoglobin concentration and therefore are pale (hypochromia).

2 *Folic acid and vitamin B_{12}* (cobalamin) are needed in the formation of the nuclei of the normoblasts and if either is deficient abnormally large cells (megaloblasts) are made instead, and they mature into large red cells (macrocytes).

3 *Vitamin C deficiency* usually causes normocytic anaemia, but is required in the metabolism of folic acid, and severe deficiency causes a megaloblastic anaemia. *Thyroxin* is a general stimulant of erythropoiesis and its deficiency (hypothyroidism) produces a normochromic normocytic anaemia; i.e. there is a reduced number of cells but the cells are normal.

4 *Protein deficiency* has to be severe to cause anaemia.

5 *Erythropoietin* is produced by the kidneys and liver and stimulates red cell production. Erythropoietin secretion is increased when there is hypoxaemia (low oxygen level in the blood), e.g. in people living at high altitudes, in emphysema and in some congenital heart diseases. This increases the red cell count above normal (polycythaemia) and the blood can then carry more oxygen.

Destruction: the red cell lives for 120 days and is then broken down by phagocytic cells in the reticuloendothelial system, especially in the spleen and bone marrow (*Fig. 5.4*). The protein of the cell and the globin of haemoglobin is broken down to amino acids which are re-used for the manufacture of protein. The remainder

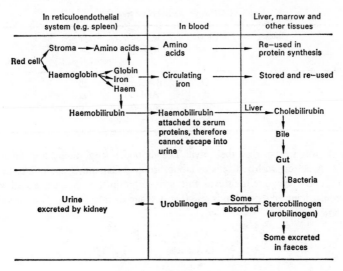

FIG. 5.4 Red cell breakdown

of the haemoglobin molecule is haem, from which the reticuloendothelial system releases iron, which is stored in the liver and marrow and used again. Bilirubin, which is not required, enters the blood (= haemobilirubin) and attaches to serum protein and therefore cannot escape into the urine. In the liver haemobilirubin is detached from serum protein and is changed into cholebilirubin, which is excreted into the bile. On entering the intestine, bacteria change bilirubin into stercobilinogen; this is partly excreted in the faeces and partly absorbed into the blood to be excreted by the kidneys into the urine, when it is called urobilinogen. Urobilinogen oxidises in air to become urobilin.

Erythrocyte Sedimentation Rate (E.S.R.). If anticoagulated blood is undisturbed the cells fall (sediment) to the bottom of the container, due to gravity. The rate of sedimentation can be measured, the normal being 0–10 mm in 1 hour (Wintrobe method). If the cells aggregate they sediment more rapidly and aggregation (rouleaux formation—not to be confused with agglutination) is caused by an increase in fibrinogen, α_2 and γ-globulins, as occurs in most infections. The sedimentation rate is increased in anaemia because there is a decreased proportion of cells to plasma, and the rate has to be adjusted to exclude any increase due to anaemia (= corrected E.S.R.).

Blood Groups. These are inherited differences in surface structure of the red cell membrane. The membrane contains a variety of antigens called agglutinogens (agglutination-producing). The most important are the ABO and rhesus agglutinogens.

The ABO Group: an individual inherits one of four ABO groups, A, B, AB or O (*Table 5.3*). Individuals also inherit antibodies in their plasma which act against red

TABLE 5.3 *ABO blood groups*

Blood group	Agglutinogen on cell	Agglutinin in plasma	Frequency in population (%)
O	O	Anti-A, anti-B	46
A	A	Anti-B	42
B	B	Anti-A	9
AB	AB	—	3

cells of groups other than their own. The antibodies (agglutinins) are anti-A or anti-B. A person with red cells of blood group A has anti-B agglutinins in his plasma, and if they are transfused with cells of group B or AB, these antibodies agglutinate (clump) the group B cells (*Fig. 5.5*) and destroy them (= incompatible

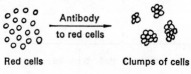

FIG. 5.5   Red cell agglutination

transfusion). Similarly a person of group B has anti-A agglutinins in the plasma which will destroy group A cells. Blood group O does not mean that there is no antigen, but the group O agglutinogens on the red cell membrane are weak, and few people have anti-O agglutinins in their serum; hence people with blood of group O became known as the 'universal donors' and can give small transfusions to patients of any blood group (the anti-A and anti-B agglutinins in the transfused plasma are diluted by the recipient's plasma and any damage caused is not obvious unless large transfusions are given).

The Rhesus (CDE) Group: the most important agglutinogen in the group is D. If it is present the person is rhesus positive, and 85% of Caucasians are rhesus positive. Africans and Japanese do not possess the D antigen and are therefore rhesus negative. If a rhesus negative person is transfused with rhesus positive (D) cells he produces anti-D antibodies in about 10 days, so if he receives a second transfusion with D positive cells a reaction follows. A rhesus negative mother may bear a rhesus positive fetus. If fetal red cells escape into the blood of the mother she produces anti-D antibodies which, if they cross the placenta in subsequent pregnancies, destroy the fetal red cells causing haemolytic disease of the newborn. Numerous other blood groups are known but are not important unless transfusions are to be repeated. They are used in the study of heredity and in paternity tests.

Blood Transfusion

Transfused blood is potentially dangerous, is expensive, and should not be used unless it is essential. Blood transfusion is used in severe shock due to acute haemorrhage, in carbon monoxide poisoning, in erythroblastosis fetalis ('rhesus babies') when an 'exchange' transfusion is given, in severe anaemia, especially aplastic anaemia and anaemia due to leukaemia, and sometimes in severe pernicious or hypochromic anaemia.

Each unit of blood contains 420 ml of blood plus 120 ml of solution containing citrate (to prevent clotting) and glucose. Concentrated blood (packed cells) is blood from which most of the plasma has been removed in order to reduce the possibility of overloading the circulation in anaemia.

Before Transfusion. In order to prevent an incompatible transfusion the blood of the patient (recipient) is grouped for ABO and rhesus groups, and tested for antibodies attached to red cells by the Coombs test. Blood taken from the patient must be labelled immediately with the patient's full name, age, record number and ward. The blood that has been donated for transfusion (donor blood) is also grouped and labelled. The patient's blood is then tested directly (cross-matched) against the bottle(s) of blood intended for him, to check that they are compatible, and the bottles are immediately labelled in the laboratory with the patient's full name, age, record number and ward. When the blood is to be given, these particulars (including the blood group) are checked against the patient's particulars. This is done for each bottle of blood that is transfused and two people should make the check.

Method: blood is stored at 4–6°C in a blood bank (not in an ordinary refrigerator) and must be used within 21 days, or packed cells within 24 hours of packing. The rate of flow is usually 40 drops a minute except in haemorrhage when transfusion may be rapid. The bottle must not be allowed to run dry; the second bottle of blood is obtained from the blood bank before the first is empty, and when the blood has reached the neck of the bottle the tube is clamped securely, the bottle unhooked and the needle of the giving-set transferred to the new bottle, the bung of which is pierced after removing the adhesive strip that protects its sterility. The needle must not be allowed to touch anything else (otherwise the blood may become contaminated). Puncture of a plastic container is avoided if it is held vertically during the insertion of the needle. The bottle is then resuspended above the patient, the clamp on the tubing opened and the rate adjusted.

Complications:

1 The drip may stop because of kinked tubing or from venous clotting or spasm which may be overcome by warming the limb or stroking along the vein towards the trunk. Any air-lock should be removed by allowing the blood to run freely through the tubing into a container before reconnecting to the needle in the vein.

2 A haematoma at the site of the needle, due to displacement of the needle out of the vein. The transfusion should be stopped and the needle re-inserted.

3 Sepsis at the site of a cannula tied into a vein.

4 Overloading the circulation with too rapid a drip may precipitate cardiac

failure, especially in anaemia. The pulse rate and venous pressure rise, the blood pressure falls, and there may be dyspnoea, cough and tightness in the chest. The speed of the drip should be reduced and a diuretic given. A fluid intake and output chart must always be kept so that any fluid retention is detected. In severe anaemia, packed cells should be given as this reduces the volume of fluid transfused.

5   Infections. Transfusion may transmit malaria, syphilis, serum hepatitis, and other virus infections. The symptoms of serum hepatitis do not appear until after 2–3 months, which is the incubation period.

6   Pyrexia and rigors due to pyrogens or to a too rapid transfusion. The cold blood passing through the temperature-regulating centre in the hypothalamus stimulates shivering and heat production. The transfusion should be slowed.

7   Allergic reaction, e.g. urticaria due to foreign protein in the blood.

8   Cardiac arrest due to excessive potassium in the plasma (hyperkalaemia). In stored blood, potassium is slowly released from the cells into the plasma. This is one reason why blood is not used after it is three weeks old. Prevention is by giving glucose and insulin which takes potassium into the cells where it belongs.

9   Repeated transfusions cause the patient to produce antibodies to red cells which makes it difficult to find compatible blood.

10 Air embolism. If the bottle runs dry air enters the vein, forming an embolism, which is likely to be fatal.

11 Incompatible transfusion is the giving of blood of the wrong group to a patient. This is prevented by cross-matching, and by ensuring that the correct bottle of blood is given to the right patient—more than one transfusion may be going on at the same time in the ward, or two patients may have similar names. All the precautions already mentioned under 'before transfusion' must be carefully followed. *Effects:* The transfused incompatible cells are agglutinated by the agglutinins in the recipient's plasma. The agglutinated cells (*Fig. 5.5*) block capillaries causing ischaemia (deficient blood supply). In the kidney this causes pain in the loin and dark red urine, in the heart it causes retrosternal pain. The clumped cells then haemolyse and release haemoglobin and potassium into the plasma. The haemoglobin passes into the renal tubules and is coagulated by the acid urine, blocking the tubules. The potassium causes hyperkalaemia. The ruptured red cell membrane causes anaphylactic shock with rigors and pyrexia. Shock causes renal tubular necrosis, anuria and renal failure. If there is any suspicion that the blood is incompatible the rate of the drip must be slowed and the label on the bottle and patient's particulars checked again. If they differ, the transfusion is stopped. If they are correct the drip is left running slowly (providing that symptoms are mild) and expert assistance called.

During transfusion. The nurse must watch for the complications listed above, and particularly for an increased pulse rate (count half-hourly), dyspnoea, 'chills', pyrexia (record temperature hourly), and pain in the loins or chest, and report any change immediately.

INVESTIGATIONS IN BLOOD DISEASE

1 *History*, especially of the diet, drugs, bleeding, ulcer symptoms. *Examination*.

2 *Blood count*. Normal levels are shown in *Table 5.2*. The haemoglobin and red cell count is low in all anaemias. The colour index and mean cell haemoglobin compare the content of haemoglobin in the blood with the number of cells. A colour index below 0·9 indicates hypochromia (low colour, i.e. low Hb), and above 1·1 indicates a large cell full of haemoglobin. The packed cell volume (haematocrit) is the total volume of red cells in 100 ml of blood and is low in any anaemia and increased in polycythaemia or dehydration. The mean corpuscular haemoglobin concentration is the average amount of haemoglobin in each cell and is below 32% in hypochromic anaemia and above 35% in macrocytic anaemia. The mean cell volume is the average volume of each cell. It is small (microcytic) in hypochromic anaemia and large in macrocytic anaemia.

3 *The reticulocyte count* is the proportion of young red cells in the blood.

4 *The white cell count* is below 5×10^9/l (5000 per mm^3) (leucopenia) often in pernicious anaemia and folate deficiency anaemia and in disorders of the white cells which are described later. The count is above 10×10^9/l, 10,000 per mm^3 (leucocytosis) in infection and other conditions such as myocardial infarction.

5 *The platelet count* is low (thrombocytopenia) in certain bleeding disorders.

6 *The osmotic fragility test:* red cells swell if placed in a dilute salt solution. The more dilute the solution the greater is the swelling, up to the point when the cell becomes spherical. Further stretching cannot occur and the cell ruptures (haemolysis). The strength of the salt solution causing haemolysis is an indication of the osmotic fragility of the cell.

7 *The Coombs test* is a test for the presence of globulin (antibody) on the surface of a red cell.

8 *Serum or plasma levels* of iron, folic acid and vitamin B$_{12}$.

9 *Bone marrow aspiration*, using local anaesthesia, from the sternum, iliac crest or tibia. A sterile dressing should cover the puncture hole for 4 days. The nucleated developing cells are examined for abnormalities in appearance and number.

10 *Faeces* for blood in gastro-intestinal bleeding. Blood is not visible to the unaided eye if bleeding is less than 100 ml a day but can be tested for chemically as occult (hidden) blood.

11 *Urine*. An increase in urobilinogen indicates that an increased amount of bilirubin is being produced, due to increased red cell destruction (haemolysis).

12   Schilling test. See vitamin B_{12} deficiency anaemia (page 103).

13   Gastric juice. After food, histamine or pentagastrin the normal stomach secretes hydrochloric acid which can be measured after aspiration through a Ryle's tube, or to avoid passing a tube an ion-exchange resin containing a dye (diagnex blue) may be used, but is not as reliable.

Method: The patient is not given anything by mouth overnight.

(*a*) *Tube test:* in the morning a Ryle's tube is passed via the nose into the stomach and the gastric contents are aspirated with a syringe. The volume of aspirate is measured, placed in a container and labelled 'fasting juice'. Aspirate every 15 minutes for 1 hour (basal secretion), give s.c. pentagastrin 6 $\mu g/kg$ body weight and aspirate every 15 minutes for another hour, each aspirate being placed in a separate container and labelled with the time and the patient's name.

Histamine acid phosphate 0·04 mg/kg preceded by mepyramine maleate (an antihistamine) 50 to 100 mg i.m. 30 minutes before the histamine, may be used instead of pentagastrin. An antihistamine has to be given to prevent the unpleasant actions of histamine, such as vasodilatation which causes headache and flushing of the skin but does not prevent its stimulation of gastric acid secretion.

(*b*) *The 'tubeless' test:* gastrotest or diagnex blue: analgesics, laxatives or substances which may colour the urine (e.g. beetroot) are not allowed for 24 hours before the test. The stomach must have been empty for 8 hours, the bladder is emptied and the urine discarded. The two white caffeine tablets are taken with 50 ml water. 1 hour later the bladder is emptied and the urine kept and marked 'control urine'. The three yellow tablets (gastrotest) or the resin granules (diagnex blue test) are now swallowed without chewing, in 50 ml of water (any granules remaining are taken with more water). $1\frac{1}{2}$ hours (gastrotest) or 2 hours (diagnex blue) later the bladder is emptied and the urine marked 'test urine'. The dye is released from the resin by acid, absorbed, and excreted in the urine. Thus blue dye in the urine indicates the presence of gastric acid. Dye is absent in achlorhydria (absence of gastric hydro-chloric acid). Achlorhydria is characteristic of pernicious anaemia, but also occurs in many patients with hypochromic anaemia and in other conditions. Pentagastrin is given 15 minutes before the resin.

DISORDERS OF THE BLOOD

Anaemia

Anaemia ('no blood') is a deficiency of haemoglobin and red blood cells. The *type* may be classified according to the appearance of the red cell in a stained blood film (a thin layer of blood on a glass slide), either according to:

1   The size of the cell: normocytic (normal size) as in anaemia due to hypo-thyroidism or chronic renal failure, microcytic (small cells) as in iron deficiency anaemia, or macrocytic (large cells) as in pernicious anaemia or folic acid deficiency; or

2   The density of the colour (= concentration of haemoglobin) of the cell: normochromic (normal colour) as in chronic renal failure or aplastic

anaemia, hypochromic (low colour) as in iron deficiency, or 'hyperchromic' (high depth of colour) as in pernicious anaemia or folic acid deficiency.

The red cells may also show anisocytosis (variation in size), poikilocytosis (variation in shape), or polychromasia, which is a bluish-grey colour (the cells normally stain pink).

Causes:

1 Deficiency of iron, folic acid, vitamin B_{12}, vitamin C, thyroxin, or protein.
2 Bone marrow disorders such as aplastic anaemia, leukaemia or myelomatosis.
3 Haemolysis, due to congenital abnormalities of the red cells, antibodies to the red cells (auto-immune anaemia), toxins or infections (e.g. malaria), hypersplenism, or drugs (sulphonamides, methyldopa).
4 Mixed causes, as in chronic renal failure, collagenoses (e.g. rheumatoid arthritis), cancer, or chronic infections.

General Symptoms and Signs of any anaemia are pallor of the skin, nail beds and mucous membranes, fatigue due to muscular hypoxia, palpitations, tachycardia, dyspnoea on exertion, light-headedness, or syncope. Pyrexia may occur in severe anaemia. *Symptoms of complications:* oedema due to congestive cardiac failure; angina pectoris due to myocardial ischaemia, especially if coronary atheroma is present.

General Treatment: if there is severe anaemia with a haemoglobin below 5 g/dl (35% of normal), rest in bed, light diet, with pulse, temperature and respirations recorded daily or more often if indicated. In mild anaemia (haemoglobin above 9 g/dl = 60%) the patient may remain at work while being treated. If the haemoglobin is between 5 and 9 g/dl the degree of rest required depends on symptoms. The diet should contain protein, green vegetables and fresh fruit.

Iron deficiency causes **hypochromic** microcytic anaemia. Iron deficiency is due to a dietary deficiency of iron-containing food such as meat, liver and eggs, achlorhydria (lack of gastric hydrochloric acid), malabsorption due to chronic pancreatitis or intestinal disease, frequent pregnancies (the fetus takes maternal iron), or chronic haemorrhage due to menorrhagia, peptic ulcer, ulcerative colitis, haemorrhoids, hookworms, or carcinoma of the rectum, colon, or stomach.

Clinically: general signs, also koilonychia (brittle, spoon-shaped nails with a hollowed centre) and glossitis (a smooth sore tongue due to loss of surface epithelium). There may be dysphagia due to atrophy of the mucosa of the pharynx, and achlorhydria due to atrophy of the gastric mucosa. Patients are usually women, since blood loss caused by menstruation reduces the iron stores of the body. The *Plummer-Vinson syndrome* is the combination of anaemia, dysphagia and glossitis.

Investigations: the blood shows a low red cell count and a greater fall in the haemoglobin, producing a low mean corpuscular haemoglobin concentration (M.C.H.C.). The serum iron is low. Achlorhydria is found in 40% of patients. Faeces for occult blood, which is positive if there is gastro-intestinal bleeding.

Treatment: rest in bed if the haemoglobin is below 5 g/dl. Ferrous sulphate 200 mg t.d.s. after meals (to prevent gastro-intestinal upset) or ferrous gluconate 600 mg t.d.s. p.c. Treatment is given for 2–3 months to replace the depleted stores of iron. Iron may be given by injection but does not increase the Hb any more rapidly than oral iron. It is used if the patient is unreliable or unable to take tablets and in malabsorption, e.g. 50–100 mg Imferon deeply i.m. or 100 mg (2 ml) Jectofer i.m., once to seven times weekly. 250 mg of iron increase the haemoglobin by 1 g/dl. Blood transfusion is used if the anaemia is severe and has to be corrected urgently, e.g. prior to operation. Well-balanced diet containing liver, meat, eggs, beans and peas. Treatment is of the cause.

Folic Acid Deficiency

This causes a macrocytic anaemia similar to pernicious anaemia but neuropathy (disorder of the nervous system) is absent. Folate deficiency occurs in pregnancy because the fetus uses large amounts of folic acid, in dietary deficiency of folate-containing foods such as dark green leafy vegetables, meat or nuts, in intestinal malabsorption as in chronic pancreatitis or coeliac disease, or may be due to certain drugs, especially phenytoin (Epanutin).

Symptoms are of anaemia in general.

Investigations: the blood count shows a macrocytic anaemia and polymorpho-nuclear leucopenia (a low white cell count due to a reduced number of polymorphs) since folate is needed in the production of all cells. The bone marrow contains megaloblasts and the serum folate level is low (below 6 ng/ml).

Treatment is of the cause; folic acid 5 mg t.d.s. orally, and a diet containing adequate green vegetables and meat.

Vitamin B$_{12}$ (Cobalamin) Deficiency

This condition causes a macrocytic anaemia. The commonest cause is pernicious anaemia, an hereditary auto-immune atrophy of the gastric mucosa. Just as amino acids are released from protein by the digestive enzymes so vitamin B$_{12}$ is released from protein by intrinsic factor secreted by the stomach, and is then absorbed from the small intestine. In pernicious anaemia intrinsic factor is absent, therefore vitamin B$_{12}$ cannot be absorbed. Deficiency also follows gastrectomy and occurs in malabsorption and in strict vegetarians, since vitamin B$_{12}$ is absent from vegetables but present in animal protein such as liver, meat and milk.

Clinically: age over 45 years. General symptoms of anaemia, also anorexia due to gastritis and a smooth, sore, raw tongue due to atrophy of the epithelium. The skin and conjunctiva are pale lemon colour due to bilirubin and there is slight splenomegaly (splenic enlargement) due to an increased rate of breakdown of the abnormally large red cells. Neuropathy may develop, and is commonly a peripheral neuritis; but there may be subacute combined degeneration of the spinal cord. Neuropathy causes numbness and paraesthesiae ('pins and needles') in the hands and feet, loss of vibration sense in the ankles, ataxia (staggering) on walking and muscular weakness or paralysis.

Complications: cardiac failure, carcinoma of the stomach, haemorrhage into the retina in severe anaemia.

Investigations: the blood shows a macrocytic anaemia with a polymorphonuclear leucopenia and the bone marrow is megaloblastic. The serum vitamin B_{12} level is low, i.e. below 105 nmol/l (140 pg/ml). The gastric juice shows a pentagastrin- (or augmented histamine-) fast achlorhydria. The urine contains an excess of urobilinogen due to the increased formation of bilirubin caused by an increased rate of breakdown of red cells. Macrocytes are 'fragile' and haemolyse easily.

The Schilling Test. The patient drinks 1 μg of radioactive vitamin B_{12} and at the same time 1000 μg of ordinary non-radioactive vitamin B_{12} is given i.m. to cause the excretion in the urine of any radioactive vitamin that is absorbed. In pernicious anaemia (P.A.) and in malabsorption, none is absorbed and therefore there is no radioactivity detected in the urine. The test is then repeated after giving intrinsic factor. A patient with P.A. will now absorb the vitamin and radioactivity will appear in the urine; whereas in malabsorption there will still be no absorption of the vitamin and the urine will not be radioactive.

Treatment: rest in bed if the haemoglobin is below 7 g/dl. Blood transfusion of packed red cells given slowly (to avoid causing cardiac failure) if the haemoglobin is under 4 g/dl. A diuretic (frusemide 40 mg orally) should be given with the transfusion. Hydroxocobalamin 1000 μg twice weekly is given for the first two weeks, then 250 μg every one to three months for life. The need for lifelong treatment should be impressed upon the patient. Iron, e.g. ferrous sulphate 200 mg t.d.s., may be needed during the phase of rapid blood regeneration. Cobalamin is continued in high dosage (1000 μg weekly) for several months if neuropathy is present. A blood count is done every six to twelve months to check that it remains normal and to make sure that the patient is continuing to have treatment.

Vitamin C Deficiency
This causes scurvy (Chapter 2) and usually a normochromic anaemia cured by giving vitamin C (ascorbic acid) 1 g daily for 1 week, then 25–200 mg daily. The patient should eat fresh fruit and vegetables as a regular part of the diet.

Hypothyroidism
In hypothyroidism (myxoedema) the anaemia is normochromic and is cured by treatment of the hypothyroidism with thyroxin. Anorexia may also cause anaemia due to folate or iron deficiency.

Anaemia due to **protein deficiency** is rare in Europe and the U.S.A., but is common in Africa and South America.

Aplastic Anaemia
Aplastic anaemia (pancytopenia) is anaemia, leucopenia (a low white cell count) and thrombocytopenia (a low platelet count) due to damage to the dividing primitive cells in the bone marrow and is caused by X-rays; drugs (chloramphenicol, sulphonamides, phenylbutazone, gold, tridione and cytotoxins); industrial chemicals

(benzene, insecticides, e.g. D.D.T. and parathion, possibly hair dyes); and viruses. These cause half of the cases, the other half are idiopathic; i.e. of unknown cause.

Clinically: general signs, also fever and a sore ulcerated throat due to infection due to the leucopenia, and haemorrhages due to the deficiency of platelets. 50% die within 1 year; 10% may recover.

Treatment: remove the cause. Blood transfusion with packed red cells for anaemia, fresh blood for haemorrhage. Corticosteroids are ineffective and should be avoided since they predispose to infection, and infection worsens the aplastic anaemia. Androgens, e.g. oxymethalone 150–300 mg daily orally, may be tried since they have a slight stimulant effect on the marrow in normal subjects, but are usually ineffective in anaemia. Antibiotics are given for infection.

Multiple Myeloma

Multiple myeloma (myelomatosis) consists of multiple tumours of abnormal plasma cells in bone, especially skull, ribs, spine and pelvis. Plasma cells are normally present in the tissues and make antibodies (γ-globulins). Abnormal plasma cells produce abnormal proteins which enter the blood (paraproteinaemia) and are mostly abnormal γ-globulins, but often Bence-Jones protein is also produced and escapes into the urine.

Clinically: age over 50 years. Tumours erode the bone and cause hypercalcaemia and spontaneous (pathological) fracture, e.g. vertebral collapse which causes pain in the back and may cause paraplegia (paralysis of both legs). There is normochromic anaemia due to malignant cells crowding the normal cells out of the marrow. The proteins precipitate in the tubules and cause renal failure. Many die of pneumonia. 50% die within 1 year; few live 5 years.

Investigations:

1 X-rays of bones show osteolytic (rarefied) "punched out" areas.
2 The blood count shows anaemia. The sedimentation rate and serum calcium are increased, serum protein electrophoresis shows abnormal proteins.
3 Sternal marrow contains abnormal plasma cells.
4 Urine may contain Bence-Jones protein.

Treatment: immobilisation of pathological fracture, spinal support (corsets and steel braces), local radiotherapy for bone pain.

Drugs: cyclophosphamide (Endoxan) 100–150 mg daily orally or 100–500 mg daily i.v. to a maximum of 7 g for any one course. The patient is warned that there is likely to be loss of hair and he may need a wig. It also may cause bone marrow depression. Melphalan (Alkeran) 5–10 mg daily orally for up to 2 weeks, then 2–4 mg daily. *Side-effects:* nausea, vomiting, bone marrow depression, oral and peptic ulceration. Prednisolone for nausea and vomiting due to hypercalcaemia.

Blood transfusion for severe anaemia.

Haemolytic Anaemia

This is anaemia due to the excessive destruction (haemolysis) of red cells. It causes enlargement of the spleen (since the spleen breaks down damaged, abnormal and old red cells) and an increased production of bilirubin (*Fig. 5.4*), hence jaundice and an increased amount of urobilinogen in the urine.

Congenital Spherocytosis (congenital acholuric jaundice) is a haemolytic anaemia due to the Mendelian dominant inheritance of abnormally thick (spherical, *Fig. 5.3*) red cells instead of the normal biconcave shape. The shape of the cells makes them osmotically fragile (osmosis; see Chapter 3) and they have a short life.

Clinically: there is slight splenomegaly, anaemia and jaundice but bile pigment is absent from the urine (= acholuric; a = no, chol = bile, uric = urine). The increased production of bile pigment may cause gall stones. Attacks of increased haemolysis (crises) may occur and are often due to infection.

Investigations: the red cell count is subnormal, the cells are rounded and show increased fragility in saline. The reticulocyte count is high (e.g. 12%). The Van den Bergh test for bilirubin shows a raised level of indirect-reacting bilirubin (= haemo-bilirubin) in the serum. Urinary urobilinogen is increased (above 2%).

Treatment: splenectomy cures by preventing the destruction of red cells. Cholecyst-ectomy for gall stones. Slow blood transfusion for severe anaemia, as in a crisis. Transfusion reactions are common and must be watched for.

Haemoglobinopathies are the inheritance of abnormal forms of haemoglobin, e.g. sickle-cell anaemia due to haemoglobin S in some Negro people, thalassaemia associated with haemoglobin F. (Normal haemoglobin is HbA.)

Haemolytic Disease of the Newborn (erythroblastosis fetalis) is due to haemo-lysis of red cells by antibodies made by the mother. The baby's red cells are rhesus (Rh) positive, i.e. they have the rhesus D antigen on their surface. During delivery some of the baby's red cells enter the mother's circulation through ruptured capillaries in the placenta. If the mother is Rh negative (i.e. she does not possess the rhesus antigen on her red cells), the foetal Rh positive cells act as a foreign protein and the mother produces antibodies (anti-D) to the rhesus factor. This does not harm the first child, since it is born before antibodies can be made; but during subsequent pregnancies antibodies will now be present and may cross the placenta and attach to the fetal red cells (if they are Rh positive) and haemolyse them, causing jaundice and anaemia. This can be prevented if Rh negative mothers who have an Rh positive baby have their blood tested (Kleihauer test) within 72 hours of delivery for the presence of fetal red cells; and if these are present she is given concentrated anti-D globulin. Anti-D globulin combines with any Rh positive (= D+) fetal cells in her circulation and destroys them before she can make antibodies.

Clinically: the infant shows increasing jaundice and anaemia and may develop kernicterus, i.e. damage of the basal ganglia and other parts of the brain causing spasticity, mental deficiency, deafness and convulsions.

Treatment of an affected infant is by exchange blood transfusion.

Autoimmune Haemolytic Anaemia (acquired acholuric jaundice) is due to the production, by the patient, of antibodies to his own red cells, and these give a positive Coombs test. (Autoimmunity is immunity against oneself.) It may occur in virus infections (e.g. glandular fever), in syphilis, and in systemic lupus erythematosus, or may be due to drugs (e.g. methyldopa). There is jaundice and often severe anaemia.

Treatment is with prednisolone 60 mg daily for 3 weeks followed by a smaller maintenance dose if there is a response; if not then immunosuppressive drugs may be tried (e.g. chlorambucil 2–10 mg daily orally). Blood transfusion may be used in severe anaemia but reactions are common. The spleen is removed if radioactive isotope testing shows hypersplenism.

Polycythaemia
Polycythaemia is an increase in the number of circulating red cells. It should not be confused with haemoconcentration which is an increased red cell count due to dehydration (e.g. due to burns, vomiting, diarrhoea or untreated diabetes). *Types:* (1) Polycythaemia vera; (2) Secondary polycythaemia.

Polycythaemia Vera. This is due to overactivity of the bone marrow which causes an increase in red cells to above $6.5 \times 10^{12}/l$ (6.5 million per mm^3), white cells above $10 \times 10^9/l$ (10,000 per mm^3), and an increase in the platelet count to above $400 \times 10^9/l$, 400,000 per mm^3.

Clinically: age over 40 years. There is insidious onset of headache, dizziness, pruritus (itching), angina pectoris and often hypertension. The face is dusky red (plethoric) or cyanosed and shows distension of the small veins and bloodshot eyes. The spleen is slightly enlarged.

Complications:
1 Thrombosis of arteries (e.g. cerebral, coronary, mesenteric, popliteal), or veins, due to the increased blood viscosity and high platelet count.
2 Cardiac failure.
3 Bronchopneumonia.

Treatment: venesection and the removal of 500 ml of blood once to four times weekly. Radioactive phosphorus is given i.v. and is effective after 5–12 weeks. It concentrates in the marrow and destroys some of the nucleated cells there. Radiophosphorus causes leukaemia in 5% of patients. Cytotoxic drugs may be used and do not predispose to leukaemia, e.g. busulphan 2–4 mg daily at first, then 2 mg every 3–7 days, or drugs which prevent the marrow from using folic acid, e.g. pyrimethamine (Daraprim).

Secondary Polycythaemia. This is caused by:
1 Hypoxia (diminished oxygen supply), e.g. in people living at high altitude; chronic pulmonary disease; and those congenital heart diseases in which blood by-passes the lungs.
2 Cushing's syndrome.
3 Certain tumours, e.g. carcinoma of the kidney which produces an excess of erythropoietin.

Treatment is of the cause.

WHITE BLOOD CELLS (LEUCOCYTES)

Leucocytes are the pale cells in the blood (leuco = white, cyte = cell). There are three main types of white cell in the blood; the polymorphonuclear leucocyte (polymorph), lymphocyte and monocyte (*Fig. 5.3*). Unlike red cells they are nucleated. The normal white cell count is $5-10 \times 10^9/l$ (5000–10,000 per mm³), and the normal differential count is shown in *Table 5.2*.

Polymorphs

The polymorphs (granulocytes) are subdivided, according to the different types of granules that they contain, into neutrophil, eosinophil and basophil. The polymorph has a multi-lobed nucleus usually of 2–4 lobes (poly = many, morph = shape). The cytoplasm of the neutrophil polymorph contains small granules which release proteolytic (protein-digesting) enzymes which destroy bacteria taken into (phago-cytosed by) the polymorph. When tissues are invaded by micro-organisms chemicals are liberated which attract neutrophil polymorphs to the area (chemo-taxis). Pus is the collection of polymorphs (pus cells), bacteria and tissue débris.

Eosinophil polymorphs (eosinophils) contain large granules which stain pink with eosin. Eosinophils limit the effects of allergy by neutralising substances such as histamine and ingest antigen–antibody complexes.

Basophil polymorphs (basophils) contain large blue-staining granules of heparin, an anticoagulant, and help to prevent the blood from clotting in normal vessels. All the polymorphs are phagocytic (phage = eat, cyte = cell), i.e. they engulf (ingest) foreign particles such as bacteria. Neutrophils are the first line of defence against invading organisms.

Polymorphs are made in the bone marrow from myelocytes, which in turn are produced by the division of myeloblasts (*Fig. 5.2*). During infection the marrow makes more polymorphs and releases them into the blood.

Lymphocytes

These have a dense spherical nucleus which almost fills the cell. Although they appear similar there are three types of lymphocyte, each with a different function. One type is the B-lymphocyte which produces antitoxins and antibodies (γ-globulins) which circulate in the plasma and provide humoral immunity. Another type is the T-lymphocyte which provides cellular immunity. Lymphocytes are made in the lymph nodes, spleen, and in the collections of lymphoid tissue in the gastrointestinal tract and tonsils. They are derived from lymphoblasts.

Monocytes

Monocytes are the largest leucocytes in the blood and have a large, irregular, and sometimes kidney-bean-shaped, nucleus. They are also present in the tissues where they are called macrophages (large phagocytes). They ingest various particles, including bacteria and tissue débris, and contain digestive enzymes similar to the neutrophil polymorph.

ABNORMALITIES OF THE WHITE BLOOD CELLS

Leucocytosis

Leucocytosis is an increase in the number of normal white cells in the blood to above $10 \times 10^9/l$ (10,000 per mm³). A neutrophil polymorph leucocytosis follows severe muscular exercise, infection, the presence of unusual proteins in the blood due to damage to tissues (e.g. after myocardial infarction the dead heart muscle is absorbed), or during the absorption of haematomas (e.g. following fractures). A lymphocytosis may be a true increase in the number of lymphocytes as in glandular fever, or a relative lymphocytosis, i.e. the lymphocyte count is high in proportion to the polymorph count, as in typhoid.

Eosinophilia

This is an eosinophil count above 4%, and occurs in allergic disease (asthma, hay fever, urticaria) and worm infections.

Leucopenia

Leucopenia is a moderate reduction in the white cell count to below $5 \times 10^9/l$ (5000 per mm³). A reduction in granulocytes (granulopenia, neutropenia) is due to tuberculosis, typhoid, some virus infections, drugs and toxins. Lymphopenia is rare and is a reduction in lymphocytes while the polymorph count remains normal.

Agranulocytosis

Agranulocytosis is a severe leucopenia due to a deficiency of polymorphs and is serious since the body is unable to combat bacterial infection. Agranulocytosis is caused by drugs; e.g. gold, phenylbutazone (Butazolidine), chloramphenicol, thiouracil, cytotoxic drugs and sulphonamides, and radiotherapy. It may be followed by aplastic anaemia. The white cell count is below $2 \times 10^9/l$, 2000 per mm³, with polymorphs less than 20% and often absent.

Clinically: the first sign is an infection, usually a sore throat and ulcerated mouth, with fever. The patient deteriorates and dies of septicaemia.

Treatment: any drugs that are being taken should immediately be stopped. Rest in bed, barrier nursed in a single room *to prevent the spread of infection to the patient.* Fresh blood transfusion. The ulcerated mouth requires special and gentle care, frequent mouthwashes with glycothymoline, and nystatin is used if there is thrush infection. Diet of fluids or soft solids since eating is painful. Adequate vitamins, minerals and protein are needed. Antibiotic is given orally after taking a throat swab for culture and sensitivity testing.

Leukaemia

Leukaemia is an increase in the white cell count due to abnormal leucocytes ('cancer of the white cells'). It may be acute or chronic.

Acute Leukaemia is the commonest cause of death from malignant disease in child-hood. It may be myeloid (of the polymorph series of leucocytes), lymphoblastic (of the lymphocyte series) or monocytic (of the monocyte series). Since symptoms and treatment are similar they are described together.

Causes:
1 Irradiation, e.g. atomic bomb explosions in Japan, patients treated with radiotherapy for ankylosing spondylitis (a disease of the spine), children whose mothers were X-rayed during pregnancy, radiologists. Irradiation causes chromosomal abnormalities in cell nuclei; this kills some cells but predisposes others to become malignant.
2 Down's syndrome (mongolism) predisposes to leukaemia. Chromosome number 21 is connected with leucocyte function and is abnormal in mongolism.
3 Certain viruses and virus-like particles. Viruses transmit leukaemia in many animals and probably also in man.

Clinically: commonly under the age of 5 years. The bone marrow is packed with abnormal leucocytes and fails to produce adequate numbers of red cells, platelets and normal leucocytes. Deficiency of red cells causes normochromic anaemia, and of platelets causes haemorrhages, e.g. purpura, epistaxis, bleeding gums. Although the white cell count in the blood may reach up to $50 \times 10^9/l$ (50,000 per mm^3), the white cells are abnormal and there is a deficiency of normal leucocytes which allows infection to occur (especially sore throat, ulcers in the mouth and pneumonia), and causes malaise and fever. Infiltration by leukaemic cells causes pain in the bones and enlargement of the spleen and liver. In lymphoblastic leukaemia there is also enlargement of the lymph nodes. Leukaemic meningitis may develop, with head-ache, drowsiness and fits. The patient dies, within a few weeks or months of onset, of infection or cerebral haemorrhage.

Sometimes only a few leukaemic cells enter the blood and the white cell count is low ('aleukaemic' leukaemia).

Investigations: (1) blood count; (2) bone marrow; (3) chest X-ray to show enlarged lymph nodes or pneumonia.

Treatment: causes a remission for 1–5 years; with intensive treatment 50% survive for 5 years. Blood transfusion, preferably fresh. Antibiotic for infection. Diet of fluid and soft solids while the mouth is sore.

Chemotherapy: a remission is induced with prednisolone 40–60 mg daily orally for 2–6 weeks plus one or more cytotoxins such as vincristine, daunorubicin, adriamycin or cystosine arabinoside; then maintenance therapy is given, using methotrexate (Amethopterin) 2–5 mg daily orally, cyclophosphamide (Endoxan) 2 mg/kg, or 6-mercaptopurine (Purinethol) 2·5 mg/kg daily orally. Craniospinal radiotherapy and intrathecal methotrexate are given to prevent meningeal leukaemia.

Immunotherapy (the injection of irradiated acute myeloid leukaemic cells) is used in acute myeloid leukaemia, in addition to the above therapy. Parents must be warned of the fatal outlook.

Chronic Myeloid (Granulocytic) Leukaemia is a malignant increase in the number of myelocytes, myeloblasts, and often of polymorphs, in the bone marrow and blood, and the white cell count may reach $500 \times 10^9/l$ (500,000 per mm^3) due mostly to abnormal cells. The concentration of the enzyme, alkaline phosphatase, is low in the polymorphs.

In some patients the leukaemia is due to radiation, such as radiotherapy to the spine in ankylosing spondylitis, the therapy of polycythaemia with radioactive phosphorus, or atomic bomb explosions. Chromosomal abnormalities are present, usually the Philadelphia chromosome.

Clinically: commonly aged 35–60 years, although the incidence is increasing in younger adults. There is fatigue and a slow onset of discomfort and enlargement of the abdomen due to enlargement of the liver and spleen by leukaemic cells, and acute pain may occur in the left hypochondrium due to infarction in the spleen. The platelet count is often high at first but later leukaemic cells crowd out the marrow and cause normochromic anaemia and haemorrhage (e.g. epistaxis). Nodules of leukaemic cells may appear in the skin. After about 3 years the patient develops fever and loses weight and dies, although some patients live longer.

Treatment considerably improves the patient's condition. Chemotherapy with busulphan (Myleran) 2–5 mg daily orally. Radiotherapy to reduce the size of an uncomfortably enlarged spleen, or splenectomy. Blood transfusion for anaemia.

Chronic Lymphoblastic (Lymphatic) Leukaemia is a malignant increase in the number of lymphocytes in the blood.

Clinically: it affects those aged 45–70 years and is twice as common in males as females. There is fatigue, weight loss, and enlargement of the lymph nodes, spleen and liver due to the presence of large numbers of abnormal lymphoid cells. Invasion of the bone marrow, and therefore anaemia, is late. The white cell count is up to $500 \times 10^9/l$ (500,000 per mm^3); mostly lymphocytes. The patient lives for an average of five years, although the elderly may survive 10 years.

Treatment is not very effective and is therefore not used if the patient has only mild symptoms. Chemotherapy with chlorambucil (Leukeran) 0·2 mg/kg body weight orally, or cyclophosphamide (Endoxana) 100 mg or more daily orally. Radiotherapy for large glandular masses. Corticosteroids for haemolytic anaemia or thrombocytopenia. Blood transfusion for anaemia. Antibiotic for infection.

PLATELETS (Thrombocytes)

Platelets are tiny cells which contain granules but no nucleus, and are made in the bone marrow from megakaryocytes. The normal platelet count in the blood is between 150 and $400 \times 10^9/l$ (150,000 and 400,000 per mm^3).

Platelets are sticky and adhere to damaged capillaries and plug them, thus stopping bleeding. They are also one of the initiators of blood clotting (the other is damaged tissue) and cause retraction (shrinkage) of clot.

Thrombocytopenia is a platelet count below $150 \times 10^9/l$ (150,000 per mm³). If the count is below $40 \times 10^9/l$, 40,000 per mm³ bleeding is likely, and the bleeding time is prolonged beyond the normal 2–7 minutes. Bleeding occurs from the nose, mouth, kidney (haematuria) and into the skin as petechiae (pinpoint spots of haemorrhage) and ecchymoses (small bruises). The clotting time is normal since only a small number of platelets are able to initiate clotting. The causes of thrombocytopenia are given under 'purpura'.

Treatment: treat the cause. Prednisolone up to 60 mg daily orally. Platelet transfusions. Splenectomy in some patients.

PURPURA

Purpura is bleeding into the skin, but bleeding may also occur into joints, eyes, brain and other organs. Purpura may consist of petechiae (tiny haemorrhages) or ecchymoses (small bruises).

Causes:
  A. *Thrombocytopenic*
    1   Drugs—quinine, quinidine, cytotoxin therapy, phenylbutazone, sulphonamides.
    2   Viruses—rubella, mumps, measles.
    3   Bone marrow disease—aplastic anaemia, leukaemia, irradiation of the marrow.
    4   Antibodies to platelets—repeated blood transfusions, auto-immune disease, e.g. systemic lupus erythematosus.
    5   Idiopathic (often follows viral infection).
  B. *Disturbed platelet function with a normal count*
    1   Scurvy (both platelets and capillaries require vitamin C).
    2   Hereditary X-linked disorder.
  C. *Vascular*
    1   Allergy—Henoch-Schönlein purpura, penicillin, sulphonamides.
    2   Senile—atrophy of elastic tissue allows small vessels to rupture easily.
    3   Prolonged therapy with corticosteroids reduces the amount of connective tissue supporting the capillaries which then rupture easily.

Idiopathic Thrombocytopenic Purpura affects children and young adults and is usually a chronic disease with relapses and remissions. There is purpura, and bleeding causes a hypochromic anaemia. The platelet count is low, the bleeding time is prolonged, and Hess's test (a sphygmomanometer cuff around the arm, inflated to just above the diastolic blood pressure for 5 minutes) is positive, i.e. petechiae are produced in excessive numbers, indicating an increased fragility of the capillaries.

Treatment: blood transfusion for anaemia, platelet transfusion to stop haemorrhage. Prednisolone 60 mg daily orally should be tried. Splenectomy benefits 75% of cases.

Henoch-Schönlein Purpura is an allergic inflammation of vessels due to infection (e.g. β-haemolytic streptococcal tonsillitis), drugs (e.g. aspirin, quinine, thiazides), or foods. It is found mostly in children, who feel ill, have fever and purpura. Bleeding into the intestinal wall causes colic, vomiting and diarrhoea with blood in the faeces. Bleeding under the periosteum of bones causes pain and swelling near joints. The urine may contain protein and blood due to nephritis. Most patients recover within 1 month.

Treatment: blood transfusion for severe haemorrhage, iron for anaemia, antibiotic if due to bacterial infection. Antihistamines or prednisolone to reduce the inflammation.

THE RETICULOENDOTHELIAL SYSTEM

The reticuloendothelial system is a scattered system of mononuclear phagocytic cells lining the endothelial vascular sinuses in the lymph nodes, spleen, bone marrow and liver. In the lymph nodes, spleen and bone marrow they are called reticular cells, and in the liver they are called Kupffer cells. They can detach themselves from the reticular tissues and become mobile cells and enter the blood as monocytes, or the tissues as histiocytes. They are all phagocytic and can take up tissue débris and bacteria and destroy old or abnormal red blood cells.

THE LYMPHATIC SYSTEM

The lymphatic system consists of lymphatic capillaries, lymphatic vessels and lymph nodes. The lymphatic capillaries consist of a single layer of endothelial cells and begin as blind tubes in the extracellular tissues (*Fig. 3.5*). The capillaries join together to form the lymphatic vessels which join others and drain into the cisterna chyli, a sac-like dilatation in front of the lumbar vertebrae. This continues upwards as the thoracic duct lying alongside the inferior vena cava and opens into the junction between the left internal jugular and the left subclavian veins. The thoracic duct conveys lymph from the lower limbs, abdomen, left arm, left half of the thorax and head, to the venous system. The right lymphatic duct conveys lymph from the right arm and right half of the thorax and head to the right subclavian vein. The lymphatic capillaries draining lymph from the small intestine absorb fat and are called lacteals. All lymphatics drain fluid and wastes from the tissues just as do the venous ends of the blood capillaries, but the lymphatics are more permeable than blood capillaries and are able to absorb the little plasma protein that escapes into the tissues, and other large molecules, including bacterial proteins. Lymph also passes through lymph nodes before entering the blood.

The Lymph Nodes are scattered throughout the body. Lymphatic tissue with the same function as lymph nodes is also present in certain sites, e.g. the tonsils and adenoids in the pharynx, and the Peyer's patches in the small intestine.

A lymph node (*Fig. 5.6*) consists of a fibrous and reticular supporting meshwork containing lymphoid follicles (groups of lymphocytes and larger cells) and is surrounded by a fibrous capsule. About four lymphatics (afferent vessels) pour

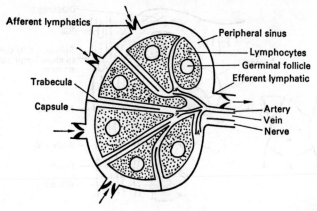

FIG. 5.6   A lymph node

lymph into the peripheral sinus of each lymph node. The lymph filters through the node and leaves through a single efferent lymphatic vessel.

The function of a lymph node is to filter off particles and prevent them from entering the blood; to break down filtered material, e.g. bacteria, and therefore act as a barrier to the spread of infection; to produce lymphocytes and to form antibodies and antitoxins.

The Spleen

The spleen (*Figs.* 5.7 and 5.8) lies in the left hypochondrium in the abdominal 'cavity' with the diaphragm above; the colon below; the stomach in front; the left kidney and adrenal behind; the pancreas on its right; and the chest wall with the ninth, tenth and eleventh ribs on its left. The spleen consists of splenic pulp and sinuses; the pulp is a reticulum of fibrous and elastic tissue containing numerous cells—red cells, lymphocytes, plasma cells, splenic cells (the phagocytic reticulo-endothelial cells) and a few granulocytes. The arterioles are surrounded by nodules of lymphoid cells (Malpighian bodies) and branch into sinuses (*Fig.* 5.9) which communicate with the pulp and return blood to the venules and splenic vein.

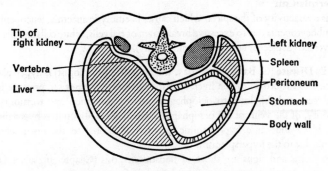

FIG. 5.7   Transverse section of the upper abdomen

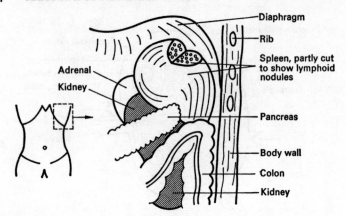

FIG. 5.8 The relations of the spleen (the stomach lies in front)

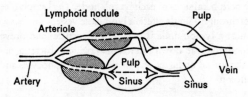

FIG. 5.9 Microanatomy of the spleen

Functions of the spleen are to remove old and abnormal red cells (*Fig. 5.4*), and to produce lymphocytes, monocytes and plasma cells which produce antibodies and antitoxins. It stores iron and filters abnormal particles from the blood.

ABNORMALITIES OF THE RETICULOENDOTHELIAL AND LYMPHATIC SYSTEMS

Hypersplenism
This is overactivity of the spleen which causes haemolytic anaemia, leucopenia and thrombocytopenia due to excessive breakdown of red cells, white cells and platelets. An overactive spleen is enlarged (splenomegaly).

Banti's Disease (G. Banti, 1852–1925, was an Italian pathologist) is hypersplenism and cirrhosis (fibrosis) of the liver. Hepatic cirrhosis increases the pressure in the portal vein and this leads to oesophageal varices (distension and tortuosity, i.e. varicosity, of the veins of the oesophagus), which are easily injured by swallowed food, bleed and cause hypochromic anaemia additional to the normochromic anaemia due to the hypersplenism.

Symptoms and signs are those of hepatic cirrhosis (Chapter 9), anaemia and leucopenia, and the treatment is of these conditions.

Splenomegaly

Splenomegaly is enlargement of the spleen, and may be due to:

1 Infection. Malaria, kala azar, glandular fever, brucellosis, bacterial endocarditis.
2 Diseases of the blood. Anaemia of any type but particularly haemolytic
   anaemia, e.g. sickle-cell anaemia, thalassaemia, acholuric jaundice; polycythaemia, leukaemia, myelosclerosis.
3 Neoplasm. Hodgkin's disease, lymphosarcoma.
4 Others. Banti's disease, Gaucher's disease (a rare hereditary disease causing
   lipoid deposition in organs), amyloidosis (the deposition of amyloid
   material in various organs).

Treatment is symptomatic (of symptoms) and of the cause.

Lymphadenitis

Lymphadenitis is inflammation of a lymph node (lymph gland). Pyogenic (septic)
inflammation results from organisms entering the node from an area of inflammation in the area drained by the node; e.g. a breast abscess may be followed by
infection of the lymph nodes in the axilla. The nodes become swollen, painful and
tender, and antibiotic therapy is needed. Severe infection may cause abscess
formation in the lymph node. An abscess requires incision and drainage.

Lymph glands may be invaded by tubercle bacilli causing 'glandular' tuberculosis,
e.g. in the cervical (neck) or mesenteric glands. The glands may be destroyed by
caseous ('cheese-like') necrosis or by granulomatous (fibrous tissue-forming)
inflammation.

Virus infections (Chapter 4), e.g. glandular fever, rubella and adenoviruses,
particularly affect the lymph glands in the neck, which become swollen and tender.

Lymphangitis

This is inflammation of the lymphatic vessels.

The Reticuloses

These are fatal diseases of the reticuloendothelial and lymphatic systems and include
the 'lymphomas' (Hodgkin's disease, lymphosarcoma and reticulosarcoma) and
myelomatosis, which is described under 'anaemia'.

Investigations: blood count to detect anaemia and abnormal cells, bone marrow may
contain abnormal cells, chest X-ray to detect mediastinal lymph node enlargement,
liver and spleen isotope scan and lymphangiography to show any involvement of
these organs, lymph node and liver biopsy to provide the diagnosis. Laparotomy
may be performed to determine the extent of the disease if curative radiotherapy is
being considered.

Hodgkin's Disease (Lymphadenoma)

Thomas Hodgkin (1798–1866) was an English physician. The cause of Hodgkin's
disease is unknown but one theory is that it may be due to a virus infecting a person
who already has an abnormality of the reticuloendothelial system.

Clinically: commonly aged 15–35, or over 70 years. The lymph nodes enlarge painlessly, often the cervical nodes at first, then those elsewhere, and may cause symptoms due to pressure on other organs; e.g. pressure on the trachea or bronchi causing dyspnoea, on the oesophagus causing dysphagia, and on the spinal cord causing paraplegia. The spleen and liver also enlarge. The patient has fever, weakness, loss of weight, pruritus, and normochromic anaemia.

Treatment: radiotherapy to lymph nodes, especially in disease localised to one group of lymph nodes, in which a 70% 5-year cure is obtained. Chemotherapy, for widespread disease, causes a remission in 25% of patients. Cyclophosphamide, mustine hydrochloride, chlorambucil, vincristine, adriamycin, and procarbazine are used in various combinations. Splenectomy if the spleen is affected.

Lymphosarcoma and Reticulosarcoma

These are similar to Hodgkin's disease except that they are more common over the age of 40 years, and patients survive only a few months.

DRUGS USED IN DISEASES OF THE BLOOD, BONE MARROW AND LYMPHATIC SYSTEM

Drugs Used in Anaemia
Iron.

1 Ferrous sulphate 200–600 mg daily orally. Each 200 mg tablet contains 60 mg of iron.

2 Ferrous gluconate 300–1200 mg daily orally. Each 300 mg tablet contains 35 mg of iron.

3 Ferrous fumarate 200–600 mg daily orally. Each 200 mg tablet contains 65 mg of iron.

4 Ferric ammonium citrate mixture 10 ml orally daily (= 400 mg iron), preferably with vitamin C. The mixture stains the teeth unless taken through a straw.

5 Ferrous aminoacetosulphate in syrup ('Plesmet') for infants and young children 10 ml t.d.s.

6 Slow-release iron causes less gastro-intestinal upset but less is absorbed.

7 Iron dextran (Imferon) 2 ml deeply i.m. (= 100 mg of iron).

8 Iron sorbitol (Jectofer) 2 ml deeply i.m. (= 100 mg of iron).

Any improvement is no quicker whether i.m. or oral iron is given and it is preferable to begin with small doses of ferrous sulphate.

Side-effects: oral iron may cause nausea, abdominal pain, constipation or diarrhoea. Intramuscular iron may be locally painful, stains the skin, and may produce headache, nausea, vomiting, a metallic taste, and shock.

Folic Acid. 5 mg t.d.s. orally daily. *Side-effects* are rare.

Vitamin B$_{12}$ (cobalamin) (1) hydroxocobalamin 100–1000 μg i.m. is retained better than cyanocobalamin; (2) cyanocobalamin 100–1000 μg i.m. Some is lost in the urine.

Antineoplastic Drugs (Cytotoxins)

Cytotoxic drugs are used in malignant diseases, often in rotation or in combination with each other, or as immunosuppressives to prevent the rejection of kidney transplants. They act not only on malignant cells but also on other rapidly dividing cells, such as bone marrow, hair follicles, gastro-intestinal tract, fetus and testis. They have similar toxic effects:

1 Bone marrow depression causing thrombocytopenia, leucopenia and eventually anaemia. Regular blood counts should be done, e.g. twice weekly at first, then weekly.

2 Alopecia, i.e. the hair may fall out.

3 Gastro-intestinal upset—nausea, vomiting (an anti-emetic is given 30–60 minutes before the cytotoxin, e.g. chlorpromazine 50 mg i.m.), diarrhoea, anorexia, ulceration of, and haemorrhage from, the gastro-intestinal tract, e.g. haemorrhagic colitis.

4 Ulceration of the mouth (stomatitis).

A. Alkylating Agents. These act by attacking the nucleic acid of the chromosomes, and alter its structure so that the nuclei of the cells cannot divide.

Busulphan (Myleran): 2–5 mg orally daily initially (for 3–6 weeks), then 0·5–2 mg daily. In addition to the above toxic effects it may cause amenorrhoea in women after four to six months.

  Use: chronic myeloid (granulocytic) leukaemia.

Chlorambucil (Leukeran): 5–15 mg orally daily initially, then 2–4 mg daily.

  Use: chronic lymphatic leukaemia, lymphosarcoma, Hodgkin's disease.

Cyclophosphamide (Endoxan, Cytoxan): 100–200 mg orally daily, or up to 1 g i.v. every three weeks. It may cause haemorrhagic cystitis.

  Use: acute leukaemia, chronic lymphatic leukaemia, chronic myeloid leukaemia, Hodgkin's disease, myelomatosis, carcinoma of ovary and breast. It is also used as an immunosuppressive in kidney transplants.

Mustine (chlorethazine): 400 μg per kg body weight i.v. single dose or divided over four days, in a fast-flowing drip.

  Use: lymphosarcoma, Hodgkin's disease, follicular lymphoma.

Melphalan (Alkeran, Sarcolysin): 2–30 mg orally daily to a total of 200 mg, or 100 mg i.v. as a single dose. Toxicity is marked.

  Use: myelomatosis, chronic myeloid leukaemia, melanoma, carcinoma of breast or ovary.

Others are ethoglucid, triaziquone, thiotepa and mitobronitol.

B. Antimetabolites. These are chemicals which are sufficiently like a normal essential substance that they combine with enzymes in place of the essential substance, but then block the action of the enzymes (*Fig. 5.10*).

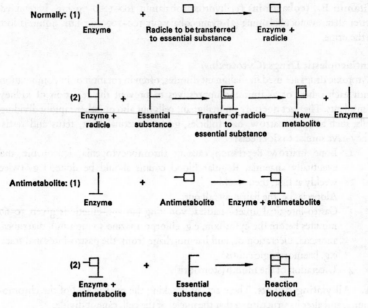

FIG. 5.10   The action of an antimetabolite

Azathioprine (Imuran): 2–5 mg per kg body weight orally daily. It is converted into mercaptopurine in the body.

Use: acute leukaemia, and also as an immunosuppressive in renal transplants and in autoimmune disease.

Mercaptopurine (Purinethol): 100–200 mg orally daily.

Use: acute leukaemia, chronic myeloid leukaemia, and as an immunosuppressive.

Cytarabine (*Cytosine arabinoside*, Cytosar): up to 4 mg per kg body weight i.v. daily for 3–15 days. It may cause conjunctivitis, keratitis and liver damage in addition to the toxic effects described above.

Use: acute myeloid leukaemia, acute and chronic lymphatic leukaemia.

Methotrexate (Amethopterin): 20–30 mg orally every fourth day. It may cause skin rash and liver damage. Bone marrow depression may be limited by giving folinic acid 3–6 mg i.m. four-hourly beginning at the same time as the methotrexate, since it is ineffective once methotrexate has been given.

Use: acute leukaemia, chorioncarcinoma, tumours of the liver, head and neck, and in psoriasis.

Others are thioguanine and fluorouracil.

C.   Alkaloids

Vincristine (Oncovin): acts by arresting the division (mitosis) of cell nuclei.

Dose: 25–150 μg per kg body weight i.v. weekly for three weeks. It is toxic and may cause peripheral neuropathy, and autonomic nerve damage causing urinary retention, constipation and paralytic ileus.

Use: acute leukaemia, lymphosarcoma, Hodgkin's disease, reticulosarcoma, neuroblastoma.

Vinblastine: is similar to vincristine but more toxic.

D. Antibiotics

Daunorubicin (Rubidomycin, Cerubidin, Daunoblastina): 2 mg per kg body weight as an i.v. infusion in saline every four to seven days. It may cause a skin rash in addition to the toxic effects described above.

Use: acute leukaemia, neuroblastoma.

Side-effects: thrombophlebitis at the site of injection.

Adriamycin (Doxorubicin): 400–800 μg per kg body weight as an i.v. infusion daily for three days a week.

Use: acute leukaemia.

Others are mithramycin and mitomycin.

E. Others

L-Asparaginase (Colaspase): an enzyme which destroys an essential amino acid (asparagine) which some malignant cells cannot synthesise and have to extract from the blood.

Dose: 200–1000 i.u. per kg body weight i.v. three times weekly.

Corticosteroids

Prednisolone 15–60 mg orally daily, is used in acute leukaemia, haemolytic anaemia, thrombocytopenia and as an immunosuppressive.

Side-effects: salt and water retention, gain in weight, hypertension, hyperglycaemia, peptic ulcer, adrenal suppression, and susceptibility to infection.

Radiotherapy

Radioactive Phosphorus (^{32}P) gives off β-rays and is taken up by the bone marrow.

Side-effects: myeloid leukaemia, anaemia, leucopenia.

Use: polycythaemia vera.

THE THYMUS GLAND

The thymus is situated behind the sternum, in front of the aortic arch and trachea, It is large in childhood but atrophies after puberty. It consists of an outer cortex packed with lymphocytes and a central medulla containing lymphocytes, reticular cells and Hassall's corpuscles, and is surrounded by a capsule.

The thymus is required for the development of immunity and in the fetus it is the main source of lymphocytes which are 'seeded' to the other lymphoid tissues.

In adults the thymus secretes a hormone, thymosin, which causes primitive lymphocytes in the lymphoid tissues to mature into T-lymphocytes (thymus-dependent lymphocytes) which are involved in the cellular type of immunity (e.g. in the rejection of foreign tissue grafts and in tuberculosis). The other type of immunity is humoral, i.e. provided by antibodies, and is not connected with the thymus.

Abnormality of the Thymus, e.g. thymoma (thymic tumour) may cause myasthenia gravis, a rare disturbance of the transmission of impulses from nerve endings to muscle which causes muscular weakness.

6 CARDIOVASCULAR SYSTEM

The cardiovascular system consists of two main parts:

1 The blood circulatory system—the heart and blood vessels.
2 The lymphatic system—the lymph glands (nodes) and lymphatic vessels (Chapter 5).

Function. The blood circulatory system is the transport system of the body. It transfers absorbed food substances from the gut to the liver and then throughout the body. It carries oxygen from the lungs to the tissues, and carbon dioxide in the reverse direction. It transports waste products from the tissues to the liver and kidneys for detoxication and excretion. The heart is the pump in this system, the blood vessels provide the route and the blood is the carrier. The route can be varied by the autonomic nervous system according to varying needs, e.g. during exercise the blood vessels to the muscles dilate to provide an increased blood flow and thus extra oxygen and glucose. The lymphatic system is for safety. Soluble molecules, e.g. glucose, can diffuse through the capillary wall and enter or leave the blood, but insoluble and larger particles, e.g. bacteria, fortunately cannot, and if they invade the tissues they enter the lymphatics and are carried to lymph nodes where anti-bodies are made and help to destroy the organisms. Lymphatics also transport large groups of molecules, e.g. chylomicrons (absorbed fat) and some proteins from the gut, and drain any extra fluid that has collected in the tissues.

THE HEART

The heart is a hollow, cone-shaped muscle the size of the owner's fist. It lies in the thoracic cavity in the mediastinum between the lungs, behind the lower part of the sternum and in front of the oesophagus, trachea, bronchi, descending aorta and thoracic vertebrae. It rests on the diaphragm below. Above it are attached the ascending aorta and pulmonary artery (*Fig. 6.1*).

Structure. The heart is composed of three layers of tissue.

The **pericardium** surrounds the heart and consists of two layers separated by the pericardial 'cavity'. In life there is no cavity and the two smooth layers are close together, separated only by a thin film of fluid which acts as a lubricant. The outer layer (the parietal pericardium) consists of a tough, fibrous membrane lined by serous membrane. The inner layer (visceral pericardium) is a serous membrane attached to the outer surface of the myocardium (myo = muscle, cardia = heart). The serous membrane secretes the pericardial fluid.

The **myocardium** consists of specialized muscle, its fibres being continuous with each other, dividing and rejoining to produce a type of mesh. It receives its blood

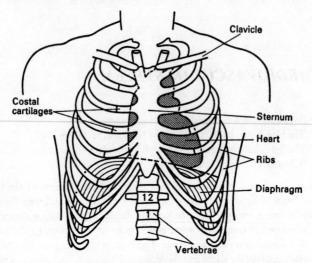

FIG. 6.1   The position of the heart

supply from the coronary arteries which are the first arteries to branch off the aorta.

The **endocardium** lines the inner surface of the myocardium, valves and papillary muscles, and is a smooth membrane of flat endothelial cells which continues into the blood vessels as their inner lining.

Interior. The heart is partitioned into right and left sides by a sheet of muscle, the septum. Each side is also divided into two by valves, forming upper chambers (atria) and lower chambers (ventricles). Therefore the heart has four chambers (*Fig. 6.2*). The valve separating the right atrium from the right ventricle is the

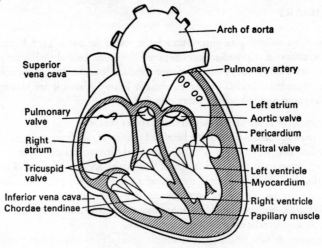

FIG. 6.2   The interior of the heart

tricuspid valve; that separating the left atrium from the left ventricle is the mitral valve. These valves are tethered to the papillary muscles (projections of the ventricular muscle) by fine tendons (chordae tendinae.) The valves prevent regurgitation of blood from the ventricles into the atria. Two other valves are present: the aortic valve, at the origin of the aorta, and the pulmonary valve, at the beginning of the pulmonary artery. These prevent regurgitation of blood from the arteries into the ventricles.

Blood Flow (*Fig. 6.3*)
From the superior and inferior venae cavae (great veins) blood enters the right atrium and passes through the tricuspid valve into the right ventricle. From the

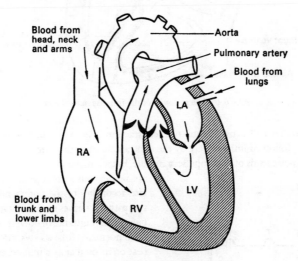

Blood from head, neck and arms

Aorta

Pulmonary artery

Blood from lungs

LA

RA

Blood from trunk and lower limbs

LV

RV

FIG. 6.3   The blood flow through the heart

right ventricle it is pumped through the pulmonary valve into the pulmonary artery the only artery carrying deoxygenated ('venous') blood. The pulmonary artery divides into right and left branches going to the right and left lungs where the blood is oxygenated (takes up oxygen) and carbon dioxide is given off. From the lungs the blood flows into two right and two left pulmonary veins (the only veins carrying oxygenated blood), then into the left atrium and through the mitral valve into the thick-walled left ventricle. From the left ventricle arterial blood is pumped through the aortic valve into the aorta and along the arterial system to the capillaries from which it returns by the venous system, entering the right atrium via the great veins.

The Heartbeat originates in the sinoatrial (S.A.) node in the atria. The S.A. node sends out regular impulses which cause contraction of the atria. Having passed through the atrial muscle the impulse reaches the atrio-ventricular (A.V.) node near the ventricles. The atrial muscle is separated from the ventricular muscle by a fibrotendinous band which prevents the direct conduction of impulses from atria to ventricles except at the A.V. node. The A.V. node is the beginning of special conducting tissue, the bundle of His, which rapidly conducts the impulse through

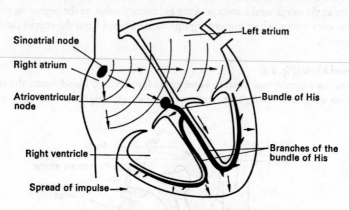

Sinoatrial node

Right atrium

Atrioventricular node

Right ventricle

Spread of impulse

Left atrium

Bundle of His

Branches of the bundle of His

FIG. 6.4   The pathway of the impulse in the heart

the ventricles and causes ventricular contraction (*Fig. 6.4*). Both atria contract together, followed immediately by the contraction of both ventricles. On its own the S.A. node sends out 60 impulses a minute, but it is under the control of the auto-

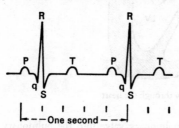

--One second--

FIG. 6.5   A normal electrocardiogram

nomic nervous system which alters this rate according to the body's needs. The sympathetic nerves speed the rate of impulses; the vagus nerve slows it. The A.V. node normally follows this rate but can beat on its own at 45 a minute, as in heart block.

The electrical changes in the heart can be detected and printed by an electrocardiogram (E.C.G.) which shows five waves called P, QRS and T. The P wave is due to the atrial impulse. Q, R and S are due to the ventricular impulse, and the T wave is due to the recovery of the muscle (*Fig. 6.5*).

THE BLOOD VESSELS

There are five types of blood vessels: artery, arteriole, capillary, venule and vein.

The Arteries

Arteries are thicker-walled than veins since they have to withstand high pressures. They transport blood away from the heart and vary in size from the largest (the aorta, which is up to 2·5 cm in diameter) to small arteries less than 1 mm in diameter.

They consist of three layers:
1   The adventitia, the outer fibrous tissue coat;
2   The media, the middle layer of smooth muscle and elastic tissue, and
3   The intima, the inner layer of endothelium (*Fig. 6.6*).

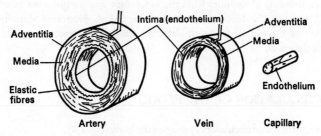

FIG. 6.6.   An artery, vein and a capillary

The tunica media contains more elastic tissue in the large arteries than in the small arteries. This is so they can expand as each heartbeat suddenly forces a volume of blood (average 70 ml per ventricle) into the aorta. After expansion the elastic recoil helps to maintain the blood pressure.

The Arterioles
These are the smallest arteries and branch into numerous minute **capillaries** which are the diameter of a red blood cell (8 μm; i.e. 0·008 mm). The wall of a capillary consists of a single layer of flat endothelial cells and is very thin, thus allowing the passage of water and other small molecules but not blood cells or proteins. Capillaries join together to form **venules**, the smallest veins. These join to form **veins** which transport blood to the heart and the wall consists of the same three layers as arteries but the media is thin. The veins in the limbs contain valves which prevent blood from flowing in the wrong direction. A **valve** is a fold of endothelium strengthened with fibrous tissue (*Fig. 6.7*).

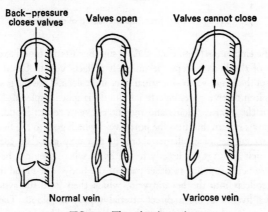

FIG. 6.7   The valves in a vein

Nerve Supply

The blood vessels, especially the arterioles, are supplied with sympathetic nerves controlled by the vasomotor centre in the medulla oblongata. The sympathetic nerves adjust the diameter of the vessels to control the blood flow through them. Increased numbers of impulses from the vasomotor centre cause vasoconstriction and this reduces the blood flow through the vessel. Decreased stimuli cause relaxation of the muscle (i.e. vasodilatation), and this increases the blood flow through the vessel.

THE CIRCULATION OF THE BLOOD

There are three blood circulatory systems in the body (*Fig. 6.8*):
1 The systemic (general) circulation;
2 The pulmonary circulation;
3 The portal system.

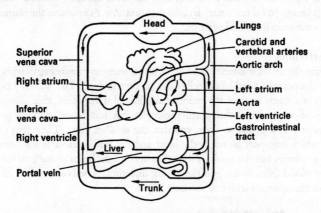

FIG. 6.8   Diagram of the circulation of the blood

The systemic circulation (*Figs. 6.9* and *6.10*) supplies arterial blood to all the organs and tissues of the body except the lungs. It collects venous blood from all the tissues except the lungs, gastro-intestinal tract and spleen. Thus the gastro-intestinal tract and spleen receive systemic arterial blood via gastric, splenic and mesenteric arteries; but the gastric, splenic and mesenteric veins return blood, not directly into the venous system, but into the portal vein which goes to the liver and breaks up into a second set of capillaries there. In this way absorbed food and other substances such as drugs go directly to the liver, where they can be modified or stored before being supplied to other parts of the body. The blood from the liver capillaries collects into the hepatic vein, which then joins the systemic venous system. The liver also has a direct arterial supply of blood. The pulmonary circulation is quite separate and is described under 'heart, blood flow'(page 123).

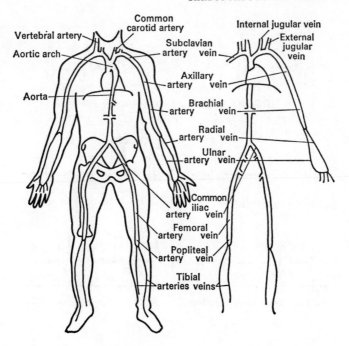

FIG. 6.9   The arterial system   FIG. 6.10   The venous system

THE PULSE

The pulse is a pressure wave transmitted in the arterial wall due to the expulsion of blood from the contracting left ventricle, and can be felt where an artery can be pressed against a bone, e.g. in the radial artery at the wrist. Recording the pulse provides information on the heart rate and rhythm, the volume of the pulse and the tension in the arterial wall. Any abnormalities are reported. The rate is counted for one minute while the temperature is being recorded.

The Rate at which the heart is beating in one minute is normally 70–75 at rest. It is increased (tachycardia, *Fig. 6.11*) by exercise, emotion, drugs (atropine, adrenaline), shock, fever, disease such as hyperthyroidism and heart failure, and is more rapid in children than in adults. It is decreased (bradycardia, *Fig. 6.12*) in hypothyroidism, heart block, liver disease, and increased intracranial pressure, e.g. cerebral tumour. If the pulse cannot be felt at the wrist, as in shock, it can be felt in the carotid artery in the neck between the larynx and sternomastoid muscle. If the pulse is irregular the heart rate should be timed by listening with a stethoscope over the apex beat in the chest, since some beats may be so weak that they cannot be felt at the wrist. The apex beat is the position of maximum impulse of the heart, normally 8·8 cm (3·5 inches) to the left of the midline in the fifth intercostal space.

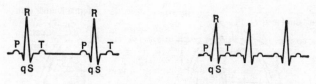

FIG. 6.11 (a) Normal E.C.G.; (b) tachycardia

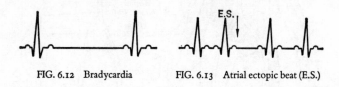

FIG. 6.12 Bradycardia   FIG. 6.13 Atrial ectopic beat (E.S.)

FIG. 6.14 Ventricular ectopic beat   FIG. 6.15 Pulsus bigeminus

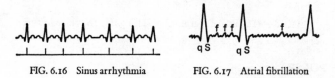

FIG. 6.16 Sinus arrhythmia   FIG. 6.17 Atrial fibrillation

FIG. 6.18 Ventricular fibrillation   FIG. 6.19 Pulsus alternans

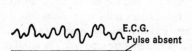

FIG. 6.20 Atrial flutter   FIG. 6.21 Complete heart block

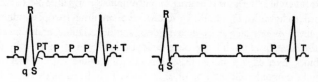

FIGS. 6.11 to 6.21 Electrocardiograms in various conditions
The arrows show the site at which the normal impulse should have arisen.

The Rhythm. The heart normally beats regularly with the same length of time between each beat.

The Volume or Strength of the beat. Moderate pressure normally obliterates the artery. The volume is increased by exercise, fever, anaemia, and increased intracranial pressure, and is lowered by shock and cardiac failure.

The Tension. The artery should feel soft and elastic, not hard and tortuous as in arteriosclerosis.

Disturbances of the Pulse

Irregular rhythm may be due to:

Ectopic Systole ('extrasystole'). This is a beat originating from an abnormal site in the heart and occurring shortly before it was normally due, followed by a longer interval than normal. Atrial ectopic beats (*Fig. 6.13*) occur in normal people, e.g. after a heavy meal, coffee, tea, tobacco. Treatment is not required, except for reassurance. Frequent ectopic beats occur in thyrotoxicosis, digitalis overdose and ischaemic heart disease. The underlying disease should be treated. Multiple ventricular ectopic beats (*Fig. 6.14*) are often a sign of impending ventricular tachycardia or fibrillation and should be reported so that lignocaine can be given.

Coupled Beats (pulsus bigeminus), *Fig. 6.15*, are ectopic beats alternating with normal beats and are due to digitalis overdose.

Sinus Arrhythmia is normal. It is an increasing pulse rate during inspiration, slowing during expiration (*Fig. 6.16*).

Pulsus Paradoxus is the reverse of sinus arrhythmia; the pulse rate slows during inspiration and increases during expiration. It occurs in pericardial effusion, constrictive pericarditis and in children with fevers.

Atrial Fibrillation (*Fig. 6.17*). Irregular contractions occur scattered throughout the atrial muscle and the atria do not contract as a single unit (*Fig. 6.22*). Irregular impulses reach the atrioventricular node so the ventricular rate is totally irregular and is 100–150 a minute. Some beats are weak and are not felt at the wrist, causing a pulse deficit (e.g. the rate may be 130 at the apex but only 105 at the wrist). To

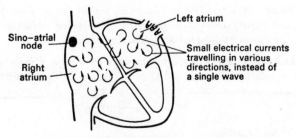

FIG. 6.22   Atrial fibrillation (compare with *Fig. 6.4*)

obtain a correct record of the pulse deficit both apex rate and pulse rate should be taken simultaneously by two people. Atrial fibrillation occurs in rheumatic heart disease (mitral stenosis), ischaemic heart disease, hypertension, and hyperthyroidism.

Treatment: **Digoxin** reduces the rate but does not cure the fibrillation. *Dose:* 1 mg i.v. or i.m., or 1·5 mg orally, then 0·25 mg one to four times daily according to the apex rate, which should be kept at 70–80 a minute. **Quinidine** may restore normal rhythm and is used if there is no underlying organic heart disease. It is used in thyrotoxicosis. It is abortifacient and cannot be used in pregnancy. *Dose:* If a test dose of 120 mg orally does not cause side-effects 200–400 mg is given orally four-hourly on the first day, then two-hourly (omitting two night doses) for two days, then a maintenance dose of 200–400 mg t.d.s. for a few days.

β-sympathetic blocking drugs will slow the rate (e.g. propranolol). The sympathetic nervous system has α-receptors and β-receptors which cause α- and β-effects. The α-effect is vasoconstriction in skin and viscera, hence increased blood pressure. The β-effect is increased heart rate, vasodilatation in muscle, and bronchial and uterine relaxation. β-blocking drugs prevent the β-effect and therefore reduce the heart rate.

Direct current (D.C.) defibrillation may be used. The cause is also treated.

Ventricular Fibrillation (*Fig. 6.18*) is fatal within two to three minutes since the ventricle does not contract as a unit and therefore there is no heart beat. It is one form of cardiac 'arrest'. It may follow myocardial infarction, digitalis overdose, adrenaline overdose, or electrocution.

Treatment: external cardiac massage, artificial respiration and defibrillation.

Pulsus Alternans (*Fig. 6.19*) consists of alternate strong and weak beats and occurs in heart failure.

Paroxysmal Tachycardia is a rate above 100 a minute, beginning and ending suddenly. It occurs in health and in heart disease. An attack lasts minutes or hours. The patient is anxious, may faint or vomit, and has palpitations (an awareness of the heart beat).

Treatment: the patient should lie down and be reassured. Breath-holding, pro-pranolol 40–80 mg t.d.s. orally, digoxin 1 mg i.v., or D.C. shock may be used.

Atrial Flutter (*Fig. 6.20*). The atria beat very rapidly (300 a minute) and the ventricles more slowly (100–150 a minute). Atrial flutter is due to heart disease from any cause. Treatment is similar to that in atrial fibrillation.

Heart Block (*Fig. 6.21*) is a failure of conduction from the atria to the ventricles and may be complete (when the pulse rate will be about 40 a minute) or partial (when every third or fourth heart-beat will be missing). It is due to ischaemic heart disease, rheumatic carditis, diphtheria, or digitalis overdose.

Stokes-Adams Attacks
If the pulse rate is very slow (e.g. 20 a minute), as in heart block, cerebral anoxia occurs and causes pallor, unconsciousness, and maybe an epileptic fit. On recovery

the skin flushes. If unconsciousness lasts more than two minutes mental damage or death may occur.

Treatment is urgent: external cardiac massage, clear airway, isoprenaline i.v. 1–5 mg in 500 ml of 5% dextrose. Artificial pacemaker, which stimulates the heartbeat electrically.

Prevention: Isoprenaline (slow-release) 30 mg t.d.s. or ephedrine 30 mg t.d.s. orally.

BLOOD PRESSURE

Physiology. Blood pressure (B.P.) is the force which the blood exerts on the wall of the vessel containing it. In the systemic circulation it is due to the discharge of blood from the left ventricle into the aorta. During ventricular contraction (systole) the pressure (systolic pressure) is increased, e.g. to 120 mmHg (millimetres of mercury). While the ventricle is resting (diastole) the pressure (diastolic pressure) is lower, e.g. 80 mmHg, i.e. B.P. = 120/80 mmHg (16/10·6 kPa).

Normal Blood Pressure. The average B.P. at the age of 20 years is 120/70 mmHg; by 45 years it is 130/85; by 60 years it is 150/90 and by 80 years it is 180/95 mmHg (24/12·6 kPa). The increase with age is due to loss of elasticity, causing increased rigidity, of the arterial walls.

Control of Blood Pressure (*Figs. 6.23* and *6.24*). Blood pressure depends on:
1 Cardiac output. This depends on the venous return and the strength of the myocardium and is the amount of blood ejected in one minute. The venous return depends on: (*a*) the position of the body—it is increased by lying down owing to the release of gravity; (*b*) muscular contractions in the limbs and abdominal wall, which squeeze veins and push blood towards the heart; (*c*) respiratory movements. Inspiration creates a relatively negative pressure ('vacuum') in the chest which assists blood flow upwards; also, the descent of the diaphragm increases the intra-abdominal pressure and forces blood towards the heart.
2 Blood volume. Blood volume is controlled by aldosterone, which causes

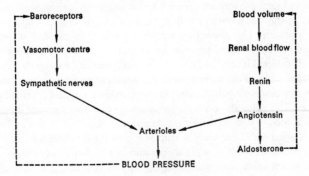

FIG. 6.23   Factors controlling the blood pressure

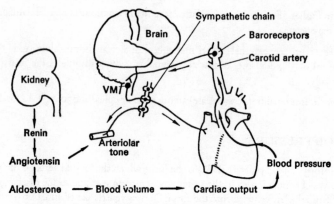

FIG. 6.24   Anatomical diagram of factors controlling the blood pressure

renal reabsorption of salt and water. If the blood pressure in the renal artery falls the kidney secretes renin. Renin is an enzyme which acts on serum angiotensinogen to produce angiotensin and this has two actions. One is to stimulate the adrenal cortex to produce aldosterone; the other is to cause vasoconstriction. Renin and aldosterone secretions are increased following, e.g. haemorrhage, burns, or dehydration due to vomiting and diarrhoea.

3 Peripheral resistance. This is the resistance of blood vessels to the blood flow and depends on the elasticity of the arterial walls and the diameter of the arterioles. The narrower the vessel the greater is the resistance to blood flow and hence the greater is the blood pressure.

In the normal person the blood pressure is largely controlled by changing the peripheral resistance by adjusting the diameter of the arterioles via the autonomic nervous system. The control centre is the vasomotor centre in the medulla oblongata which normally sends out a small continuous stream of impulses down the sympathetic nerves to the muscular layer of the arteries and arterioles to maintain a small degree of contraction in the vessels. This vasoconstriction (tone) can be increased to increase the blood pressure, or decreased to reduce the blood pressure. Changes in blood pressure are detected by baroreceptors (pressure-sensitive nerve endings) in the carotid artery and aortic arch and these send impulses to the vasomotor centre. This centre then accordingly adjusts the number of impulses it sends out, e.g. fall in blood pressure due to standing up from the sitting or lying position is detected immediately by the baroreceptors and reduces the number of stimuli these send to the vasomotor centre. This causes the vasomotor centre to send out more impulses, which cause vasoconstriction and return the blood pressure to normal. This reflex also occurs in haemorrhage and other forms of shock, and it is vasoconstriction which causes the pale and cold skin seen in shock. The vasomotor centre, besides receiving information from the baroreceptors, also receives other information on, for example, the presence of pain, hypoxia or excess of carbon dioxide, which affect vasomotor tone, e.g. sudden pain or fear elevate the blood pressure.

In emergencies sympathetic stimulation releases noradrenaline from the adrenal medulla and this is another cause of vasoconstriction.

Measuring the Blood Pressure. This may be done by palpation, auscultation or may be done electronically. In the auscultatory method the sphygmomanometer (sphygmo = pulse, mano = 'pressure', meter = measure) is placed level with the heart and the cuff is wrapped around the upper arm, neither loosely nor tightly, and inflated until the artery is occluded and no sound heard with a stethoscope over the brachial artery in front of the elbow. The pressure is slowly lowered, and at the point at which the systolic pressure in the artery just exceeds the cuff pressure a spurt of blood passes through with each heartbeat and is heard. As the cuff pressure is lowered further the sounds become louder, then dull and muffled, and finally disappear. The diastolic pressure is that at which the sound becomes muffled. A false high reading will be obtained if the patient is not relaxed, if the cuff is small, or the arm is fat. An electronic sphygmomanometer is used with an inflatable cuff but the pressure levels are gauged electronically.

Hypertension (High Blood Pressure)

A rough guide to a normal systolic blood pressure in mmHg is 100 plus age. Hypertension may be present if the pressure is 120 (or more) plus age or the diastolic pressure above 105. In pregnancy a level of 140/90 mmHg (18·7/11·9 kPa) or more suggests the possibility of complications, e.g. pre-eclampsia.

Causes

A   Essential (Idiopathic); the cause is unknown but there is an hereditary predisposition to increased vasoconstriction and a tendency to emotional tension. It is not due to an excess of renin.

B   Secondary:

1   Renal disease: polycystic kidneys, renal artery stenosis, diabetic nephropathy, chronic nephritis. These cause renal ischaemia which releases renin from the kidney, causing hypertension.

2   Coarctation of the aorta (stenosis of the arch of the aorta, *Fig. 6.25*).

3   Endocrine: Cushing's syndrome (adrenal cortical tumour or hyperplasia), primary aldosteronism (Conn's syndrome), phaeochromocytoma (tumour of the adrenal medulla).

4   Eclampsia (toxaemia of pregnancy).

5   Drugs: monoamine oxidase inhibitors, which are used in depression, e.g. iproniazid, if taken with amphetamines, ephedrine or foods containing amines (cheese, Bovril, Marmite). Amines, which increase the blood pressure, are normally destroyed by monoamine oxidase. If monoamine oxidase is inhibited the amines are not destroyed and they therefore elevate the blood pressure.

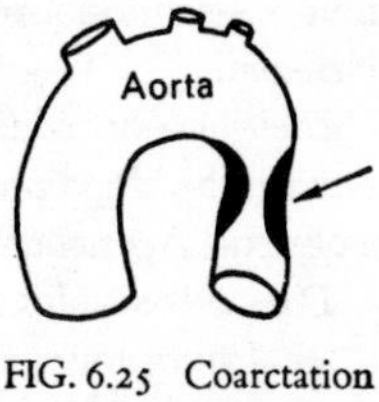

FIG. 6.25 Coarctation of the aorta

Note: Although the systolic pressure rises after meals and in pain and thyrotoxicosis, this is not considered to be hypertension.

Types:

1   *Benign:* does not cause renal failure.

2   *Malignant:* there is retinopathy and renal failure and the *diastolic* pressure is over 140 mmHg (18·7 kPa). The B.P. is often 250/150 mmHg (33·3/20 kPa) and the patient is likely to die within three years.

Either the benign or malignant type is due to any of the above causes.

Clinically: mild or moderate benign hypertension may be symptomless and the patient lives to old age—unless he is told that he has a high blood pressure, then he worries about it and develops headaches, fatigue and poor memory. In severe hypertension the symptoms are those of complications.

Complications:
  1   Left ventricular failure: breathlessness, at first on exertion, later at rest. Paroxysmal nocturnal dyspnoea (attacks of breathlessness at night).
  2   Cerebral haemorrhage.
  3   Hypertensive encephalopathy. This is acute focal cerebral oedema and ischaemia due to high blood pressure and causes confusion, transient paralysis and paraesthesiae, fits and unconsciousness, but without permanent disability.
  4   Renal damage is absent or mild (albuminuria) in benign hypertension but uraemia due to renal failure occurs in malignant hypertension.
  5   Ischaemic heart disease ('coronary thrombosis').

Investigations to Determine the Cause: Renal function tests, urine for albumin, casts (nephritis), pus and organisms (pyelonephritis), specific gravity (low in chronic renal failure). Intravenous pyelogram if a renal cause is likely. Chest X-ray, E.C.G.

Observations: symptoms, weight, blood pressure, pulse, urine.

Treatment: adequate rest and sleep. Learn the art of relaxation. Moderate exercise (walking, golfing) but avoid sudden stress. Anxious boredom and situations involving emotional upset should be avoided. The occupation may need to be changed.

Diet: weight reduction, if obese, reduces the strain on the heart. A low-salt diet reduces the blood pressure but is not practical and it is easier for the patient to take a diuretic. Aperient for constipation, to avoid straining.

Drugs: Tranquilliser, such as phenobarbitone 30–60 mg t.d.s.

Antihypertensives are used if symptoms and signs are present. The aim is to reduce the standing blood pressure to 160/100 mmHg (21·2/13·3 kPa) and so avoid complications.
  1   Ganglion-blocking drugs block both sympathetic and parasympathetic ganglia. Parasympathetic block is not required and causes *side-effects* such as blurred vision due to paralysis of accommodation, dry mouth, and constipation, thus ganglion-blocking drugs are used only if sympathetic blockers fail and in malignant hypertension, since they are powerful. **Mecamylamine** 2·5 mg t.d.s. increasing by 2·5 mg daily to 15 mg t.d.s.

Hexamethonium is given in hypertensive encephalopathy or pulmonary oedema. *Dose:* 5–500 mg i.m. or 2–50 mg i.v.

2 Sympathetic blocking drugs block the peripheral sympathetic nerves. **Guanethidine** (Ismelin): begin with 10 mg daily, increasing by 10 mg every five days to the desired blood pressure, e.g. 30–100 mg daily. *Side-effects:* postural hypotension, nasal congestion, muscular weakness, diarrhoea, tolerance. **Debrisoquine** (Declinax) is similar. **Bethanidine** (Esbatal) 5 mg b.d., increasing to 5 mg per dose daily up to e.g. 250 mg daily. **Methyldopa** (Aldomet) 250 mg eight-hourly increasing by 250 mg every two days, up to 2–4 g daily. *Side-effects:* dry mouth, malaise, postural hypotension, tolerance. **Clonidine** (Catapres) 100 μg t.d.s., increasing by 50 μg every two days to the desired blood pressure. *Side-effects:* constipation, dry mouth. **Propranolol** (Inderal) 5 mg q.i.d., increased every two weeks up to 20–1000 mg daily. *Side effects:* cardiac failure, asthma.

3 **Vasodilators:** diazoxide, guancycline, minoxidil, hydrallazine, or prazosin.

Diuretic may be used alone in mild hypertension or given with another antihypertensive drug. Bendrofluazide 5 mg t.d.s. or hydrochlorothiazide 50 mg t.d.s., with potassium chloride 500 mg t.d.s.

The Cause is treated, e.g. surgery for certain renal diseases and coarctation of the aorta. *Associated conditions* are treated, e.g. angina pectoris with glyceryl trinitrate (trinitrin) 500 mg dissolved slowly in the mouth.

Shock and Acute Circulatory Failure

Shock is general depression of bodily functions due to a deficient blood flow to the tissues caused by a fall in cardiac output and a low blood pressure (acute circulatory failure).

Types and Cause of Shock

1 **Primary (Neurogenic).** Pain or emotion may cause a vasovagal reflex. This is a reflex stimulation of the vagus nerve which slows the heart rate, reducing cardiac output. There is also capillary dilatation in the gastro–intestinal (splanchnic) vessels, thus blood collects (pools) here and less is available in the systemic circulation, thus causing a fall in blood pressure. The patient faints due to a reduced blood supply to the brain. Recovery occurs within minutes on lying down.

2 **Secondary**

(a) Acute cardiac failure, i.e. a weak pump, as in myocarditis, myocardial infarction, arrhythmia, pericardial effusion (causing cardiac tamponade, i.e. a fall in cardiac output due to failure of filling of the heart with blood owing to compression of the heart by fluid in the pericardium).

(b) Pulmonary embolism, obstructing the circulation in the pulmonary artery.

(c) Hypovolaemic ('surgical', 'established') shock. Due to a low blood volume from haemorrhage, loss of plasma (exudation) in burns, peritonitis, pancreatitis, and anaphylactic reaction, and from loss of water and electrolytes (dehydration) in vomiting, diarrhoea, Addison's disease, heatstroke, and renal tubular disease.

(d) Bacteraemic shock. Certain bacteria, e.g. *E. coli* and *Proteus*, during septicaemia, release endotoxin which causes a fall in blood pressure.

Physiology: fall in blood pressure stimulates the baroreceptors in the carotid artery and aortic arch, which cause the vasomotor centres in the medulla to send impulses directly along sympathetic nerves; these in turn cause vasoconstriction in the skin and splanchnic area and cardiac acceleration, to compensate for the fall in blood pressure. Stimulation of the sympathetic nerves to the adrenal medulla releases catecholamines (adrenaline and noradrenaline) which also cause skin and splanchnic vasoconstriction and tachycardia. Deficiency of the circulation leads to ischaemia and hypoxia of the tissues, and metabolites accumulate in them. Some of these metabolites are acids, such as lactic acid, which normally are oxidised to carbon dioxide and water. Their accumulation causes acidosis (metabolic acidosis).

Clinically: the skin is pale, cold (vasoconstriction) and clammy. There is fall in blood pressure which causes giddiness, apathy, nausea, muscle weakness and oliguria. The pulse is rapid and of poor volume (thready) and respiration is shallow. The eyebrows are furrowed with anxiety, the pupils dilated (adrenaline) but react to light, and consciousness may be lost due to the reduced blood supply to the brain.

Complications: shock may become irreversible (decompensated) if vasoconstriction is inadequate to compensate for the degree of shock. Irreversible shock is usually due to metabolic acidosis. Acidosis causes vasodilatation; the blood pressure rapidly falls and the pulse rate rises still further.

Observation: the degree of shock—facial appearance, colour and temperature of the skin, state of venous filling as seen in the jugular and other superficial veins (it is reduced in shock), blood pressure and pulse rate, volume and rhythm, recorded every 15–60 minutes. The volume of the urinary output, hourly.

Prevention: removal of the cause—arrest of haemorrhage with pressure bandage or suture, immobilisation of fractures, relief of pain (e.g. morphine for burns), reassurance. Pre-operative measures: treat dehydration with oral or intravenous fluids or rectal drip, and maintain fluid balance (chart). Avoid purgation, which causes dehydration. Plasma or blood transfusion if needed.

Treatment: removal of the cause. Reassurance. Position: horizontal on the side, with the foot of the bed raised to aid the venous return to the heart by gravity. The head is low by 10° and not more than 20° (which would cause the internal organs to press on the diaphragm and impede respiration).

Warmth: blankets are used but external heating (such as hot water bottles) is avoided since only moderate heat may cause burns and gangrene because vaso-constricted skin, unlike normal skin, cannot carry heat away in its poor circulation. In addition, external heat causes dilatation of the blood vessels in the skin; this is undesirable since it lowers the blood pressure still further, thus worsening the shock.

Oxygen for cyanosis, clear airway if in coma, artificial respiration for severe respiratory depression.

Sedation: morphine 15–20 mg i.v. or i.m. (absorption is delayed if given s.c.), methadone (Physeptone) 10 mg s.c., barbiturate, or paraldehyde 10 ml i.m. (rarely used). Restoration of blood volume—isotonic ('normal') saline for dehydration, plasma for burns, blood transfusion for haemorrhage. Plasma expanders such as dextran (Macrodex) in an emergency. Overtransfusion may cause cardiac failure and pulmonary oedema. The *minimum* basic fluid requirement is 2 litres daily (= the losses in urine, faeces, perspiration and respiration) plus the amount lost (e.g. by vomiting, diarrhoea, and aspirations from the stomach). The average is 3 litres daily and comprises 600 ml isotonic saline plus 2400 ml 5% glucose. Fluid balance records are essential.

Note: Noradrenaline, a vasoconstrictor, is dangerous and is no longer used. Hydrocortisone 100 mg i.v. is sometimes given in severe shock.

Haemorrhage

Haemorrhage may occur from arteries, veins or capillaries.

Arterial. Pulsatile, spurting, bright red, and largely issues from the end of the vessel nearest the heart.

Venous. Flows, dull red, and both ends bleed but the one away from the heart bleeds most.

Capillary. Oozes, bright red.

Types:
1 Primary: occurs at the moment of wounding.
2 Reactionary: occurs after 12–24 hours and is due to recovery causing rise in blood pressure as it returns to normal and dislodges clots or slips a ligature.
3 Secondary: occurs at 7–10 days and is due to infection.

Causes:
1 Injury.
2 Inflammation, e.g. pulmonary tuberculosis causing haemoptysis.
3 Neoplasms, e.g. a tumour of the bladder causing haematuria.
4 Degenerative, as in ruptured aortic aneurysm.
5 Blood diseases such as hypoprothrombinaemia (deficiency of vitamin K caused by obstructive jaundice or interference by drugs such as Dindevan), haemophilia, thrombocytopenia (low blood platelet count).

Effects depend upon:
1 The site of the haemorrhage: (*a*) external; (*b*) internal (fluid and iron is still available for reabsorption).
2 The volume of blood lost. It is possible to lose one litre of blood without shock if other factors are satisfactory.
3 The speed of loss. A more rapid haemorrhage causes more severe symptoms.
4 The previous haemoglobin. The effect of haemorrhage is more marked in anaemia.
5 The degree of hydration. If there is dehydration there is less tissue fluid available to make up the blood volume and restore blood pressure.

6   Circulatory responses maintaining an adequate blood flow to vital organs.
7   The general condition of the patient.

Clinically:

Local Signs: external haemorrhage is visible from the respiratory tract (haemo-ptysis), gastro-intestinal tract (haematemesis and melaena—melaena stools may take 24 hours to be passed), uterus (menorrhagia), urinary tract (haematuria), and the nose (epistaxis). Internal haemorrhage may be due to cerebral haemorrhage, a ruptured spleen, haemarthrosis (haemorrhage into a joint).

General Signs: shock occurs if more than one litre of blood is lost and causes a pale, cold, clammy skin, tachycardia, fall in blood pressure, restlessness, muscular weakness, oliguria, thirst, and giddiness, and there may be loss of consciousness.

Treatment: as for shock. Loss of up to one litre of blood does not normally require i.v. therapy. Loss of over two litres requires blood transfusion. Loss of one to two litres may need transfusion, depending on blood pressure, haemoglobin and pulse rate, and whether bleeding is likely to continue or not. Apply pressure to the bleeding spot, raise the affected part, and lower the head unless the head is bleeding.

MAJOR SYMPTOMS AND SIGNS IN HEART DISEASE

Dyspnoea ('hard breath') is shortness of breath—on exertion in mild disease, at rest in severe disease. It is due to pulmonary congestion or pleural effusion.

Orthopnoea (upright breath) is dyspnoea on lying flat, relieved by sitting up. It is due to severe pulmonary congestion or pulmonary oedema.

Cyanosis is a dark blue discolouration of the skin of the cheeks, ears and lips, due to the presence of an increased amount (at least 5 g/dl) of Hb (haemoglobin) which is not carrying oxygen (the normal Hb is 14·8 g/dl = 100%), therefore cyanosis cannot occur if the Hb level is below 5 g/dl (= about 30%).

Palpitations are an awareness of the heartbeat and may occur in normal subjects and in heart disease.

Tachycardia and other changes in the pulse have already been discussed.

Pain. Cardiac pain is a retrosternal tightness, and may radiate into the arms, neck, jaw and epigastrium.

Oedema (swelling) is due to fluid in the tissues due to several causes (*see* Chapter 3), including congestion of the veins due to cardiac failure. It appears first in the dependent parts due to the effect of gravity.

Cerebral Symptoms are due to cerebral hypoxia (low oxygen) and include loss of memory, restlessness, confusion and delirium.

INVESTIGATIONS IN HEART DISEASE

1   Pulse and apex rate and rhythm, sleeping and waking.
2   Temperature.
3   Blood pressure. Sitting (and standing if on hypotensive drugs).
4   Auscultation with a stethoscope.
5   Phonocardiography records heart sounds and murmurs.
6   Electrocardiography (E.C.G.) records the electrical activity of the heart.
7   Radiography shows the shape and size of the heart.
8   Angiography is the injection of radio-opaque material which outlines the cardiac chambers and blood vessels. Coronary angiography outlines the coronary arteries.
9   Cardiac catheterisation. A flexible catheter is introduced into a vein in the arm and pushed upwards until it enters the superior vena cava and then the right atrium, the right ventricle, and the pulmonary artery. Pressures are measured and blood is taken at various points.
10 Blood enzymes. Serum transaminase, lactic dehydrogenase and creatine kinase (see under 'myocardial infarction').
11 Blood count to detect anaemia and leucocytosis.
12 Blood cholesterol and other fats are often increased in ischaemic heart disease, especially if it is due to diabetes mellitus or hypothyroidism.
13 Blood Wassermann, Kahn or Meinicke to detect syphilis as a cause of aortic aneurysm or aortic incompetence.

DRUGS USED IN HEART DISEASE

Digitalis

Actions:
1   Direct stimulation of heart muscle, increasing its efficiency.
2   Depression of the conducting tissue of the bundle of His, slowing the ventricular rate.
3   Increased activity of the vagal nerve, which slows the heart rate (bradycardia).

Use: cardiac failure, atrial fibrillation, paroxysmal tachycardia, atrial flutter. *Side-effects:* nausea, vomiting, bradycardia. Higher doses increase myocardial excitability, which leads to arrhythmias such as ventricular ectopic beats, ventricular fibrillation, and atrial tachycardia. Alternation of ventricular ectopic beats with normal beats is called pulsus bigeminus (coupled beats).

Preparations:
1   Digoxin 1–1·5 mg stat. (if digitalis drugs have not been taken for two weeks) then 0·5 mg six-hourly for two doses then 0·25 mg one to four times daily according to the apex rate.

2 Digitoxin is cumulative, i.e. collects in the body; toxic effects are therefore not easily reversed.

3 Lanatoside C (Cedilanid) is similar to digoxin but not as powerful. It is used if digoxin causes vomiting. *Dose:* 3 mg stat. (if digitalis has not been taken for two weeks) then 0·5 mg one to four times daily according to the apex rate.

4 Oubain (strophanthin-G) is more rapidly acting and is used in an emergency. *Dose:* 0·25–1 mg i.v. It is not used orally owing to erratic absorption.

5 Digitalis folia is obsolete. It is a crude preparation and is cumulative.

6 Medigoxin (Lanitop) 0·2 mg t.d.s. for 2–4 days for rapid digitalisation, then 0·1 mg b.d. or t.d.s., according to the apex rate.

Aminophylline

Action: relieves paroxysmal dyspnoea due to left ventricular failure. It acts by relaxing the smooth muscle of the veins so that blood collects in the veins and relieves pulmonary congestion. *Dose:* 10 ml containing 250 mg i.v. slowly.

Diuretics

Action: they prevent the tubular reabsorption of salt and water which are therefore excreted by the kidneys.

Use: (1) To remove excessive fluid from the body in, e.g., cardiac failure, hepatic cirrhosis, nephrosis. (2) To reduce the blood pressure in hypertension. Oral diuretics are given in the morning since their action lasts for six to twelve hours. *Side-effects:* all cause the loss of potassium in the urine, and hypokalaemia (low blood potassium) increases the toxicity of digitalis, therefore potassium chloride 0·5 g orally t.d.s. is also given. They may cause nausea, rash, hyperglycaemia (reversible diabetes mellitus), hyperuricaemia (high blood uric acid), agranulocytosis and thrombocytopenia.

Thiazides. Bendrofluazide (Neo-naclex) 10 mg daily, chlorothiazide (Saluric) 1 g daily, hydrochlorothiazide (Hydrosaluric) 25–100 mg daily, hydroflumethiazide (Naclex) 100 mg daily.

Similar to thiazides are: frusemide (Lasix) 40–80 mg daily, which is powerful and rapidly acting but expensive, and is used if other diuretics fail or in an emergency (i.e. for acute pulmonary oedema). Ethacrynic acid (Edecrin) 50–200 mg daily is also powerful and rapidly acting. *Side-effects:* anorexia, nausea, vomiting, diarrhoea and rash. Chlorthalidone (Hygroton) 100–200 mg daily.

Spironolactone (Aldactone-A) 25–50 mg q.i.d. antagonises aldosterone (aldosterone is secreted by the adrenals and causes retention of sodium and water and loss of potassium), but has to be given with a diuretic to be effective. It is used in cardiac failure, hepatic cirrhosis and the nephrotic syndrome in which there is an increased aldosterone activity. It reduces the potassium loss caused by diuretics.

Organic Mercurials, e.g. mersalyl, are toxic to the kidney and have to be injected and are no longer used.

Triamterene (Dytac) 50–200 mg daily is a weak diuretic but retains potassium and may be used with a thiazide to counter the potassium loss caused by the thiazide.

Amiloride (Midamor) 10 mg daily acts similarly to triamterene.

Metolazone (Zaroxolyn) is long-acting. It may be used in chronic renal failure since it is still active when there is a low glomerular filtration rate. *Dose:* 5–50 mg orally daily.

Bumetanide (Burinex) is rapidly acting. *Dose:* 1–4 mg orally daily.

Anti-arrhythmic Drugs

Lignocaine (Xylocaine) dampens myocardial excitability (the ability of the heart muscle to conduct an 'electrical' impulse). *Dose:* 100 mg i.v. followed, if necessary, by a slow infusion of 500 mg in 500 ml 5% dextrose. *Side-effects:* confusion, sweating, drowsiness, fits. Disopyramide acts similarly.

Procainamide (Pronestyl) depresses myocardial excitability and strength of contraction, and may cause hypotension. *Dose:* 0·5-1 g six-hourly orally, or 100 mg i.v. *Side-effects:* rash, pyrexia, hypotension, sudden death.

Quinidine acts similarly to procainamide. Arrhythmias are preferably corrected using D.C. shock, which is safer. *Dose:* 200 mg t.d.s. May begin with 200 mg two-hourly for five doses. *Side-effects:* nausea, vomiting, diarrhoea, headache, tinnitus, blurred vision, rash, hypotension, sudden death.

Phenytoin (Epanutin). *Dose:* 250 mg i.v. then 100–400 mg six-hourly orally. *Side-effects:* rash, bradycardia; hypotension with overdose.

β-Sympathetic Blockers are used to slow the tachycardia due to thyrotoxicosis, and to reduce the blood pressure in hypertension.

Propanolol (Inderal) 10–40 mg t.d.s. orally. *Side-effects:* cardiac failure, bronchial spasm. **Oxprenolol** (Traiscor) is similar. **Atenolol** (Tenormin) 100 mg daily orally.

Isoprenaline increases the ventricular rate in heart block. *Dose:* 2 mg in 500 ml isotonic saline or 5% dextrose, given at 20–40 drops a minute according to the response, or 30 mg six-hourly orally.

Vasoconstrictors

These are generally dangerous since they may cause gangrene or anuria and are now used only during anaesthesia.

Anticoagulants

These are discussed under 'phlebothrombosis'. Oral anticoagulants prevent the liver from making prothrombin from vitamin K; the blood prothrombin level falls and this reduces the ability of the blood to clot.

Analgesics

Morphine-like Drugs

1 Morphine 10–20 mg i.m. or i.v. (absorption from s.c. injection is slow in shock). It is given to relieve pain in myocardial infarction, and to relieve dyspnoea and anxiety in acute pulmonary oedema. *Side-effects:* Vomiting

(relieved by cyclizine 50 mg i.m.), respiratory depression which may be serious in patients with chronic lung disease, constipation, tolerance (an increasing dose is necessary to be effective), addiction.

2 Diamorphine (heroin) is similar to morphine but causes less nausea and vomiting.

3 Pethidine is similar to morphine but weaker. *Dose:* 100 mg i.m. or orally.

4 Methadone (Physeptone) 15–30 mg orally, 5–10 mg s.c. *Side-effects:* nausea, dry mouth, sweating, respiratory depression, dizziness.

Pentazocine (Fortral) does not allay anxiety, unlike morphine-like drugs. *Dose:* 50–100 mg four-hourly p.c.

Codeine, Aspirin and **Paracetamol** do not relieve anxiety, and morphine-like drugs are more powerful in relieving pain.

DISORDERS OF THE HEART

CARDIAC FAILURE

Cardiac failure is failure of the heart to supply an adequate output for the needs of the tissues. There may be failure of the left ventricle, the right ventricle, or both left and right ventricles. Congestive cardiac failure refers to general congestion of the tissues and is due to failure of the right ventricle. There may or may not be left ventricular failure also. *Pure* acute left ventricular failure, although it causes pulmonary congestion, does not cause general congestion of the body and it is not usually called congestive cardiac failure.

CONGESTIVE CARDIAC FAILURE (C.C.F.)

Is due to:

1 Left ventricular failure. Persistent pulmonary congestion increases the work of the right ventricle. If the right ventricle fails, congestion of the systemic venous system (C.C.F.) occurs.

2 Ischaemic heart disease.

3 Rheumatic heart disease, e.g. mitral stenosis.

4 Chronic lung disease, e.g. chronic bronchitis and emphysema, pneumo-coniosis. Cardiac failure due to lung disease is called **cor pulmonale**.

5 Severe anaemia.

6 Thyrotoxicosis.

7 Congenital heart disease, e.g. pulmonary stenosis, patent ductus arteriosus, atrial septal defect.

8 Infective endocarditis.

9 Myocarditis.

10 Beri Beri. The 'wet' type is due to thiamine (Vitamin B_1) deficiency.

11 Excessive administration of i.v. fluid.

Mechanism of Symptoms: failure of right ventricular output causes deficiency of blood going through the lungs to the systemic arteries, hence a reduced blood flow to the tissues, and an increased build-up of blood behind the right ventricle in the veins, causing venous congestion and an increased venous pressure throughout the body. This reduces the reabsorption of fluid into the blood capillaries from the tissues, causing oedema.

Clinically: there is dyspnoea, at first on exertion, later at rest. Cyanosis (blueness of the lips and the skin of the extremities) is due to hypoxia (low oxygen supply) and venous stagnation. The increased venous pressure causes distension of the jugular veins, an enlarged tender liver, anorexia, nausea, fatigue, epigastric discomfort, albuminuria, and oedema. Oedema is the collection of fluid in the tissues, which show 'pitting' if pressed with the fingers. Owing to gravity oedema collects at the lowest part of the body—in the legs on standing and over the sacrum and genitals on sitting. In chronic or severe failure fluid collects (an effusion) in the peritoneal, pleural and pericardial 'cavities', causing ascites, hydrothorax and pericardial effusions.

The diminished blood supply to the organs causes weakness, insomnia, loss of memory, mental confusion, and oliguria. Nocturia (increased urinary output at night) is due to the reabsorption of tissue oedema fluid at night aided by the complete rest provided by sleep.

Complications:
1 Deep venous thrombosis due to the sluggish circulation caused by C.C.F. and predisposed by rest in bed. It may cause pulmonary embolism.
2 Bronchopneumonia.

Observations: any change in symptoms and signs, especially oedema and cyanosis, and the appearance of new ones, should be reported. Apex and pulse rate, rhythm and volume. Temperature, respirations, blood pressure. Fluid balance chart. Urine for albumin. If the patient's state permits he is weighed each morning; changes represent fluid retention or loss.

Treatment: rest the body and the heart—in bed for three weeks or longer. Complete rest at first, sitting up with a back-rest and pillows. A cardiac bedframe is better for severe dyspnoea since it causes fluid to collect in the legs rather than in the lungs.

Rest the mind by reassurance, explanation, avoidance of excitement, sedation with diazepam (Valium) 2–10 mg t.d.s. and a hypnotic for adequate sleep, e.g. chloral 0·5–2 g o.n. (hypnotics cause confusion in the elderly). Well-ventilated but warm room, near the lavatory. Socks on cold feet, bed cradle to keep the weight of the bedclothes off the legs. Smoking should be avoided. Oxygen, via a ventimask or nasal spectacles, for cyanosis.

Diet: Three evenly balanced small meals daily, eaten slowly. Large meals should be avoided since they distend the stomach which then presses on the heart. Low energy diet (3·2–4 MJ, 800–1000 kcal. daily) if obese. Low in salt—no salt is added at the table or in the cooking. This reduces the intake to 3 g daily (from the normal 10 g daily). Avoid salty foods (e.g. ham), and medicines containing sodium (e.g. sodium bicarbonate), or causing the retention of sodium, such as biogastrone. A salt-free diet is impractical. If the patient is on a low-salt diet, fluid is not restricted except in severe oedema not responding to diuretics. Vitamins B and C.

Paracentesis (draining) of large effusions if they cause dyspnoea. Acupuncture (needle-pricking) may be used if oedema resists other treatment; the patient's legs hang down from one to three days to collect fluid and are then drained, using aseptic precautions, by inserting Southey's tubes into the skin or by applying Lassar's paste (to prevent maceration of the skin by fluid draining from punctures) followed by making multiple punctures in the skin. Afterwards the legs are elevated to allow the punctures to heal. Attention to pressure areas.

Avoid constipation, since it causes straining on defaecation, by using a mild aperient or suppository (Dulcolax). A bedside commode may be easier to use than a bedpan since it is difficult to balance on a bedpan on a soft mattress and to use a toilet roll simultaneously.

Drugs: Digoxin 1·5 mg orally (if none has been taken during the previous two weeks) then 0·5 mg six-hourly for 2 doses, then 0·25 mg b.d. or t.d.s. according to the apex rate which should be 70–80 a minute. *Side-effects:* anorexia, nausea, headache, bradycardia, 'extrasystoles', coupled beats, vomiting, diarrhoea.

Diuretic: Bendrofluazide 10 mg or chlorothiazide 0·5–2 g orally on alternate days. Frusemide (Lasix) 40–80 mg orally if the less powerful diuretics fail. Plus potassium chloride 0·5 g t.d.s. on the days the diuretic is not given. In resistant oedema spironolactone (Aldactone-A), which inhibits aldosterone, is given (25 mg q.i.d. orally) with a diuretic.

Linctus codeine 5 ml for cough. Vasodilators e.g. prazosin.

Treat the cause, for example surgery (valvotomy) for mitral stenosis.

Convalescence: The patient should sleep downstairs if dyspnoea is present on going upstairs. Adequate rest—a minimum of eight hours in bed. May need to rest for 30–60 minutes after meals or exercise.

Activity is gradually increased and some exercise is desirable, such as walking, but undue and sudden exertion should be avoided. A degree of exercise is allowed that does not cause symptoms.

The health visitor gives advice and assesses the need for a home help.

COR PULMONALE

This is congestive cardiac failure due to lung disease. In chronic lung disease there is destruction of lung tissue and the number of capillaries in the lung is reduced. This puts extra work on the right ventricle in its attempt to force blood through the smaller vascular bed and the ventricle may fail.

LEFT VENTRICULAR FAILURE

Is due to:
1 Hypertension.
2 Coronary arterial disease with or without myocardial infarction.
3 Aortic valvular disease (stenosis or regurgitation).

Mechanism of Symptoms: inadequate left ventricular pumping reduces the output of blood into the aorta and causes the collection of blood in the lungs (pulmonary congestion) since the right ventricle continues to pump blood normally. If the pulmonary congestion is severe the blood capillaries lining the alveoli (air-sacs) are so distended that plasma leaks out of them into the alveoli (pulmonary oedema), reducing the air space in the lungs, and this reduces oxygen uptake into the blood. Some of the distended blood capillaries may rupture, releasing red cells into the alveoli and staining the oedema fluid pink.

Clinically: pulmonary congestion causes:
1 Dyspnoea, with rapid shallow respiration, on exertion in mild failure, at rest in severe failure.
2 Orthopnoea—dyspnoea on lying down, relieved by sitting or standing.
3 Cyanosis (a blue colour).
4 Tightness in the chest, with palpitations.
5 The pulse is rapid (tachycardia) and thready.

In more severe failure there is pulmonary oedema which causes all these symptoms and also
6 Cough with frothy pink-stained sputum (haemoptysis).
7 Confusion due to cerebral hypoxia; agitation, anxiety.
8 Pale cold extremities (shock) due to the poor output of blood into the aorta.
9 Cheyne-Stokes respiration in severe cases, i.e. alternate phases of rapid deep respiration diminishing to shallow slow respirations, due to hypoxia of the respiratory centres.
10 Paroxysmal nocturnal dyspnoea ('cardiac asthma') is pulmonary oedema occurring when the patient is asleep. The patient awakes dyspnoeic and suffocating, sits up or rushes to the window for air, has tightness in the chest, cough and frothy sputum.

Treatment: rest in the sitting position, with a bed-table covered with a pillow to lean forward on to help breathing. Reassurance. Sedation with morphine 15–20 mg i.v. or i.m. to relieve agitation and overbreathing. Aminophylline 500 mg i.v. lowers the venous pressure and temporarily reduces the *right* ventricular output; this reduces pulmonary congestion.

Venesection—removal of one pint of blood, or pressure cuffs (tourniquets) around the thighs for 30-minute periods, also reduce the venous return to the heart by allowing blood to accumulate in the legs. These are used if drugs, especially diuretics, are not available.

Digoxin 1 mg i.v. or 1·5 mg orally (if digoxin has not been taken for 14 days previously).

Diuretic: frusemide (Lasix) 20 mg i.v. or 40–80 mg orally, then bendrofluazide 10 mg or chlorothiazide 1–2 g alternate days. Plus potassium chloride 0·5 g t.d.s. on the day the diuretic is not given.

Diet: low in calories if the patient is obese. Meals should be small without added salt. Fluid intake need not be reduced if a diuretic is being given. Sputum carton within easy reach.

Treat the cause, e.g. hypertension.
Observations and nursing care are as for congestive cardiac failure.

RHEUMATIC HEART DISEASE

This is due to recurrent rheumatic fever. The mitral and aortic valves are those most commonly affected and may be stenosed (constricted) or regurgitant.

Mitral Stenosis

This is the commonest valvular lesion. The mitral valve is narrowed by fibrosis. To force blood through the narrowed valve the left atrium has to pump harder. If it fails to pump out all the blood it receives from the lungs it dilates (stretches) and pressure builds up behind the atrium in the lung capillaries, so the lungs become congested, as in left ventricular failure (but the left *ventricle* is not failing in mitral stenosis).

Symptoms: at this stage symptoms are similar to left ventricular failure, with dyspnoea, cyanosis, orthopnoea, haemoptysis, tachycardia and a small pulse volume.

Complications:
1 Pulmonary congestion increases the pressure in the right ventricle which eventually fails, causing congestive cardiac failure.
2 The dilated atrium may fibrillate.
3 A fibrillating atrium does not contract as a unit, and clotting occurs in it (*Figs. 6.22* and *6.26*).
4 Pieces of clot may break off to form emboli which travel through the left ventricle into the aorta and any of its branches such as the carotid artery (causing hemiplegia), or femoral artery (causing gangrene of a leg).
5 Infective endocarditis (infection of the damaged valve.)

Treatment: reduction of exertion to tolerable levels in mild cases. *Surgery:* mitral valvotomy (division of the stenosed valve), or artificial valve insertion for severe cases.

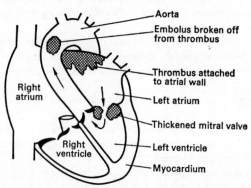

FIG. 6.26   Thrombus in fibrillating atrium in mitral stenosis

Anticoagulants then digoxin for rapid atrial fibrillation. Penicillin 'cover' for dental or surgical operations as there is a risk of infective endocarditis if organisms enter the blood during these procedures, e.g. organisms from a dental abscess.

Aortic Stenosis leads to weakness and fainting owing to the reduced cardiac output, and to angina due to poor coronary filling. It may require surgical division or artificial valve insertion.

Aortic Regurgitation. May need valve replacement with an artificial one.

ISCHAEMIC HEART DISEASE

This is cardiac damage due to an inadequate blood supply to the myocardium. It is usually due to narrowing of the coronary arteries by atheroma, but may be due to aortic valve disease, severe anaemia or syphilitic aortitis. It may cause:

1 Angina of effort.
2 Myocardial infarction.
3 Arrhythmias.
4 Cardiac failure.

Anatomy. The heart receives its blood supply from the right and left coronary arteries, which are the first branches of the aorta (*Fig. 6.27*).

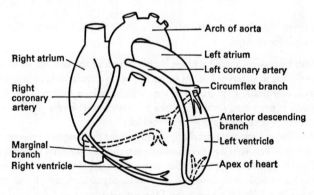

FIG. 6.27 The coronary arteries

Atheroma is the deposition of fat under the intima of an artery (*Fig. 6.28*). It does not occur in veins. It is caused by several factors:

1 Heredity.
2 Androgens; atheroma is commoner in males than in females.
3 Excessive intake of food.
4 Excessive intake of saturated (animal) fat—butter, lard, cheese, milk.
5 Diseases causing a high blood cholesterol—diabetes mellitus, hypothyroidism.
6 Hypertension.
7 Cigarette smoking.
8 Lack of regular physical exercise—sedentary occupation.

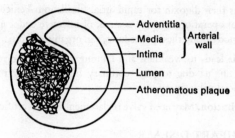

FIG. 6.28   Atheroma

Angina of Effort (Angina pectoris)

Angina of effort is due to ischaemic heart disease, usually coronary atheroma. The blood supply to the myocardium (heart muscle) is sufficient at rest but inadequate for exertion.

Clinically: pain is produced by physical effort, excitement, cold weather or a heavy meal, and is relieved by a few minutes rest. The pain lasts a few minutes and feels like a tightness in the chest, retrosternally, and may spread (radiate) to the arms, especially the left arm, and to the neck, jaw and epigastrium. The patient appears pale.

Investigations: E.C.G. before and after exercise. The E.C.G. taken after exercise shows ischaemic changes.

Treatment: the patient should arrange his life to reduce the number of attacks. He should have regular exercise but not enough to bring on an attack. During an attack he should remain still. Explanation of the cause, to relieve anxiety. Stop smoking, but alcohol is permitted since it is a general vasodilator. Reducing diet if obese, since extra weight increases the work of the heart.

Drugs: Glyceryl trinitrate (trinitrin) 0·5 mg under the tongue or chewed slowly so that it is absorbed from the buccal mucous membrane. The drug should always be carried by the patient so that it may be taken as necessary, for example immediately before he has to walk or do work which would bring on an attack. Up to 30 tablets may be taken in a day if necessary and the patient is reassured that they will not cause any harm or addiction, but he should be warned of tachycardia and flushing of the face, and of headaches which occur at first. Trinitrin acts by relaxing the smooth muscle of all blood vessels, dilating the arterioles and thus reducing the blood pressure; hence it reduces the work of the heart and therefore its need for oxygen.

Amyl nitrite 0·2 ml inhaled after crushing the glass capsule. Perhexiline (Pexid), nifedipine (Adalat), and long-acting nitrates, such as pentaerythritol tetranitrate, are usually ineffective but may be tried if angina is frequent.

Sedatives for anxiety, e.g. phenobarbitone 30 mg t.d.s. or diazepam 5 mg. t.d.s. β-adrenergic blocking drugs: these inhibit sympathetic activity which occurs with exercise or emotion. Propranolol (Inderal) 10–40 mg t.d.s. and oxprenolol (Trasicor) 20–120 mg t.d.s. are similar. *Side-effects:* cardiac failure should be watched for.

Treatmènt of any predisposing cause such as anaemia.

Surgical improvement of the blood supply to the myocardium, for example a graft by-passing the atheromatous segment of the coronary artery, is used if angina is incapacitating.

Prevention: diet low in animal (saturated) fat. Avoid excessive calorie intake. No smoking. Treatment of predisposing disease such as diabetes mellitus or myxoedema.

Clofibrate (Atromid-S) 500 mg t.d.s lowers the serum cholesterol and may prevent further atheroma, but a low-fat diet is preferable.

Myocardial Infarction ('Coronary Thrombosis')

Myocardial infarction is death of a portion of heart muscle due to loss of its blood supply by obstruction of a coronary artery, by atheroma alone or by thrombosis (blood clot) on an ulcerated patch of atheroma. The dead muscle heals by forming a fibrous scar (*Fig. 6.29*).

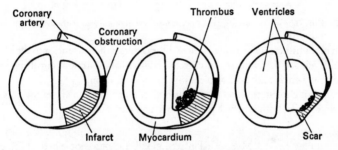

FIG. 6.29   The heart in myocardial infarction

Clinically: it usually affects males over 45 years of age and often occurs while the patient is at rest (unlike angina of effort) but may occur any time. The pain is severe and lasts for hours. It is a retrosternal 'crushing' or 'tight' sensation, and may radiate to the neck, jaw, arms and epigastrium. Pain may cause reflex nausea and vomiting.

The patient is anxious, restless and shocked. Shock and fall in blood pressure cause reflex vasoconstriction and the release of noradrenaline into the blood, which produce a pale, cold, sweating skin; and there is oliguria. The pulse is feeble and may be rapid because of shock, or slow or arrhythmic due to infarction of conducting tissues. There may be dyspnoea and cyanosis due to pulmonary congestion, and a pericardial friction rub due to the infarct. Dead cardiac muscle causes pyrexia, a raised erythrocyte sedimentation rate and a leucocytosis, and releases enzymes causing a rise in serum aspartate aminotransferase (glutamic oxaloacetic transaminase, S.G.O.T.), lactic dehydrogenase (L.D.H.), and creatine kinase (C.K.).

Investigations: electrocardiogram (E.C.G.), *Fig. 6.30.* The blood count shows a polymorph leucocytosis. The erythrocyte sedimentation rate is raised above 10 mm in one hour.

Serum enzymes: the serum levels of transaminase, lactic dehydrogenase and creatine kinase are raised. These enzymes are present not only in heart muscle but

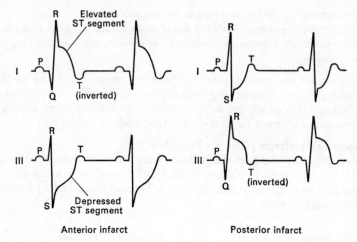

FIG. 6.30   The electrocardiogram in myocardial infarction. Q = Pathological q wave

also in other tissues, and damage to these tissues releases the enzymes into the blood. Raised levels are therefore not specific for myocardial infarction, but if the levels are normal there has not been a recent myocardial infarction.

The serum cholesterol level is often increased, especially in diabetes mellitus and hypothyroidism, both of which predispose to coronary atheroma.

Complications:

1   It may be fatal. Myocardial infarction kills 140,000 people in the U.K. each year.
2   Recurrence.
3   Congestive cardiac failure.
4   Arrhythmia.
5   Rupture of the dead area of heart muscle releases blood into the pericardium (haemopericardium).
6   Angina of effort.
7   Deep venous thrombosis due to poor circulation and rest in bed.
8   'Frozen shoulder'—pain and stiffness in the shoulder, which recovers completely.
9   Bronchopneumonia.
10   Embolism. Pulmonary embolism is due to deep venous thrombosis or to clot in the right side of the heart. Systemic embolism arises from a clot in the left side of the heart. This passes into the aorta and may lodge in a cerebral artery causing hemiplegia, or in a popliteal artery causing gangrene of a limb, or elsewhere.

Observations:

1   In order to detect arrhythmia the E.C.G. should be monitored, using an oscilloscope with a warning device, for the first 24 hours when arrhythmia is common.

2   If monitoring is not available the pulse should be recorded ½-hourly at first.

3   Sudden loss of consciousness and pallor (cardiac arrest) require immediate treatment.

4   Blood pressure is recorded hourly at first.

5   The onset of oedema and dyspnoea is watched for in order to detect cardiac failure.

Treatment: at first the patient is treated in a unit where cardiac rhythm can be monitored, since arrhythmia (*Figs. 6.11–6.20*), particularly ventricular fibrillation, is a common cause of death in the first 24 hours. In severe infarction with marked shock the patient should be recumbent at absolute rest in bed for the first few days, then gradually increase activity and may be allowed up after two to six weeks. Rest is required in order to allow a firm scar to form in the damaged area of heart muscle. The amount of rest required depends on the severity of the infarct. In a mild attack with only a small infarction the patient may rest in an armchair.

Smoking should be stopped.

Diet: light, 1000 kcal. (4·2 MJ) a day, low in animal fat. Reduce weight if obese. Constipation is avoided by giving an aperient if necessary. A bedside commode is preferable to a bedpan since it requires less effort to sit on.

Physiotherapy: Passive exercises to prevent stiff joints.

Drugs: Morphine 15–20 mg i.m. to relieve pain and anxiety, repeated if necessary, or pentazocine (Fortral) 30–60 mg i.m. relieves pain but not anxiety. Oxygen for cyanosis or dyspnoea.

Anticoagulants do not affect the coronary atheroma, but may be given to prevent deep venous thrombosis and pulmonary embolism. They are not necessary in mild attacks if the patient is being mobilised early. They are not given to patients liable to bleeding, such as patients with peptic ulcer, or to the elderly. Heparin 150 mg i.v. then 100 mg i.v. six-hourly for four doses (it may be given i.m. but may cause a painful haematoma). This covers the first 24 hours. Since oral anticoagulants take 24–36 hours before they are effective they are begun at the same time as the first dose of heparin. Phenindione (Dindevan) 150–300 mg stat. then 25–50 mg. b.d., or warfarin (Marevan) 30–60 mg stat. then 3–15 mg daily, according to the blood prothrombin time. *Side-effects:* haemorrhage from, e.g. kidney, stomach, or nose. Anti-arrhythmic drug e.g. disopyramide or lidocaine.

Convalescence: Gradual increase in activity and return to work in three months. Diet low in animal fat. No smoking. Reducing diet if obese. Advice to patient and relatives as to how much the patient may do. If symptoms develop on increasing his activity, activity should be reduced by one stage for a while, e.g. 2 weeks.

CARDIAC ARREST AND RESUSCITATION

Cardiac arrest is the cessation of an effective heartbeat, and may be due to ventricular asystole or ventricular fibrillation. Irreversible brain damage occurs after three to four minutes, and may occur before this.

Causes:

1 Anoxia, e.g. respiratory obstruction, drowning.
2 Ischaemia due to sudden fall in blood pressure (haemorrhage), coronary air embolism (intravenous drip run out), or pulmonary embolism.
3 Myocardial damage, for example infarction.
4 Toxins and drugs—poisons, cyclopropane, chloroform, adrenaline, excessive potassium given i.v.
5 Electrocution.

Clinically: there is sudden loss of consciousness, absent carotid pulse, the pupils dilate, respirations are gasping then cease, and the patient appears to be dead.

Treatment is by urgent cardiopulmonary resuscitation. The aim is to provide the brain with oxygenated blood immediately. Cardiac massage and mouth-to-mouth respiration are given (mouth-to-mouth breathing is not new since it was used by Elisha in 800 B.C.).

The patient is placed on his back on a hard surface, or a board is placed behind his chest. Cardiac massage is given by placing one hand on top of the other over the lower one-third of the sternum (*Fig. 6.31*) and compressing the heart between

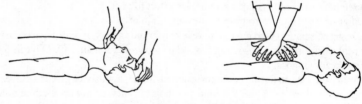

FIG. 6.31   External cardiac massage

the sternum and spinal column, then quickly releasing, 60 times a minute. The sternum should move about 4 cm. This empties blood from the ventricles and provides a circulation. The force must be sufficient to produce a carotid or femoral pulse, but not so much as to break ribs. The legs should be elevated to aid venous return. The patient's head is fully extended and the nostrils closed with the fingers; one respiration is given to every five chest compressions (= 12 a minute) and the chest should be seen to expand (if not, there is airway obstruction or faulty technique). When help arrives the airway is aspirated, a cuffed endotracheal tube is passed and mechanical ventilation is applied using oxygen and an air-bag.

If ventricular fibrillation is present (E.C.G.) electrical defibrillation is tried after applying electrode jelly (to prevent burning the skin). If this fails 5 ml 10% calcium chloride is given into the heart or i.v. then 100 mg lignocaine intracardiac (or i.v.) or procainamide 25 mg, and defibrillation repeated after three minutes.

If asystole is present and does not respond to intracardiac calcium chloride it is converted to fibrillation with 5–10 ml of 1:10,000 adrenaline into the heart, then defibrillated. Cardiac arrest is followed by acidosis which requires treatment with 150 ml 8·4% sodium bicarbonate (= 150 mmol, 150 mEq) i.v. followed by 70 ml every 10 minutes if required. Oxygen is given for at least 24 hours after recovery.

Complications: circulatory arrest causes: (1) cerebral damage; (2) renal damage, therefore urinary output should be recorded.

Cerebral oedema may be reduced with 180 ml 60% magnesium sulphate by slow rectal infusion b.d., or a diuretic.

CONGENITAL HEART DISEASE

Congenital heart disease is heart disease present at birth and is due to failure of the normal development of the heart and major blood vessels. Development takes place during the first eight weeks of fetal life, except for closure of the foramen ovale (oval hole) between the right and left atria, and closure of the ductus arteriosus (a channel between the aorta and pulmonary artery), which close at birth.

Congenital heart disease is due to:

1 Virus infection, e.g. German measles or influenza in the mother in the first eight weeks of pregnancy.
2 Genetic abnormality, e.g. Down's syndrome.
3 Drugs—thalidomide, aminopterin.

Diagnosis: (1) cardiac catheterisation; (2) radiography.

Persistent (Patent) Ductus Arteriosus (*Fig. 6.32*). The channel between the aorta and pulmonary artery allows blood to pass directly from the pulmonary artery to the aorta in the fetus and thus by-pass the functionless fetal lungs. If the

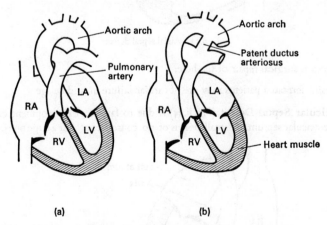

FIG. 6.32   (*a*) Normal heart and vessels; (*b*) patent ductus arteriosus

ductus fails to close at birth there is a 'shunt' of blood from the aorta into the pulmonary artery (the reverse to that in the fetus) thus oxygenated blood re-enters the pulmonary circulation and increases the work of the left ventricle.

Treatment: the ductus should be tied and divided in childhood.

Prognosis: untreated patients die before the age of 40 years. Following treatment the life expectation is normal.

Coarctation of Aorta (*Fig. 6.25*). This is a congenital narrowing of the aorta at the junction of the arch with the descending aorta. It causes hypotension in the arteries below it and hypertension in the carotid and subclavian arteries which are above it.

Treatment is surgical at the age of seven to 15 years.

Prognosis: untreated patients die of cerebral haemorrhage, left ventricular failure or bacterial endocarditis. Surgical treatment is curative.

Atrial Septal Defect (Patent foramen ovale) (*Fig. 6.33*). Some blood is pumped from the left atrium (where the pressure is higher) into the right atrium and goes through the lungs for a second time.

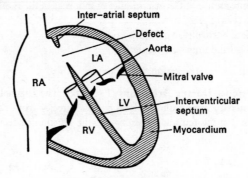

FIG. 6.33   Atrial septal defect

Treatment is surgical repair of the hole.

Prognosis: untreated patients may die of cardiac failure in middle age.

Ventricular Septal Defect (*Fig. 6.34*) is due to failure of development of the interventricular septum. A small hole is of no consequence, but a large one causes

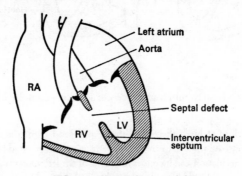

FIG. 6.34   Ventricular septal defect

congestive cardiac failure and is liable to bacterial endocarditis; surgical repair is required.

Fallot's Tetralogy (*Fig. 6.35*) is pulmonary stenosis, ventricular septal defect, enlarged right ventricle, and the aorta over-rides both ventricles. Blood by-passes

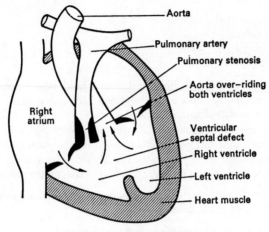

FIG. 6.35   Fallot's tetralogy

the lungs into the aorta so that there is cyanosis (blue baby), clubbing of the fingers and toes, and failure to thrive. Surgical operation is necessary. Untreated patients die in childhood.

INFECTIVE ENDOCARDITIS

Infective endocarditis is infection of the endocardium, the inner lining of the heart.

Causes:

1 Subacute bacterial endocarditis is due to bacteria growing on valves previously damaged, for example by rheumatic fever, or on congenital abnormalities such as patent ductus arteriosus. The commonest organism is *Streptococcus viridans* which is normally harmlessly present in the mouth but may enter the circulation, e.g. after tooth extraction.

2 Acute bacterial endocarditis is due to staphylococci and other organisms which attack normal valves, and occurs in drug addicts.

3 Endocarditis may also be due to fungi.

Note: Fibrin is deposited on infected valves and forms vegetations ('warty' outgrowths). A portion of vegetation may break off into the circulation as a small septic embolus.

Clinically: there is malaise, fatigue, anorexia, pyrexia, finger clubbing, splenomegaly, brownish ('café-au-lait') pigmentation of the skin, anaemia, leucocytosis and a raised erythrocyte sedimentation rate. Petechial haemorrhages into the skin, conjunctiva and retina, and haematuria, are due to small emboli.

Diagnosis: blood culture is taken BEFORE any antibiotic is given, since a single dose of antibiotic may prevent the growth of bacteria in culture.

Complications:
1 Congestive cardiac failure.
2 Renal failure.
3 Hemiplegia.
The last two are due to emboli.

Treatment: complete rest in bed. Frequent changes of bedclothing if sweating.
Diet: High protein, high calorie, vitamins B and C. Abundant fluids.
Urine testing daily for albumin and blood.
Antibiotic is given, for a minimum of six weeks, according to the sensitivity of the organism. Usually benzylpenicillin 600 mg (1 Mu) is given six-hourly until apyrexial then phenoxymethylpenicillin 500 mg four-hourly orally with probenecid. Streptomycin 0·5 g i.m., b.d. may also be given for the first two weeks.

Treatment of complications, e.g. digoxin and diuretic for heart failure. Follow-up for several months afterwards to detect any relapse.

Prevention: patients with rheumatic or congenital heart disease should be given antibiotic such as procaine penicillin 600 mg b.d. on the day of any dental or surgical operation and on the following three days.

PERICARDITIS

Inflammation of the pericardium may be:
1 Acute (*a*) dry (fibrinous); (*b*) with effusion (fluid in the pericardial sac).
2 Chronic (constrictive), i.e. with fibrosis and maybe calcification.

Causes:
1 Sterile—rheumatic fever, myocardial infarction, malignant invasion (e.g. from carcinoma of bronchus), uraemia, collagenosis.
2 Infected: (*a*) benign pericarditis, due to virus infections; (*b*) pyogenic from septicaemia or pneumonia; (*c*) tuberculous.

Clinically: the inflamed pericardial surfaces are rough because of fibrin deposition and rub together with each heart–beat, causing retrosternal pain. A friction rub may be heard through a stethoscope or felt by palpation, and there is pyrexia and dry cough.

An effusion (*Fig. 6.36*) separates the layers of the pericardium and takes up space in the pericardial sac, reducing the venous inflow into the heart.

In constrictive pericarditis the two surfaces adhere and do not glide over one another; this limits cardiac expansion during diastole and reduces the venous inflow of blood into the heart. Thus in severe effusion and in constrictive peri-

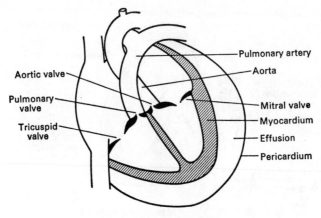

Aortic valve

Pulmonary valve

Tricuspid valve

Pulmonary artery

Aorta

Mitral valve

Myocardium

Effusion

Pericardium

FIG. 6.36   Pericardial effusion

carditis there is increased venous pressure causing signs similar to congestive cardiac failure; i.e. dyspnoea, distended jugular veins, hepatic congestion, ascites and oedema.

Investigations:
1. Chest X-ray.
2. Ultrasonic detection of effusion.
3. Diagnostic tapping of the effusion to confirm its presence and for bacteriology. Only a small amount need be taken for diagnostic purposes.

Treatment: rest in bed. Treatment of the cause, for example an antibiotic for infection, sedation for restlessness, analgesic for pain—morphine if necessary.
    Paracentesis (tapping) of large effusions if interfering with cardiac function.
    Surgical: pericardectomy in constrictive pericarditis.

ACUTE PULMONARY EMBOLISM

Acute pulmonary embolism is obstruction of the pulmonary artery by blood clot which has detached from the right side of the heart or from a large vein in the leg or abdomen. From the vein the clot passes up the inferior vena cava, through the right atrium and ventricle and into the pulmonary artery where it lodges and obstructs the pulmonary blood supply, causing pulmonary infarction.

Causes (Fig. 6.37): thrombus forms in: (1) the atria in atrial fibrillation; (2) the ventricle in myocardial infarction; and (3) the deep veins in prolonged rest in bed or pelvic operation. Thrombus in the right, but not the left, side of the heart causes pulmonary embolism.

Clinically: massive embolism—the patient asks for a bedpan because of stimulation of the vagus nerve, and suddenly dies.
    Smaller emboli cause shock (pale, cold, clammy skin, tachycardia, fall in blood

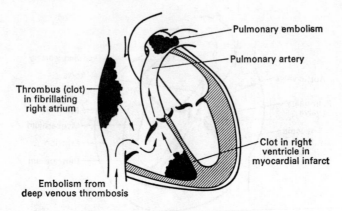

Pulmonary embolism

Pulmonary artery

Thrombus (clot) in fibrillating right atrium

Clot in right ventricle in myocardial infarct

Embolism from deep venous thrombosis

FIG. 6.37   Sources of pulmonary embolism

pressure, faintness), dyspnoea (rapid shallow breathing), retrosternal discomfort, mild pyrexia, haemoptysis, and pleuritic pain. Right ventricular failure may occur.

Investigations:
1 E.C.G.
2 Pulmonary arteriography.
3 Isotope scanning of the lungs.

Treatment: the patient is nursed flat during shock. Oxygen for cyanosis, morphine 15–20 mg i.m. for anxiety and pain. Anticoagulants to prevent further deep venous thrombosis or extension of coagulation on the embolus: Heparin 15,000 u (150 mg) i.v., then 100 mg i.v. six-hourly for four doses. An oral anticoagulant is begun at the same time as the first dose of heparin. Streptokinase or urokinase may be injected, via a catheter, into the pulmonary artery and will dissolve recently formed fibrinous clot. Streptokinase may cause haemorrhage or an allergic reaction. Urokinase is expensive. Surgical embolectomy, using cardiopulmonary by-pass, may be performed if the patient is in a cardiothoracic centre, but this has a high mortality rate. Pulse and blood pressure are recorded every 15 minutes at first.

Prevention: patients in bed should have passive leg movements, or active movements if possible. If deep venous thrombosis occurs anticoagulants should be given. If these fail to prevent further pulmonary embolism then the iliac vein or inferior vena cava may need to be partially tied. This leaves sufficient space for blood to flow but stops clots from passing beyond the ligatures.

DISEASES OF ARTERIES

Atheroma (Atherosclerosis)

This is the commonest arterial disease. It is a patchy deposition of lipid (fat) in the intima (*Fig. 6.28*). The patches thicken and partially or completely block medium and small arteries such as the coronary or cerebral arteries, causing ischaemia (deficient blood supply) in the organ supplied by the obstructed artery. The atheromatous plaque may ulcerate and thrombus form on it (*Fig. 6.38*) and a portion of thrombus may break off to form an embolus. Plaques may calcify, making the artery hard and rigid.

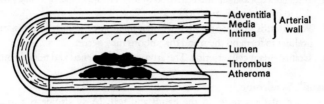

FIG. 6.38   Thrombus on an ulcerated atheromatous plaque

Causes: atheromatous patches occur at the sites of greatest stress in an artery such as the origin of branches from the aorta. It is increased by over-eating, by a diet containing animal (saturated) fat (butter, milk, fatty meat), lack of physical exercise (sedentary occupation, riding instead of walking), cigarette smoking (the incidence of ischaemic heart disease is four times that of non-smokers), diseases causing hyperlipidaemia (high level of fat in the blood, e.g. diabetes mellitus), and hypertension. Males are more commonly affected than females, and at an earlier age— atheroma is already present by the age of 40 years in males, but the same degree of atheroma does not appear in women until the age of 60 years, unless they have a predisposing disorder such as diabetes mellitus. Food processing may be a factor; for example in its manufacture margarine becomes saturated fat. There is a familial tendency, but the environment is more important; thus Africans and Asians have a higher incidence of ischaemic heart disease if they become more prosperous and live in the U.S.A. or Europe than if they live in their native country.

Effects:
1   Ischaemic heart disease (angina of effort, myocardial infarction).
2   Cerebrovascular disease (stroke, senile dementia).
3   Claudication or gangrene of the legs.

Treatment: reducing diet if obese. Diet low in saturated (animal) fat and the use of vegetable (unsaturated) oil instead. Stop smoking.

Surgical: removal of an atheromatous segment of artery and its replacement with a graft.

Arteriosclerosis (hardening of the arteries)
This is thickening of the arteries with fibrous connective tissue from any cause. Non-atheromatous arteriosclerosis is due to, e.g. hypertension or old age and, unlike atheroma, it (1) affects both media and intima; (2) is generalised, not in plaques; (3) is not due to fat; (4) causes only slight narrowing of vessels which is not sufficient to cause ischaemia; (5) arteriosclerosis due to hypertension affects arteries but particularly involves the arterioles.

Note: Pure (uncomplicated) atheroma does not harden the arteries, but the arteries are hardened if fibrosis also occurs (= atherosclerosis).

Arteritis (inflammation of arteries)

This is due to:

1 Syphilis, which weakens large arteries causing aneurysmal dilatation.
2 Buerger's disease, an inflammation of arteries and adjacent veins, probably due to hypersensitivity to tobacco.
3 Polyarteritis nodosa, an allergic inflammation of smaller arteries, causing nodules to form on them and thrombosis may occur.
4 Cranial (giant cell) arteritis. The arteries are thickened and may thrombose.

Raynaud's Syndrome

This is spasm of the arteries in the hands and feet. (A syndrome is a group of symptoms and signs having several causes).

Causes:

A *Primary* (i.e. Raynaud's disease).

B *Secondary* to organic disease:
1 Collagenoses, for example scleroderma.
2 Cervical rib.
3 Occupational in people using vibrating tools.
4 Certain blood disorders.
5 Syringomyelia.

Raynaud's Disease is spasm of the arteries due to hypersensitivity to cold in young women. It begins in childhood.

Clinically: in an attack the hands, fingers and feet are cold, white and pulseless, with loss of sensation and clumsiness. When the spasm wears off the part becomes blue, then red and tingling and throbs. The tips of the fingers may develop superficial ulceration. Major gangrene is rare.

Treatment: cold water should be avoided, gloves worn in cold weather, heated by a battery if necessary. Warm clothing. Vasodilators may be tried but are seldom effective, e.g. tolazoline (Priscol) 25–50 mg t.d.s. orally.

Arterial Obstruction in the Lower Limb

1 *Acute:* (a) embolism; (b) thrombosis.

2 *Chronic:* (a) atheroma; (b) Buerger's disease.

Acute Arterial Obstruction is due to: (a) an embolus detached from the left side of the heart in atrial fibrillation, bacterial endocarditis or myocardial infarction or from a clot on an atheromatous patch in the aorta (*Fig. 6.39*); or to (b) thrombus forming on an atheromatous patch in the artery to the affected part.

Clinically: there is sudden pain and absent arterial pulse in the affected part. The skin is suddenly cold, pale and numb.

Treatment: rest in bed with the head-end elevated to increase the blood flow to the

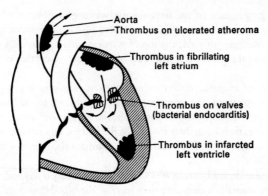

Aorta
Thrombus on ulcerated atheroma
Thrombus in fibrillating left atrium
Thrombus on valves (bacterial endocarditis)
Thrombus in infarcted left ventricle

FIG. 6.39 Sources of systemic embolism (compare *Fig. 6.37*)

legs. The affected part is kept cool (local hypothermia) by exposing it to the atmosphere and blowing air over it using a fan. This reduces its metabolism and therefore reduces its need for blood, while the rest of the body is warmed to promote reflex vasodilatation. A woollen sock is worn on the unaffected leg.

Drugs: anticoagulants to prevent extension of clot. Streptokinase or urokinase to dissolve fresh clot.

Surgery: embolectomy. Amputation for established gangrene.

Chronic Arterial Obstruction is due to: (*a*) atheroma, with or without thrombus formation on the atheromatous plaque, the commonest cause; or to (*b*) Buerger's disease (thromboangiitis obliterans), an inflammation of the arteries and adjacent veins which occurs only in smokers and may be due to an allergy to tobacco. The inflammation narrows the lumen causing arterial obstruction.

Clinically: the limb is cold and numb with inelastic, shiny, dry, pale skin and brittle nails. Intermittent claudication ('lameness') may occur. This is cramp-like pain in the calf or foot on walking, relieved by resting. Pain at rest indicates severe ischaemia and may be relieved by hanging the leg out of bed so that gravity increases the blood flow to the part.

Complications:
  1 Ulceration and infection of the skin due to minor injury.
  2 Dry gangrene (death of tissue), which begins as a blue discolouration.

Investigations:
  1 Urine for sugar (atheroma is common in diabetes mellitus).
  2 Temperature of the limb.
  3 Arterial pulses are measured (plethysmography) and are absent or diminished in the affected limb.
  4 Arteriography.
  5 Blood count (anaemia increases symptoms).
  6 E.C.G. (myocardial ischaemia is likely).

Treatment: proper care of the feet: regular washing, avoidance of tight shoes, careful cutting of nails and corns since minor injury precipitates infection and gangrene. Avoidance of cold; the use of warm clothing, woollen socks changed daily, bedsocks at night. Raising the heels of the shoes reduces the work of the calf muscles.

Correction of anaemia, cardiac failure, obesity. Smoking is stopped. Exercise improves the collateral circulation but should be restricted to the limits permitted by pain. Exercise to improve the circulation: the leg is raised above the horizontal for one minute, then hung over the side of the bed for one minute while the toes and ankles are exercised. The health visitor examines the domestic circumstances and gives advice.

Drugs: general vasodilators are of no value since the artery is physically obstructed, and they are contraindicated since they increase the blood flow to all the parts of the body except that supplied by the narrowed vessel; but vasodilators e.g. tolazoline (Priscol) may be injected directly into the affected vessel to encourage a collateral circulation, i.e. the dilatation of adjacent vessels which may then provide an adequate circulation. Analgesic for pain.

Surgery: lumbar sympathectomy (ganglionectomy) improves skin nutrition by removing sympathetic tone and causing skin vasodilatation, but does not affect claudication. Disobliterative endarterectomy is excision of the material obstructing the artery. Arterial reconstruction using a by-pass graft (*Fig. 6.40*). Amputation, if necessary.

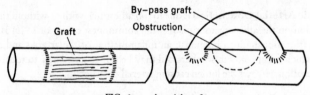

FIG. 6.40   Arterial grafts

Threatened Gangrene

Aim: to reduce the oxygen need of the tissues by keeping the limb cool; to dilate arteries and to avoid injury and infection.

Treatment: rest in bed with the affected limb exposed; a fan may be used to keep it cool. The head of the bed is raised to allow gravity to increase the blood in the limb. Sheepskin pads under the ankles prevent pressure on the heels.

Aneurysm

This is a local dilatation of a vessel.

Types (Fig. 6.41):

1   Saccular. Part of the arterial wall bulges.
2   Fusiform. The whole circumference of a segment of vessel is dilated.
3   Dissecting aortic aneurysm is due to degeneration of the media. Blood enters a tear in the intima and passes along the degenerate media separating

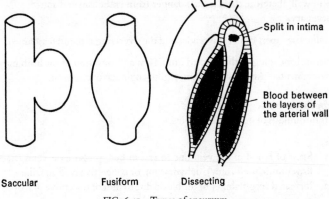

Split in intima

Blood between
the layers of
the arterial wall

Saccular   Fusiform   Dissecting

FIG. 6.41   Types of aneurysm

the layers of the vessel, then ruptures either through the adventitia (when the patient usually dies), or through the intima back into the lumen.

Causes:
1   Degeneration such as atheroma, or medial degeneration.
2   Infection, e.g. syphilis.
3   Injury.
4   Congenital weakness of the arterial wall, as in aneurysm of the circle of Willis in the skull.

Clinically: symptoms are due to pressure on vertebrae, ribs (causing pain), oesophagus (dysphagia), and trachea (dyspnoea).

Treatment: treat shock and the pain of the ruptured aneurysm. Treatment of hypertension. Surgery.

CHILBLAINS
Chilblains are due to cold causing vasoconstriction in the fingers and toes followed by vasodilatation. The circulation is deficient and the skin becomes painful, shiny, oedematous and purplish-red.

Treatment: protection from cold with warm clothing and adequate heating.

DISEASES OF VEINS

Thrombophlebitis
This is thrombosis (clotting of blood in a blood vessel) of veins due to inflammation of the wall, usually of a superficial vein.

Cause: injury, intravenous infusion of irritant chemicals, varicose veins, Buerger's disease (inflammation of artery and adjacent vein). It may affect first one vein then another (thrombophlebitis migrans). The inflammation makes the clot adherent to the vein wall, therefore there is little danger from embolism and anticoagulants are not necessary.

Clinically: the superficial vein is tender and the overlying skin often inflamed.

Treatment: bandaging of the affected limb. Rest and elevation of the limb may help but is not essential. Analgesic for pain, e.g. phenylbutazone, aspirin.

Phlebothrombosis
This is thrombosis of normal deep veins.

Cause:

1 Stasis of blood in the vein due to rest in bed, pressure on veins (fractured lower limb, pregnancy), dehydration, or congestive cardiac failure.
2 Increased coagulability of the blood due to the contraceptive pill, operation, or certain cancers, e.g. carcinoma of the pancreas.

Clinically: many cases are symptomless, others show mild pyrexia, oedema and increased temperature of the part, usually the leg, due to obstruction to the venous return. Pain, tenderness and a positive Homan's sign (calf pain on dorsiflexion of the foot).

Investigations: daily examination of patient's legs for signs of thrombosis. The temperature chart shows a spike of fever.

Radiofibrinogen uptake test—the fibrinogen becomes part of the clot and its radioactivity is detected. It is not used in pregnancy owing to the possibility of radiation damaging the fetus.

Doppler ultrasound detects changes in speed of blood flow.

Phlebography (venography)—radio-opaque material is injected into a vein, and X-rayed to show the obstruction.

Complications: pulmonary embolism and infarction. A large embolus causes sudden death.

Prevention: prevent dehydration. Breathing exercises to aid the venous return to the heart. Avoid tight bandages and faulty position of the limbs. Active exercises of the limbs in bed, and early mobilisation.

Treatment: rest in bed with the foot-end elevated 23 cm (9 inches), with elastic bandages applied firmly from toe to groin. As soon as acute symptoms subside the patient should get up. Prolonged rest is undesirable since it encourages stasis and further thrombosis.

Drugs:

1 *Anticoagulants to prevent further coagulation.* Heparin 40,000 units in i.v. drip over 24 hours, or 15,000 u (150 mg) stat. then 10,000 u (100 mg) six-hourly i.v. for 24–36 hours. At the same time oral anticoagulants are given (these take 24–36 hours to act and this is why heparin has to be given), either phenindione (Dindevan) 150–300 mg stat. orally then 25–50 mg b.d. or Warfarin (Marevan) 30–60 mg stat. then 3–15 mg daily from the third day. *Side-effects:* Rash, haemorrhage.

Heparin levels are controlled from the clotting time and an overdose is neutralised with protamine sulphate 50 mg i.v. (acts immediately) for every 5000 u of heparin.

The dose of oral anticoagulant is determined from the blood prothrombin level which should be kept at 20–30% of normal. Overdose is neutralised by vitamin K_1 (phytomenadione) 10–20 mg i.v. (acts slowly).

2 *Fibrinolytic drugs (dissolve fibrin clot).* Streptokinase 600,000 u in 250 ml of dextrose-saline plus 100 mg hydrocortisone (to prevent allergy) given i.v. in 30–60 minutes, repeated six-hourly for three days. NOT given if there is a history of peptic ulcer or other possible cause of haemorrhage, or with anticoagulants since this may cause haemorrhage. *Side-effects:* Allergic reaction, pyrexia. Aminocaproic acid (Epsicapron) is kept available to reverse the effects of streptokinase if bleeding occurs.

Varicose Veins

Varicose veins are dilated tortuous veins (*Fig. 6.7*). They may occur in the lower end of the rectum (piles, haemorrhoids) or oesophagus (oesophageal varices) but the following applies to those which occur in the legs. These are due to a congenital deficiency of the valves and walls of the veins or to conditions impeding venous return (tight garters, prolonged standing, pregnancy, deep venous thrombosis). The superficial veins are not supported by muscles and if they are stretched the valves do not close properly. This causes an increased pressure on the valve below, which then gives way and causes an increased pressure on the next valve, and so on. The tissues become congested, interfering with their nutrition, thus the skin easily breaks down.

Clinically: there are dilated and tortuous veins and oedema of the leg after standing.

Complications: chronic venous congestion causes:
1 Varicose eczema: a chronic scaling and pigmentation of the skin.
2 Varicose (gravitational) ulcer: ulceration of the skin above the ankle.
Ulceration of a vein causes:
3 Rupture, causing haemorrhage which is easily controlled by elevation of the limb or local pressure on the bleeding point.
4 Phlebitis and thrombophlebitis.

Treatment: elastic stocking or crêpe bandages; avoid standing for long periods of time. Varicosities have a psychological effect on women and these patients need reassurance that their veins are not as obvious as they think they are. Sclerotherapy —injection of ethanolamine into the vein. This causes clotting and obliteration of the lumen. Surgical ligature or excision (stripping) of the vein.

Varicose Ulcer: rest with elevation of the limb above the level of the heart whenever possible, and a raised foot-end of the bed at night to reduce the congestion in the leg Local dressing e.g. tulle gras. Protection from injury and cold with bandages applied from the toes to below the knee. Avoidance of medicaments on the healing edge of the ulcer. Antibiotic for infection, according to sensitivity.

7 THE RESPIRATORY SYSTEM

ANATOMY AND PHYSIOLOGY

The function of the respiratory system is to take air into the lungs and allow the absorption of oxygen into the blood and the excretion of carbon dioxide from the blood into the alveoli and the air. The respiratory tract is artificially divided into upper and lower parts. The upper respiratory tract (U.R.T.) includes the nose, nasopharynx (nasal cavity and pharynx) and larynx. The lower respiratory tract includes the trachea, two bronchi, two lungs (bronchioles and alveoli) and pleura. The respiratory tract is supported by bone and cartilage to keep it open, and is lined with vascular mucous membrane of ciliated columnar epithelium which ensures that the inspired air enters the lungs fully saturated with water vapour at body temperature. In the mucous membrane are cells which secrete mucus onto its surface. Mucus is sticky and traps particles, including bacteria. The cilia waft the mucus towards the throat to be swallowed. The mucous membrane is supported by a thin layer of surrounding fibrous tissue, and around this, from the pharynx to the bronchioles, is a layer of muscle.

The Nasal Cavity (Fig. 7.1)
The roof of the nasal cavity is formed by the base of the skull; the floor by the roof of the mouth (the maxillary and palatine bones and soft palate); the medial wall by the nasal septum (ethmoid bone, vomer and cartilage); the anterior (front) wall by the nasal bones and cartilage covered with skin; the lateral (side) wall by the superior maxillary bones and the superior, middle and inferior conchae which increase the surface area of the mucosa and cause eddies in the inspired air which help to trap particles and assist in warming and moistening the air; and the posterior (rear) wall is formed by the pharynx. The anterior nares are the nostrils, the anterior opening into the nasal cavity. The posterior nares open into the pharynx.

The Nasal Sinuses
These are air cavities which make the skull lighter and give resonance to the voice. The frontal and sphenoidal sinuses open into the roof of the nasal cavity, the ethmoidal and maxillary sinuses open into the lateral walls of the nasal cavity. Through these openings they may become infected from the nose.

The Pharynx (Fig. 7.1)
The pharynx is common to the respiratory system and the alimentary tract. It extends from the base of the skull to the larynx and oesophagus at the level of the sixth cervical vertebra. In front is the nasal cavity and the mouth; behind are the six cervical vertebrae. Into the nasopharynx open the right and left Eustachian tubes

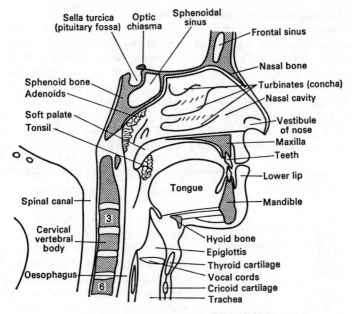

FIG. 7.1 The nasal cavity, pharynx and larynx

which allow air to pass along them to the middle ear, since air on both sides of the tympanic membrane has to be at the same (atmospheric) pressure (*Fig. 7.2*). The adenoids are on the posterior wall of the nasopharynx, and lower down are the tonsils. The tonsils and adenoids consist of lymphoid tissue and are the first antibody-producing defences in throat infections. Surrounding the mucous membrane and its supporting fibrous tissue are the constrictor muscles of the pharynx which are important in swallowing. The pharynx helps to separate food from the airway during swallowing.

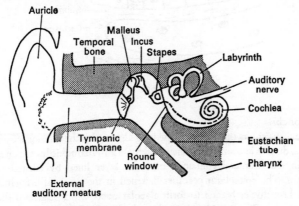

FIG. 7.2 The relations of the middle ear

The Larynx ('voice box', 'Adam's apple')

This extends from the root of the tongue and the hyoid bone to the trachea. It consists of the epiglottis and the thyroid, cricoid and arytenoid cartilages which are attached to each other by ligaments and membranes, and is supplied by the laryngeal and recurrent laryngeal nerves which are branches of the vagus nerves. Within the larynx are the vocal cords, two folds of mucous membrane which are silent when relaxed but can be pulled together by the adjacent muscles; when air is forced through the narrowed space between the cords they vibrate and produce sound. Speech is produced by altering the shape of the mouth and the position of the tongue, lips and facial muscles. During swallowing the larynx rises so that it can be closed by the epiglottis. The larynx, by the cough reflex, prevents large particles from reaching the lower respiratory tract.

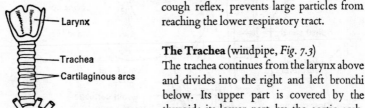

FIG. 7.3   The trachea and bronchi

The Trachea (windpipe, *Fig. 7.3*)

The trachea continues from the larynx above and divides into the right and left bronchi below. Its upper part is covered by the thyroid; its lower part by the aortic arch. The oesophagus and vertebral column are behind and the lungs are on each side. The trachea, main bronchi and smaller bronchi are supported by C-shaped incomplete rings of cartilage with the gap behind. They are lined by ciliated epithelium containing goblet cells which secrete mucus (*Fig. 7.4*).

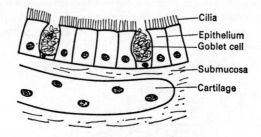

FIG. 7.4   Microscopic section of trachea

The Bronchi

Each bronchus enters the hilum of the lung along with the pulmonary artery and veins, and divides into smaller bronchi and these into **bronchioles** which are about 1 mm in diameter and contain a muscular layer lined by ciliated columnar epithelium. The epithelium becomes flattened in the terminal bronchioles. The terminal bronchioles branch to form alveolar ducts which lead into the alveoli (minute air sacs, *Fig. 7.5*). Alveoli consist only of a thin layer of flattened epithelial

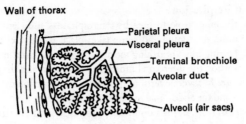

Wall of thorax

Parietal pleura
Visceral pleura
Terminal bronchiole
Alveolar duct
Alveoli (air sacs)

FIG. 7.5   Microscopic section of lung

cells which are surrounded by blood capillaries and here oxygen and carbon dioxide are exchanged by diffusion.

The Lungs (*Fig. 7.6*)

The right and left lungs are separated by the mediastinum which contains the pericardium, heart, aorta, pulmonary vessels, venae cavae, trachea, bronchi and

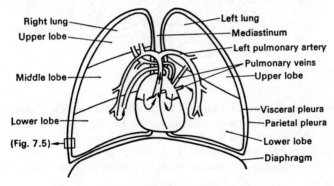

Right lung
Upper lobe
Middle lobe
Lower lobe
(Fig. 7.5)

Left lung
Mediastinum
Left pulmonary artery
Pulmonary veins
Upper lobe
Visceral pleura
Parietal pleura
Lower lobe
Diaphragm

FIG. 7.6   Diagram of the lungs and their blood supply

oesophagus. The lungs rest on the diaphragm which separates them from the abdomen. The right lung has three lobes; the left has two.

The lung consists of bronchi, bronchioles, respiratory bronchioles, alveolar ducts and alveoli. The pulmonary artery conveys deoxygenated blood to the lungs and divides and subdivides into the capillary network surrounding the alveoli. The capillaries join to become venules and these join to form pulmonary veins conveying oxygenated blood to the left atrium of the heart.

The Pleura

Each lung is surrounded by a serous membrane, the pleura, which is composed of flattened epithelial cells and has two layers (*Fig. 7.5*): the visceral pleura which is attached to the lung, and the parietal pleura lining the thoracic wall and upper surface of the diaphragm. Both layers are normally in contact and are lubricated by a thin film of serous fluid secreted by the cells of the pleural membrane. The pleural cavity is the potential space between the two layers.

Mechanism of Respiration

Ventilation of the lungs is performed by the respiratory muscles. The respiratory cycle of inspiration, expiration and pause takes place at the rate of 12–16 times a minute at rest. During quiet breathing the diaphragm is the main muscle of respiration. During exertion the intercostal muscles are also used and the respiratory rate and depth increase. In severe exertion or bronchial obstruction the sternomastoids assist inspiration and the abdominal muscles assist expiration.

The **diaphragm** (*Fig. 7.7*) is a dome-shaped muscle with a central tendon and it separates the thoracic and abdominal cavities. It is attached to the lower ribs, sternum

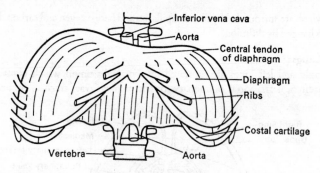

FIG. 7.7   The diaphragm

and vertebral column and is supplied by the phrenic nerves. On contraction its central tendon is pulled downwards, elongating the thoracic cavity and causing inspiration. The intercostal muscles raise the ribs and increase the diameter of the thorax. When the diaphragm relaxes it is drawn upwards by the elastic recoil of the lungs; thus expiration is a passive movement, unlike the active contraction of inspiration.

Gaseous Exchange between the alveoli and the blood capillaries takes place continuously. The pressure of oxygen (PO_2) is higher in the alveoli than in the blood so oxygen passes into the capillaries. The pressure of carbon dioxide (PCO_2) is higher in the blood and so diffuses into the alveoli and is exhaled. Atmospheric air contains oxygen 21%, nitrogen 78%, carbon dioxide 0·04%, other gases nearly 1%. Expired air contains 16% oxygen, 80% nitrogen, and 4% carbon dioxide.

The Control of Respiration (*Fig. 7.8*) is by chemical and nervous stimuli. The respiratory centres in the pons and medulla oblongata send regular impulses along the phrenic nerves to the diaphragm and along the intercostal nerves to the intercostal muscles. The muscles contract, causing inspiration. When the lung expands stretch-receptor nerve endings in the bronchioles send impulses via the vagus nerve to the respiratory centre in the medulla; these impulses inhibit the centre (Hering-Breuer reflex) and cause relaxation of the respiratory muscles and hence expiration. The respiratory centres are also controlled by the level of carbon dioxide and oxygen in the blood. An increase in the blood carbon dioxide concentration stimulates chemoreceptor nerve endings in the carotid body which is in the wall of the common carotid artery. Impulses pass via the vagus and glossopharyngeal nerves to the respiratory centre and stimulate it to increase respiration and thus drive off

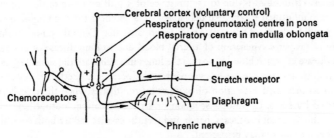

FIG. 7.8 The control of respiration

the excess carbon dioxide. Oxygen lack in the blood (hypoxaemia) has a similar but smaller effect and its effect is overridden by carbon dioxide. The respiratory centres can be controlled voluntarily for a short period by the cerebral cortex.

The Rate and Depth of Breathing. The work of respiration is increased when the lungs are more rigid (less compliant) due to pulmonary oedema or fibrosis, or when the chest wall cannot expand properly as in ankylosing spondylitis or severe kyphosis ('hump-back'), and these cause rapid shallow breathing. Rapid breathing, airway obstruction (asthma, chronic bronchitis, bronchial tumour) and emphysema also increase the work of the respiratory muscles and their need for oxygen. Shallow breathing wastes energy, and therefore oxygen, since the air inspired into the nose, pharynx, larynx, trachea, bronchi and bronchioles is not used in gaseous exchange and is 'dead space'.

Normal quiet ventilation takes 500 ml of air in each breath; 150 ml of this is dead space and 350 ml functions for gaseous exchange. Shallow respiration may take in only 350 ml, but the dead space is unaltered, leaving only 200 ml for gaseous exchange. Underventilation is present in chronic bronchitis and emphysema, respiratory depression by narcotics, anaesthetics or intracranial disease, respiratory muscle paralysis, and chest deformity. Local ventilation in the lung is impaired by pulmonary collapse, consolidation, fibrosis, or oedema. Overventilation occurs in anxiety, hysteria, mild asthma, interstitial lung disease, and pulmonary embolism, and is protective in metabolic acidosis. Overventilation removes carbon dioxide ($\equiv$ carbonic acid) from the body, thus the blood becomes more alkaline (respiratory alkalosis).

Internal (Cell) Respiration. Oxygen from the alveoli enters the blood and attaches to haemoglobin to form oxyhaemoglobin. When this circulates to the tissues oxygen diffuses from the blood, where it is at a higher concentration, to the tissues where the concentration is low. Carbon dioxide, being at high concentration in the tissues, diffuses into the blood where the concentration is low, and is carried to the lungs to be exhaled.

SYMPTOMS AND SIGNS

Cyanosis (Blueness) is due to the presence of 5 g/dl or more of deoxygenated haemoglobin caused by oxygen deficiency. It is absent if the haemoglobin is less than 5 g/dl (= 30% of normal), i.e. in severe anaemia. Central cyanosis is due to failure of proper oxygenation of arterial blood due to lung disease or congenital heart disease in which blood by-passes the lungs in a veno-arterial shunt (*Fig. 6.35*). The mouth and tongue are as cyanosed as the periphery. Peripheral cyanosis is due to an increased extraction of oxygen by the tissues when the circulation is impaired by stasis, by vasoconstriction or by a low cardiac output, and is best seen in the lips, nail beds, ears, hands and feet. In cardiac failure both central and peripheral cyanosis may be present.

Hypoxaemia is a reduced amount of oxygen in the arterial blood.

Hypercapnia is an increase in the carbon dioxide content of the arterial blood.

Shallow Respiration may be due to pulmonary disease, to pleural or abdominal pain which is increased if breathing is deep, or to depression of respiratory centres by morphine.

Tachypnoea is an increased rate of respiration. It is caused by pyrexia, pulmonary congestion (pneumonia, pulmonary oedema due to heart failure), or acidosis.

Deep Breathing (Hyperpnoea) is produced by stimulation of the respiratory centre by excess of acid (metabolic acidosis), e.g. in diabetic coma, uraemia, exertion.

Stertorous (Snoring) Breathing is caused by the vibration of paralysed parts such as the cheek and throat in, e.g. a stroke.

Irregular Breathing, e.g. Cheyne–Stokes respiration, is due to medullary damage or ischaemia caused by congestive cardiac failure, uraemia or increased intracranial pressure.

Orthopnoea is difficulty in breathing (except in the upright position).

Dyspnoea is difficulty in breathing and occurs in heart and lung disease. The hyperpnoea of exercise is not dyspnoea.

Apnoea is cessation of breathing.

Wheezing is a musical sound, more likely to be present on expiration when the airway narrows most; it is caused by narrowing of the bronchi due to oedema of the mucosa, bronchial muscle spasm, or material such as mucus or pus in the lumen.

Stridor is a crowing noise heard on inspiration and is due to obstruction of the major airway (larynx, trachea).

Cough is due to stimulation of the vagal nerve endings in the respiratory tract by foreign particles, mucus or inflammation, and serves to expel obstructing material. The vocal cords are closed and pressure builds up behind them until they are opened and the air is expelled violently. A dry cough, i.e. cough without sputum, should be suppressed if severe. A productive cough (cough with sputum) should be encouraged in order to remove secretions which may cause complications.

Sputum is the coughed-up secretions of the respiratory tract combined with foreign material such as dust and organisms. It is mucoid if it is due to chronic irritation of the trachea and bronchi, e.g. cigarette smoking. In infection it becomes mucopurulent or purulent (containing pus). In lung abscess or bronchiectasis the sputum may have a foul odour owing to stagnation and putrefaction. It is watery in pulmonary oedema. The volume and appearance of the sputum should be noted. It should be collected in a sterile labelled container on waking.

Haemoptysis is the coughing-up of blood and is found in acute bronchitis, pulmonary congestion (as in mitral stenosis), bronchiectasis, pulmonary infarction due to embolism, pulmonary tuberculosis, carcinoma of the bronchus, and bleeding diseases such as leukaemia. Haemoptysis must be distinguished from haematemesis, the vomiting of blood. In haemoptysis there is a history of lung or heart disease and the coughing-up of bright red frothy blood mixed with sputum which has an alkaline reaction. In haematemesis there is a history of abdominal disease or the ingestion of tablets such as aspirin, and the vomiting of dark red or dark brown (altered, 'coffee-grounds') blood with an acid reaction and mixed with food.

Note: coughed-up blood may be swallowed and then vomited.

Treatment: for severe haemorrhage, rest in bed, sedation: morphine 15 mg s.c. or i.m. allays anxiety, restlessness and cough. Morphine should not be used in chronic bronchitis and emphysema since it may cause serious respiratory depression. Blood transfusion if hypotensive. In mild haemoptysis: reassurance and explanation of the cause.

Chest Pain may be a retrosternal ache, worse on coughing, due to tracheitis, or sharp (stabbing), worse on deep breathing and coughing, and caused by inflammation of the parietal pleura as in pleurisy, pneumonia and pulmonary embolism. It may be non-respiratory in origin, e.g. cardiac or oesophageal.

INVESTIGATIONS

Breathing. The rate in one minute, depth, and the presence of wheezing or dyspnoea are noted and any abnormality reported. The nurse should not let the patient know she is counting respirations, otherwise he may alter their frequency.

Sputum
1 Consistency. Whether watery (pulmonary oedema) or tenacious (asthma).
2 Colour. Colourless (mucoid), green or yellow (purulent), rusty (pneumonia), blood-streaked.
3 Quantity. Sputum is copious in bronchiectasis and lung abscess.
4 Odour is normally absent, but is foul in bronchiectasis and lung abscess.
5 Laboratory examination for pus, organisms, including tubercle bacilli, and malignant cells ('cytology').
Note: saliva is not sputum.

Blood. The white cell count is increased, due to an increase in the number of polymorphs, in bacterial (pyogenic) infections, but is normal or shows an increase in lymphocytes in viral infections. **Serology** (examination for antibodies in the serum) in viral infection.

Chest Radiology
1　Plain X-rays.
2　Tomography—radiographs (X-rays) focused to show different depths in the lungs—demonstrates tumours and cavities.
3　Bronchogram. Radio-opaque material is poured into one bronchus and the lung X-rayed; the material is then drained off and the test repeated on the other side. It is used in the diagnosis of bronchiectasis.
4　Screening demonstrates the position and movement of the diaphragm.

Pleural Fluid is examined for malignant cells (cytology) and for evidence of infection (pus cells, lymphocytes, organisms).

Laryngoscopy is inspection of the larynx and detects tumours, foreign bodies, and the movement of the vocal cords.

Bronchoscopy is inspection of the bronchi for, e.g., tumour or distortion by tuberculous inflammation or external pressure.

Thoracoscopy. The pleura is inspected via a thoracoscope inserted through an intercostal space.

Mediastinoscopy is inspection of the mediastinum via the neck.

Biopsy of lymph node, pleura or lung in obscure conditions.

Pulmonary Function Tests
1　The vital capacity is the amount of gas that can be expelled from the lungs after a full inspiration. The average normal is $4 \cdot 8$ l in males and $3 \cdot 2$ l in females.
2　After full inspiration the amount of air that can be forced out of the lungs in one second is the forced expiratory volume (F.E.V.$_1$), and the normal is 75% of the vital capacity and averages $3 \cdot 2$ l. It is low in airway obstruction (chronic bronchitis, asthma).
3　Peak expiratory flow is measured with a Wright peak flow meter. The normal is above 500 l a minute. The patient takes a deep breath and blows as hard as he can into the mouthpiece.
4　Arterial gas (carbon dioxide and oxygen) analysis.

Skin Tests. The tuberculin test is positive in tuberculosis (*see* Chapter 4). The Kveim test is positive in sarcoidosis. An extract of sarcoid material is injected into the skin, and six or more weeks later a papule appears and a biopsy of it is examined microscopically for the changes of sarcoidosis. Pollen and dust sensitivities are positive in allergic diseases such as hay fever and asthma. Extracts of different pollens, feathers, moulds, dusts, tobacco and foods are placed on the skin and a scratch made through them. Twenty minutes later a papule with a red margin indicates an allergic response. Extracts may be inhaled and the production of symptoms indicates a positive test. Inhalation (provocation) tests cannot be performed during an attack of asthma since symptoms are already present. They may be dangerous at any time; therefore adrenaline and hydrocortisone or prednisolone must be ready for use if a severe attack of asthma is precipitated.

DRUGS USED IN RESPIRATORY DISEASE

Antibiotics are discussed in Chapter 4.

Expectorants are intended to loosen sticky mucus, and include ammonium chloride, ammonium bicarbonate, potassium iodide, ipecacuanha, squill, and bromhexine (Bisolvon).

Cough Suppressants may be used for persistent useless (unproductive) cough, and include linctus codeine and linctus pholcodine, dose 5 ml. Proprietary preparations mostly act as sedatives and include Actifed, Benylin, Phensedyl and Tixylix.

Respiratory Stimulants may be used if ventilation is depressed; e.g. nikethamide 2–10 ml of 25% i.v. or i.m. *Note:* Nalorphine (Lethidrone) is not a respiratory stimulant but is an antidote to morphine and pethidine. *Dose:* 5–10 mg i.v., repeat as necessary up to a total of 40–100 mg. 1 mg may be injected into the umbilical vein of the newborn whose mother has received pethidine or morphine during labour.

Drugs Relieving Airway Obstruction

A Bronchodilators. These act by relaxing the smooth muscle of the bronchi:
1   Sympathomimetics: isoprenaline 10 mg, orciprenaline (Alupent) 20 mg or salbutamol (Ventolin) 2 mg tablet sublingually or aerosol, adrenaline up to 1 ml s.c., ephedrine 30 mg orally. One of these, 1–4 times daily.
2   Aminophylline 250 mg in 10 ml i.v. slowly, or choline theophyllinate (Choledyl) 200–400 mg t.d.s. orally.

B Anti-inflammatory. Corticosteroids reduce inflammation and hence reduce the narrowing of bronchi due to mucosal oedema.
1   Prednisolone 15 mg six-hourly at first, reducing the dose over the next few days.
2   Hydrocortisone succinate 100–200 mg i.v. four-hourly in status asthmaticus.
3   Tetracosactrin (Synacthen, Cortrosyn) 0·25 mg i.m.

C Anti-allergic. These drugs prevent the allergic inflammation from taking place: sodium cromoglycate (Intal, Rynacron) 20 mg inhalation two to six times daily. Ketotifen 1–2 mg (base) b.d.

Antihistamines. Partly act by sedation and partly by preventing the inflammatory action of histamine after it has been released by the antigen-antibody reaction. They are useless in asthma.

Diphenhydramine (Benadryl, Histex) 25 mg b.d. to 50 mg q.i.d. orally. Mepyramine (Anthisan) 100–200 mg t.d.s. orally. Promethazine (Phenergan, Avomine) 10–75 mg b.d. orally. Dimenhydrinate (Dramamine) 25–100 mg two to four times daily. Chlorpheniramine (Piriton) 4–8 mg t.d.s. orally. Tripelennamine (Pyribenzamine) 50–100 mg t.d.s. orally. Chlorcyclizine (Histantin) 50–200 mg t.d.s. orally. Phenindamine 25–50 mg t.d.s.

Side-effects: all except phenindamine cause sedation, and commonly a dry mouth and constipation.

OXYGEN THERAPY

Oxygen is required if there is hypoxaemia (a low oxygen level in the arterial blood). *Note:* hypoxia = low oxygen; anoxia = no oxygen. Hypoxia is caused by impaired ventilation of the lungs due to respiratory muscular paralysis, drug overdose depressing the respiratory centre, pulmonary oedema or infection, and cardiac failure, and occurs in some congenital heart diseases ('blue babies'). These all cause central cyanosis in which the blood is not saturated with oxygen when it leaves the left side of the heart. It is often advisable to give oxygen even when there is no cyanosis since oxygen may be deficient in the absence of cyanosis. Before giving oxygen the nostrils must be cleaned. Smoking is not allowed on the ward during oxygen therapy. The oxygen supply must be checked daily.

A high concentration of oxygen of 40–80% is used in acute illness such as carbon monoxide poisoning, pulmonary oedema, and myocardial infarction and is provided by masks which fit closely to the face and have a reservoir bag which fills with oxygen during expiration. The Polymask and Pneumask allow rebreathing of expired air, the Portogen mask has a valve which prevents rebreathing. Oxygen is given at 6–10 l per minute. The oxygen does not need to be humidified with these appliances.

Oxygen tents usually supply less than 60% owing to leakage, and they have to be carefully tucked in to prevent this. They are seldom used now, except for small children. The tent sleeves must be kept closed and inlet and outlet pipes connected to a drum of soda lime or caustic soda which absorb carbon dioxide; ice is placed in another container from which water is released at intervals via a drainage tube.

In chronic bronchitis and emphysema a high concentration of oxygen cannot be used since in this condition the respiratory centre relies on oxygen-lack for its stimulation and is insensitive to carbon dioxide, which is normally the main respiratory stimulus. If hypoxia is abolished by giving a high concentration of oxygen, ventilation is reduced and carbon dioxide builds up and may cause carbon dioxide narcosis (coma). Thus a low concentration of oxygen (30%) is given and a rebreathing bag is not used since it would contribute to carbon dioxide retention and narcosis. A Venturi mask (ventimask) delivers 24%, 28% or 35% oxygen. An Edinburgh mask acts similarly. Masks need to be removed for eating and sputum ejection. Plastic twin nasal catheters, with the tips in the anterior nares, do not become hot, do not obscure vision and are more comfortable than masks and 1 l of oxygen a minute delivers 25–30%, 2 l per minute delivers 30–35% of oxygen, which should be humidified to prevent dryness of the nasopharynx.

Toxic effects of oxygen: retrolental fibroplasia (retinopathy causing blindness) may result from high concentrations of oxygen in premature infants and the concentration in incubators should not be more than 35%. In adults and children, breathing pure oxygen for more than a few hours damages the alveoli in the lungs.

TRACHEOSTOMY

Tracheostomy is the opening of the trachea by an incision in the midline of the neck below the cricoid cartilage, and the insertion of a plastic or metal tracheostomy tube so that air enters the trachea directly and not through the nasopharynx. Its aim is to improve the air supply to the lungs.

Use

1 To by-pass an obstruction in the pharynx or larynx, for example a foreign body impacted in the pharynx or larynx; laryngeal diphtheria when the diphtheritic membrane causes obstruction; laryngeal tumours; laryngeal or pharyngeal oedema due to inflammation such as scalds or syphilis.
2 Throat operations.
3 When there is poor ventilation of the lungs, as in poliomyelitis or deep coma (head injury, chest wall injury, stroke, barbiturate poisoning).

Tracheostomy halves the respiratory 'dead space', i.e. the inhaled air in the nose, pharynx and larynx, which does not reach the lungs. It therefore reduces the effort of breathing and improves ventilation (*Fig. 7.9*).

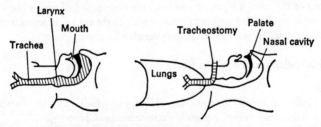

FIG. 7.9   Respiratory 'dead' space (shaded): (*a*) Normal; (*b*) with tracheostomy

A tracheostomy tube consists of four main parts: an outer tube, an inner tube, an introducer (pilot), and a collar to which tapes are attached and are tied around the neck of the patient to keep the tube in place. Tubes are made in various sizes, therefore all parts must be of the correct fit. The tracheostomy tube used with positive pressure respiration has an inflatable cuff.

Care. The inner tube must be kept clean by removing it and cleaning it in sodium bicarbonate solution every one to three hours, or more frequently at first. It must be removed carefully so that the outer tube does not come out of the trachea. A displaced outer tube must be reported immediately. The tube acts as a foreign body and causes the secretion of excessive mucus which must be removed by suction, the sucker being inserted into each main bronchus. Noisy breathing, restlessness, dyspnoea or cyanosis are indications that there is obstruction to the airway. The patient should be encouraged to cough. The orifice is kept covered with gauze moistened with sodium bicarbonate and a humidifier or steam kettle used to humidify the air near the patient (but not so near that he might knock it over). Oxygen is given for cyanosis *after* clearing the airway. The patient is unable to speak and should be given a writing pad and pencil for communication. An emergency tray should always be at hand containing spare tubes and tracheal dilators.

DISORDERS OF THE RESPIRATORY SYSTEM

Epistaxis (nose bleeding)

Causes:

1   Acute nasal infection e.g. coryza.
2   Injury to the nose, nose-picking, fracture of the base of the skull.
3   Hypertension.
4   Tumours in the nose.
5   Bleeding diseases, e.g. leukaemia.

Treatment: the patient should sit up to reduce the venous pressure in the nose. A little blood-letting in hypertension does no harm. The nostrils are firmly squeezed between finger and thumb for five to ten minutes and the patient breathes through the mouth. This will stop most bleeding, which is usually from a small area near the front of the nose. If bleeding continues the nose is packed with ribbon gauze which must be removed within 24 hours owing to the risk of infection. Repeated epistaxis is treated by sealing the bleeding vessels with electric cautery.

Rhinitis (inflammation of the nose)

Causes:

1   Infection, usually the common cold (coryza) which is an infection with one of the many viruses, especially rhinoviruses (*see* Chapter 4).
2   Allergy to pollens or dusts (hay fever), which is inherited.
3   Pungent odours or chemical irritants.

Clinically: The nose pours out watery secretions and the mucous membrane becomes oedematous and swollen, causing nasal obstruction. Irritation causes sneezing. The conjunctiva also may be inflamed. The sense of smell is lost; sleep is disturbed by mouth-breathing, and the patient awakes with a dry mouth and throat.

In **Coryza** the discharge often becomes mucopurulent due to secondary bacterial infection. Obstruction of the Eustachian tube by inflammation causes headache and partial deafness. Complications are due to spread of infection or secondary infection and include sinusitis, pharyngitis, laryngitis, tracheitis, bronchitis and pneumonitis.

Treatment: a day or two in a warm room helps to prevent both complications and spread of virus to others, and may shorten the disease. 1% ephedrine nasal drops improve the airway. Analgesics, e.g. aspirin, for headache.

Allergic Rhinitis. In allergic rhinitis ('hay fever') the nasal discharge contains eosinophils.

Investigation: skin prick or nasal instillation testing for allergens.

Treatment: antihistamine orally or by nasal spray, 1% ephedrine nasal drops, hydrocortisone snuff, or intranasal cromoglycate (Rynacron). Removal of nasal polyps. Diathermy of the inferior concha to relieve oedematous obstruction. Desensitisation: a series of injections of the offending allergen, e.g. pollen, is given before the 'hay fever' season.

Vincent's Angina
This is an inflammation of the gums, mouth and throat, due to a spirochaete and a bacillus.

Treatment: penicillin or metronidazole.

Sinusitis
Sinusitis is inflammation of a nasal sinus (*Fig. 7.10*).

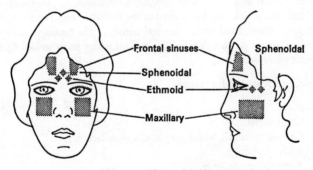

FIG. 7.10 The nasal sinuses

Acute Sinusitis. In acute sinusitis the mucous membrane is inflamed and oedematous and may block the opening into the nose. Pus forms in bacterial sinusitis.

Cause: common cold, allergy, infected water forced into the sinus during diving.

Clinically: there is a stuffy nose, nasal discharge, and headache which is worse on stooping. Tenderness is present over the inflamed sinus, and pain occurs in the sinus if its outlet is blocked. Referred pain may be felt in nearby teeth.

Treatment: rest in bed in a warm room. Nasal decongestant spray or drops, e.g. ephedrine, and steam inhalations, four-hourly. Analgesic, e.g. aspirin, for pain. Antibiotic for pyogenic infection.

Chronic Sinusitis. This may follow acute sinusitis, especially if there is a physical defect in the nose such as polypi, deviated septum or enlarged turbinate bone. Maxillary sinusitis may be caused by a dental abscess in the upper jaw.

Clinically: headache and nasal catarrh.

Treatment: the sinus should drain freely and a hole is made in it if necessary. A deviated septum is straightened, polypi and enlarged turbinates are removed.

Investigations in Sinusitis: transillumination of the sinus and X-ray show opacity due to thickened mucous membrane, fluid or pus.

Complications: post-nasal drip may cause laryngitis and bronchitis. Frontal and ethmoidal sinusitis may cause infection of the orbit, meningitis, cerebral abscess, cavernous sinus thrombosis or osteomyelitis.

Tonsillitis

Causes: (1) β-haemolytic streptococci; (2) glandular fever; (3) adenovirus infections. It is important to distinguish these from diphtheria.

β-Haemolytic Streptococcal Tonsillitis

Clinically: there is sore throat with difficulty in swallowing, pyrexia up to 40°C (104°F) and pain which may be referred to the ear. The lymph nodes in the neck are enlarged, inflamed and tender (cervical adenitis). The tonsils are enlarged and inflamed and exude pus which is easily wiped off with a swab, unlike diphtheritic membrane which adheres.

Investigation: throat swab for culture.

Complications:
1 Otitis media.
2 Chronic tonsillitis, which may require tonsillectomy.
3 Acute nephritis.
4 Acute rheumatic fever.
5 Quinsy (peritonsillar abscess), which may need opening to allow drainage.

Treatment: rest in bed. Aspirin for pain. Antibiotic, preferably benzylpenicillin 300 mg̀ (0·5 Mu) i.m. six-hourly, to prevent nephritis and rheumatic fever. Warm pad to the neck for painful glands. Adequate fluids (minimum of 2·5 l daily), semi-solid diet because of painful swallowing. Ice or ice cream relieves sore throat.

Adenoids (nasopharyngeal tonsils)
Adenoids are lymphoid tissue in the posterior wall of the nasopharynx (*Fig. 7.1*).

Clinically: chronic infection causes the adenoids to enlarge, obstructing the posterior part of the nose and causing mouth-breathing, a 'nasal' voice, snoring and coughing. Enlarged adenoids block the opening of the Eustachian tube causing earache and deafness, and predispose to otitis media and bronchitis.

Treatment: surgical removal of the tonsils (which are also enlarged) and adenoids. Improve general health with good food, vitamins and fresh air.

Pharyngitis

Although streptococcal tonsillitis and glandular fever cause inflammation of the pharynx they are usually considered separately from pharyngitis. The other causes of pharyngitis are usually viruses, especially Coxsackie-A viruses which cause herpangina.

Clinically: the throat is sore and inflamed and there is anorexia, headache, malaise and fever. In herpangina there are vesicles, which become ulcers, present on the fauces.

Treatment: antibiotics are ineffective against viruses. Local anaesthetic lozenges, e.g. benzocaine Co. lozenges, relieve pain, and codeine compound tablets relieve headache.

Laryngitis

Inflammation of the larynx may be due to:

1 Virus infections, e.g. common cold, measles.
2 Pulmonary tuberculosis.
3 Trauma—auctioneers, singers, lecturers, politicians.
4 Inhalation of irritant gases, smoking.
5 Chronic nasal infection.
6 Allergy may cause oedema of the respiratory tract which is especially serious in the larynx.
7 Tumours.

Clinically: the voice is hoarse, whispering, or may be lost. Speaking is painful; the throat is dry and there is a non-productive cough. Narrowing of the larynx by oedema in children causes 'croup'.

Treatment: rest in bed in a warm room, using a humidifier or a steam kettle nearby to keep the air moist. Speaking is avoided and the patient communicates using signs, whispering or writing. Smoking is prohibited. Linctus codeine 5 ml for cough.

Tracheitis

Inflammation of the trachea is due to infection, irritants or allergy and causes pyrexia, headache, and cough. *Treatment* is as for laryngitis.

Acute Bronchitis

Acute inflammation of the bronchi is caused by viruses (influenza, measles), bacteria (whooping cough, *H. influenzae*), or irritant gases. Secondary pyogenic infection with bacteria (streptococci and others) may follow upper respiratory infections due to a virus, e.g. the common cold. Bronchitis is predisposed by cold, damp and fog.

Note: acute bronchitis due to allergy is called asthma.

Clinically: irritating dry cough and upper retrosternal aching is followed by pyrexia, malaise, tightness in the chest, dyspnoea and mucoid (virus infection) or mucopurulent (bacterial infection) sputum which may be streaked with blood. Recovery takes a few days.

Complications:
1   Bronchiolitis, which is one cause of 'cot' death in infants.
2   Bronchopneumonia.
3   Bronchiectasis.
4   Chronic bronchitis.

Treatment: rest in bed in a warm room, humidified with a steam kettle or Mistogen humidifying machine or steam inhalations taken. Abundant fluids (at least 2·5 l daily). Oxygen for cyanosis. Bronchodilator, e.g. isoprenaline, for bronchospasm. Linctus codeine is given to suppress a dry cough, but not a productive one. Sedation at night. Antibiotic for bacterial infection (purulent sputum).

Chronic Bronchitis

Cause: chronic bronchitis is due to prolonged irritation of the bronchial mucosa, commonly by tobacco smoke but also by the dusts and fumes of general atmospheric pollution in industrial areas. Fog, dampness and sudden change in temperature are predisposing. Sometimes there is a familial predisposition, e.g. deficiency of anti-trypsin in the serum. Anti-trypsin normally prevents excessive damage to lung and other tissues by proteolytic enzymes released by bacteria and leucocytes during infection.

The irritation causes the bronchi to secrete an excess of mucus.

Clinically: repeated attacks of 'winter' or 'smoker's' cough increase in duration and severity until cough is present for most of the year. There is wheezing, dyspnoea and tightness in the chest, especially in the morning, improved by coughing up sputum, occasionally streaked with blood. Acute exacerbations due to bacterial infection cause pyrexia and cyanosis and the sputum becomes purulent. Patients may die in a few years from complications; others survive for 20 years with varying degrees of incapacity.

Complications: (1) Bronchopneumonia; (2) emphysema; (3) cardiac failure (cor pulmonale).

Prevention: smoking must be discontinued. Avoid badly ventilated, crowded places where respiratory infection is likely to be spread. Sleep in a warm bedroom. Avoid fog, go out in fog only if it is essential to do so, and then wear a well-fitted mask. Windows should be kept closed in foggy weather. Avoid dusty occupations—this may involve a reduction in income. Live away from industry. Spend as much time as possible, especially in winter, in a warm climate. Prevent atmospheric pollution.

Treatment: stop smoking. Breathing exercises to expand all lung tissue. Bronchial antispasmodic, e.g. ephedrine 60 mg b.d. orally; isoprenaline inhalation (excessive use may cause death from ventricular fibrillation); aminophylline, orciprenaline, salbutamol. Linctus codeine 5 ml orally to prevent unproductive cough at night and allow sleep, but not during the day since secretions will be retained in the lungs, worsen the infection, and obstruct bronchi, causing atelectasis. Steam inhalation four-hourly may loosen tenacious sputum. Oxygen 28% via a Venturi type of mask. Above 30% of oxygen is dangerous in chronic bronchitis and emphysema since it depresses respiration and may cause carbon dioxide narcosis and death for the reasons given under 'oxygen therapy'. Bromhexine (Bisolvon) 8–16 mg six-hourly orally, is said to liquefy secretions, then postural drainage with percussion to the chest. Antibiotic for five to seven days for infection according to sensitivity tests, e.g. tetracycline 250 mg six-hourly orally or co-trimoxazole. It is no longer advised to take an antibiotic throughout the winter since it does not prevent infection—resistant organisms readily cause infection, and antibiotics have side-effects—sore mouth, diarrhoea, superinfection.

Emphysema

Emphysema is unnatural distension with air which may enter the tissues anywhere, e.g. in the mediastinum or in the subcutaneous tissues (penetrating wound, post-operatively) where it gives a crackling sensation.

Pulmonary Emphysema

Pulmonary emphysema is overdistension of alveoli and occurs in bronchial asthma, obstruction of bronchi by tumours, mucus, foreign body (obstructive emphysema), and in chronic bronchitis. It causes impaired ventilation and exertional dyspnoea.

In emphysema due to chronic bronchitis the alveolar walls are destroyed, producing bullae (*Fig. 7.11*). This reduces the area over which blood can be oxygenated.

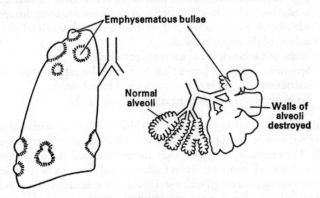

FIG. 7.11 Pulmonary emphysema

The muscular effort of breathing is increased, the ribs are raised causing the chest to become deeper (barrel-shaped), and the accessory muscles of respiration, e.g. the sternomastoids, are used. The loss of alveolar walls and their capillaries increases the pressure in the pulmonary artery and strains the right ventricle, leading to right ventricular failure, a common cause of death in chronic bronchitis and emphysema. Heart failure due to lung disease is called cor pulmonale.

Complications:

1 Ventilatory failure, causing hypoxaemia (a low oxygen concentration in the arterial blood) and hypercapnia (a high carbon dioxide concentration in the arterial blood).
2 Right ventricular failure.
3 Pulmonary bullae (large, thin-walled sacs) may rupture causing spontaneous pneumothorax.

Treatment is of the associated chronic bronchitis.

Bronchial Asthma

Bronchial asthma consists of recurrent attacks of dyspnoea and wheezing due to temporary narrowing of bronchi by bronchial muscle spasm, mucosal swelling and partial obstruction with viscid secretions. The narrowing is worse on expiration, it increases the work of breathing and reduces pulmonary ventilation. It must not be confused with cardiac 'asthma' which is acute pulmonary oedema due to cardiac disease.

Causes:

1 Allergic asthma is an hereditary abnormal reaction to allergens. The patients also have other allergies, e.g. hay fever, urticaria, eczema. The allergen is usually inhaled, e.g. dusts, house mites, pollens, spores of fungi, animal dandruff, hair (cats, dogs) or feathers (pillows, eiderdowns, pet birds), or biological detergents. Less often the allergen is ingested: fish, eggs, milk, chocolate, or drugs. Asthma due to inhaled or ingested allergens is called *extrinsic asthma.* This begins in childhood and often disappears in adolescence. Asthma in which there is no known allergen is called *intrinsic asthma* and this begins in middle age.
2 Bronchitic asthma is due to infection (bronchitis).
3 Spasmodic asthmatics have a history of psychological disturbance causing overaction of the vagus nerve, which causes bronchospasm.
4 β-adrenergic receptor blocking drugs e.g. propranolol.

Clinically: asthma affects any age, including children. There are attacks of sudden onset of tightness in the chest, dyspnoea and wheezing. Expiration is especially difficult. The respiratory and pulse rates are increased and the patient uses the accessory muscles of respiration. He is frightened and fears that he is suffocating. There is a dry cough or a cough with viscid mucoid sputum unless there is infection (bronchitic asthma) when the sputum is purulent. Cyanosis is central in type, and hypoxaemia may cause disturbances of consciousness.

Status Asthmaticus is asthma persisting for over 24 hours and it causes exhaustion.

Investigations:

1 Skin or inhalation sensitivity tests.
2 Chest X-ray.
3 Pulmonary function tests.

4 Blood may show an eosinophilia (increased number of eosinophil polymorphs) in allergic asthma.
5 Sputum may also contain eosinophils.

Complications:
1 Spontaneous pneumothorax.
2 Chronic bronchitis.
3 Emphysema.
4 Atelectasis.
5 Respiratory failure.

Treatment: Rest in bed propped up. Oxygen for cyanosis, using the M.C. mask or
polymask, which provide 60% oxygen if oxygen is given at four to six litres a
minute. Tranquilliser or mild sedative, e.g. diazepam 5–10 mg i.m., o.n., but heavy
sedation should be avoided since it may depress respiration, and morphine should
never be given.

Sympathomimetic drugs: isoprenaline aerosol or 20 mg sublingually; ephedrine
30 mg q.i.d. orally; adrenaline 0·1–0·5 ml of 1:1000 s.c. slowly, repeated after 30–60
minutes if necessary; salbutamol (Ventolin) aerosol or 4 mg q.i.d. orally, orciprenaline (Alupent) aerosol or 20 mg q.i.d. orally. The patient should be instructed not
to continue the use of a sympathomimetic drug unless relief is obtained, since excessive use may cause ventricular fibrillation and sudden death. In using an aerosol
the patient is taught to exhale, inhale from the spray and hold his breath, and to
expect tachycardia.

Antihistamines are usually ineffective and are undesirable since they dry the
respiratory secretions. Aminophylline 500 mg may be given slowly i.v., or as a
rectal suppository. Disodium cromoglycate (Intal) must be taken regularly to be
effective since it is said to act by preventing the release of histamine. 20 mg of
powder is inhaled two to eight times daily using an insufflator (spinhaler). It is not
absorbed from the gut. Ketotifen 1–2 mg (base) b.d.

Corticosteroids are used if sympathomimetics and theophylline fail and are given
for seven to fourteen days only owing to their serious side-effects, e.g. prednisolone 15 mg six-hourly on the first day, reducing the dose over seven to fourteen
days, or inhaled beclomethasone. Corticotrophin may be used in children.

Bromhexine (Bisolvon) 8–16 mg six-hourly may liquefy mucus.

Abundant fluids to prevent dehydration (which increases the viscosity of the
sputum). Antibiotic if infection is present. Change of clothing after sweating during
an attack. The correction of poor posture, and breathing exercises to prevent chest
deformity in children. Desensitisation may be tried, especially for pollen and house
mite allergy. Explain the cause and reassure the over-protective and anxious parents
of the asthmatic child.

Prevention: avoid allergens, e.g. feathers (use latex pillows and Terylene eiderdowns),
animal dandruff (the family pet is given away), certain foods and drugs (antibiotics,
antidepressants and aspirin may cause allergy). Vacuum-cleaning of the house, including mattresses (mites). Early treatment of respiratory infection. Psychotherapy:
hypnosis helps some patients.

Pneumonia

Pneumonia is inflammation of the lung. The inflamed areas become airless and solid (consolidated).

Causes: infection may be due to bacteria (pneumococci, streptococci, staphylococci, *H. influenzae*, rickettsiae), viruses (chickenpox), and rarely fungi. Lobar pneumonia is usually due to pneumococci and occurs in previously healthy people. Bronchopneumonia usually has a predisposing cause such as chronic bronchitis, and is caused by many different organisms.

Acute Lobar Pneumonia (pneumococcal pneumonia)

Acute lobar pneumonia is usually due to the pneumococcus which is spread by droplet infection. Usually only one lobe of the lung is affected (*Fig. 7.12*).

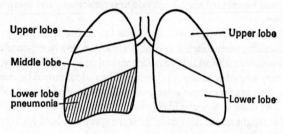

FIG. 7.12   Lobar pneumonia

Clinically: any age is affected but it is most common in young adults. The onset is sudden, with a rigor which causes a pyrexia of 39·5°C (103°F), and there may be vomiting and convulsions in children. There is malaise, anorexia, headache, generalised aching, and cough which is dry at first but viscid sputum follows and is rust-coloured due to blood. Pleurisy is due to inflammation spreading to the parietal pleura, and causes a stabbing pain in the chest wall; this pain is worse on coughing and deep breathing. Respirations are particularly rapid: usually 35 a minute in adults and 50 a minute in children. Respirations are shallow and painful. There is tachycardia, a hot dry skin, flushed face, cyanosis, restlessness, and there may be delirium. Herpes labialis is common and produces vesicles around the lips. If untreated at the end of about one week the patient sweats profusely, the temperature suddenly falls over a few hours, and the patient recovers, but chronic alcoholics or the elderly may die owing to a poor resistance.

Investigations: sputum contains pneumococci. The blood shows a polymorph leucocytosis, the white cell count being 15,000–30,000 per mm³ $(15-30\times 10^9/l)$.

Complications:
1   Pleural effusion, which may need aspirating.
2   Lung abscess.
3   Empyema (pus in the pleural cavity) needs surgical drainage.
4   Spread to other lobes.

5   Pneumococcal pericarditis.
6   Pneumococcal meningitis due to septicaemia. Rare.
7   Delayed resolution. Resolution usually takes two weeks but may be de-
    layed, to e.g. four weeks, if there is underlying bronchiectasis or carcinoma
    of the bronchus.
8   Cardiac failure is shown by a fall in the blood pressure, a rising pulse rate
    and increasing cyanosis.

Treatment: rest in bed in a well-ventilated room, sitting propped up on a back-rest.
The temperature, pulse and respiratory rate are taken four-hourly. Sponging with
tepid water is required if the temperature exceeds 39·5°C (103°F). Attention to the
dry mouth. Diet: semi-solids—milk, fruit juice, custard, junket, eggs, broth,
flavoured glucose solution. Fluid intake and output is recorded. Oxygen for
cyanosis. Antibiotic, e.g. benzylpenicillin 300 mg i.m. eight-hourly for 24 hours
then penicillin V 250 mg six-hourly orally. Occasionally streptomycin i.m. may
need to be added, or tetracycline given, according to the sensitivity of the organism.
Suppositories for constipation, e.g. bisacodyl (Dulcolax). Analgesic for pain, e.g.
pethidine 100 mg, and warm wool or an electrically heated pad may be applied to
the chest. Kaolin poultices are comforting but are messy. Linctus codeine 5 ml for
cough. Hypnotic, e.g. barbiturate or chloral at night. The patient is allowed up
when the temperature has been normal for two to four days.

Bronchopneumonia

Cause: bronchopneumonia usually has a predisposing cause such as:
1   Chronic bronchitis, in which the bronchi are already damaged and there
    is excessive mucus which obstructs smaller bronchi. Whenever there is
    obstruction of a tube, infection is common behind it.
2   Left ventricular failure. Organisms can grow more easily if there is fluid
    in the lungs and the patient's resistance is low.
3   Viral infections, e.g. following measles, when the patient's general health
    is reduced and the virus has also damaged the airways, making it easy for
    secondary infection with bacteria.
4   Hypostatic pneumonia follows operations or coma. Secretions accumulate
    in the bases of the lungs and become infected.
5   Aspiration of foreign material, e.g. pus from the sinuses in sinusitis, or
    secretions or vomit, e.g. during coma, draws infected material directly into
    the bronchi and lungs.
6   Bronchial obstruction, e.g by carcinoma, causes retention of bronchial
    secretions which become infected.
Bronchopneumonia is patchy and usually affects both lungs (*Fig. 7.13*). It may be
caused by many different types of organism, either by a single type of organism or
as a mixed infection.

Clinically: bronchopneumonia is commonest in children, the elderly and chronic
bronchitics. There is a history of the predisposing cause, e.g. acute bronchitis. The
pulse rate and temperature rise and there is dyspnoea, cyanosis, cough and purulent

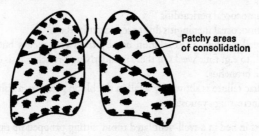

FIG. 7.13   Bronchopneumonia

sputum. Haemoptysis and pleurisy may occur and the patient may die from tox-aemia or cardiac failure.

Investigations: sputum for pus, types and sensitivities of organisms. Chest X-ray shows patchy shadowing. The blood shows a polymorph leucocytosis.

Treatment is as for lobar pneumonia except that the organisms are seldom sensitive to penicillin alone, therefore penicillin and streptomycin, tetracycline or other antibiotics are used according to the sensitivity of the organism. Expectoration is encouraged and cough suppressants are avoided.

Prevention: the elderly should not be confined to bed unless it is essential and then should be mobilised as soon as possible. Post-operatively patients should not smoke, should perform deep breathing exercises and should be given only the minimum amount of morphine since it causes respiratory depression which predisposes to hypostasis and atelectasis. Unconscious patients should be turned from one side to the other every one to two hours so that secretions drain from the bronchi into the trachea where they can be sucked out. Percussion applied to the chest, with postural drainage, helps to remove secretions.

Tuberculous Pneumonia may be lobar or bronchopneumonic. It is discussed under 'infectious diseases'.

Lung Abscess
A lung abscess is a localised collection of pus in the lung due to destruction of lung tissue (*Fig. 7.14*).

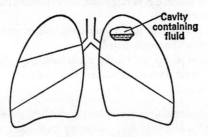

FIG. 7.14   Lung abscess

Causes:
1 Pulmonary tuberculosis.
2 Pneumonia, especially staphylococcal.
3 Bronchial obstruction and infection, e.g. bronchial stenosis, carcinoma of the bronchus, foreign body.
4 Inhaled septic material, e.g. from a dental or nose and throat (E.N.T.) operation, or vomit.
5 Infection of an area of previously damaged lung: bronchiectasis, necrotic malignant tissue.
6 Septicaemia may cause multiple small abscesses.
7 Extension from an adjacent infected organ such as oesophagus, mediastinal glands, or subphrenic abscess.

Clinically: there is cough with foetid, often bloodstained sputum if the abscess communicates with a bronchus; pyrexia; shivering; sweating; malaise; weight loss; finger clubbing; there may also be pleuritic pain. The patient is very ill and is likely to die if untreated.

Complications:
1 Spread of organisms via the blood may cause cerebral abscess or meningitis.
2 Spread through the lung causes pleurisy, empyema, or pericarditis.

Investigations: the blood shows a polymorph leucocytosis of $15-25 \times 10^9/l$, 15,000–25,000 per mm^3. Chest X-ray shows a cavity with a fluid level. Bronchoscopy to detect carcinoma of the bronchus. Sputum for organisms, especially T.B.

Prevention: precautions during E.N.T. operations to prevent the inhalation of blood and fragments of tissue. Removal of secretions by suction in a comatose patient.

Treatment: postural drainage; bronchoscopic aspiration; antibiotic, e.g. penicillin and streptomycin. General treatment as for pneumonia. Lobectomy (surgical removal of the affected lobe) if the abscess does not heal with medical treatment.

Bronchiectasis
Bronchiectasis is abnormal dilatation of bronchi.

Causes:
1 Pulmonary collapse due to obstruction of small bronchi. The collapsed tissue causes neighbouring bronchi to stretch to take up the space previously occupied by the collapsed portion of lung.
2 Bronchial distension by pus beyond an obstruction.
3 Congenital abnormality of the bronchi.
4 Damage to the bronchial wall by infection, e.g. whooping cough, measles, pneumonia, tuberculosis.

Clinically: bronchiectasis usually begins in childhood. The dilated bronchi are easily infected, causing cough with a large amount of purulent and sometimes foetid sputum (up to 350 ml daily), worse in the morning, with haemoptysis, pyrexia, malaise, weight loss, finger clubbing (the ends of the fingers become bulbous), and often anaemia. The foul smell of the sputum is due to stagnation of sputum in the bronchiectatic cavities which allows organisms to grow which cause putrefaction.

Complications:

1   Lung abscess.
2   Empyema.
3   Bronchopneumonia.
4   Pericarditis.
5   Septicaemia, which may cause abscesses anywhere e.g. in the brain.
6   Amyloidosis.

Investigations:

1   Bronchogram: X-ray after the injection of radio-opaque material into the bronchi.
2   Sputum. Volume, appearance, presence of organisms, especially T.B., odour.

Treatment: postural drainage for 10 minutes twice or three times daily. The patient is placed with the pelvis higher than the head so that gravity aids the drainage of sputum (*Fig. 7.15*). Physiotherapy includes slapping the chest wall over the affected

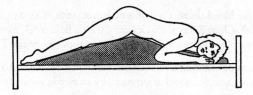

FIG. 7.15   Postural drainage

area, the encouragement of coughing and breathing exercises. Antibiotic. The diet must include adequate protein, i.e. 80–120 g daily, and vitamins. Bronchoscopic suction to empty the cavities. Associated infection, such as sinusitis, requires treatment. *Surgical treatment:* segmental resection of the lung or lobectomy.

Atelectasis (pulmonary collapse)

Atelectasis is partial or complete collapse of a lung, which becomes airless, contracted and solid (*Fig. 7.16*).

Causes:

1   Bronchial obstruction by inhaled foreign body, viscid mucus, tumour, blood clot from the upper respiratory tract, or pressure on a bronchus by enlarged lymph nodes. The air in the alveoli is absorbed and the lung collapses.
2   Pressure on the lung from a pleural effusion (hydrothorax) or air in the pleural sac (pneumothorax).
3   Decreased respiratory movements: poliomyelitis, injury, tight bandage around the chest, post-operative sedation, or pain.

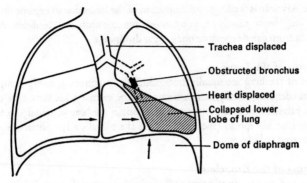

FIG. 7.16   Pulmonary atelectasis

4   Failure of the lung to expand in the fetus at birth due to over-sedation of the mother, the sedative depressing the fetal respiratory centres, or to abnormality of the lung, e.g. hyaline membrane disease.

Clinically: collapse of small segments of lung may be symptomless. In extensive atelectasis there is dyspnoea and cyanosis.

Complications:
  1   Infection of the collapsed part, which may become an abscess.
  2   Fibrosis and bronchiectasis.

Prevention: avoidance of heavy sedation, turning the unconscious patient to drain secretions from the bronchi, bronchial suction, breathing exercises, early ambulation. No smoking. Encouragement in coughing. The patient should sit up using a back-rest and not be slumped with an unexpanded chest.

Treatment: treatment of the cause, e.g. bronchial suction or postural drainage to remove secretions. Antibiotic for infection. Oxygen for cyanosis.

Occupational Lung Diseases
In certain occupations dust and fumes may be inhaled and cause damage to the lungs.

Pneumoconioses are diseases caused by mineral dusts which cause fibrosis of the lungs, e.g. silicosis in quarry workers and stone masons, coal-miners' pneumoconiosis (due to silica and coal dust), asbestosis due to asbestos dust. These are industrial diseases and disablement benefits are paid to sufferers and death benefits to widows.

Clinically: there is dyspnoea on exertion, slowly increasing over 10–30 years and the patient may die of respiratory or cardiac failure. Cough and sputum are due to bronchitis. Pulmonary tuberculosis may complicate silicosis or coal-miners pneumoconiosis.

Prevention: wearing of masks, damping the dust, efficient ventilation.

Treatment: the patient must change his occupation.

Allergic Alveolitis is allergic inflammation of the lungs due to organic dusts, e.g. farmer's lung due to mouldy hay, byssinosis due to cotton dust, bird-fancier's lung due to dust from dried pigeon or budgerigar droppings.

Neoplasms of the Lung

Tumours of the lung are usually malignant (e.g. carcinoma), rarely benign (e.g. bronchial adenoma). Malignant tumours may be primary, i.e. they arise directly from the bronchus or lung, or may be a deposit in the lung secondary to a cancer elsewhere that has spread (metastasised) via the blood or lymphatics, e.g. from breast, thyroid or kidney.

Carcinoma of the Bronchus

Carcinoma of the bronchus causes 40% of deaths from malignant disease in males. It spreads via the lymphatics to the supraclavicular, mediastinal and axillary lymph nodes and pleura, and via the blood to the liver, brain, adrenals, bones, skin and kidneys.

Cause: it is five times commoner in men than women, and most cases are due to cigarette smoking. Heavy smokers are forty times more liable to carcinoma of the bronchus than non-smokers, even if they live where there is no other form of atmospheric pollution, as in Iceland. It occasionally occurs in people working in industries using chromium, nickel and asbestos.

Clinically: cough is dry at first but later may produce bloodstained sputum; there is wheezing due to obstruction of the bronchus by the tumour, and weight loss. Infection in the lung behind the obstruction causes recurrent pneumonia and dyspnoea.

Pleurisy or pleural effusion may occur and is due to spread of infection from the pneumonia or to spread of the growth to involve the pleura. Pain in the chest due to involvement of nerves is late. Symptoms are also caused by spread of the tumour to other organs, e.g. brain. Most cases are untreatable and die within nine months. 25% of patients who are treated early live for five years.

Complications:
1 Spread to pleura, brain, liver, adrenal, bone, or lymph nodes.
2 Pneumonia (infection in secretions retained behind the obstruction).
3 Collapse of lung due to bronchial obstruction.
4 Lung abscess due to infection of the lung supplied by the obstructed bronchus, or to degenerating tumour.
5 Obstruction of the superior vena cava causing headache, dilated veins, and oedema of the head and arms.
6 Metabolic effects—neuropathy, Cushing's syndrome.

Investigations: sputum for malignant cells. Bronchoscopy. Chest X-ray. Lymph node biopsy.

Treatment: surgical—lobectomy or pneumonectomy. Radiotherapy alleviates symptoms in superior vena caval obstruction but is not curative. Antimitotic (cytotoxic) drugs are usually ineffective.

Prevention: stop smoking. Even those people who have smoked for years have a better chance of escaping from carcinoma of the bronchus if they give up smoking.

Sarcoidosis

Sarcoidosis is a disease affecting many organs in the body including the lungs, eyes, lymph nodes, spleen, liver, parotid glands and bones. The tissue shows fibrosis and follicles resembling those in tuberculosis but there is no caseation. It is sometimes due to toxins, e.g. beryllium, but most cases are of unknown cause. Treatment is often unnecessary, but corticosteroids are given if sarcoidosis involves the eyes.

Cystic Fibrosis

Cystic fibrosis (mucoviscidosis) is an hereditary disease due to an autosomal recessive gene in which glandular secretions are excessively viscid.

Clinically: there is chronic bronchial and pulmonary infection, pancreatic insufficiency causing steatorrhoea, and a high level of sodium in the sweat. Concentrated secretions block the bronchial, pancreatic and other ducts.

Treatment: antibiotic for infection. Dietary fat is reduced and pancreatin is given with each meal.

Haemothorax

Haemothorax is blood in the pleural cavity. The haemorrhage causes shock, and there may be sudden death. Treatment is by aspiration of clot and serum, blood transfusion, and thoracotomy (surgical opening of the chest) to attend to bleeding points if necessary.

Pneumothorax

Pneumothorax is the entry of air into the pleural cavity. This releases the elastic tension of the lung which then collapses.

Causes:

1 Trauma. A penetrating wound of the chest wall allows air to enter the pleural cavity (*Fig. 7.17*).
2 Diseased lung may rupture (= spontaneous pneumothorax) and air enters the pleural cavity through the hole in the lung, e.g. ruptured emphysematous bulla, congenital cyst of the lung, or tuberculous focus.
3 Therapeutic pneumothorax was once used in the treatment of pulmonary tuberculosis.

Clinically: there is usually a sudden onset of acute pain in the chest with cyanosis, rapid and shallow breathing, and shock—rapid feeble pulse, pale, cold, clammy skin. The affected lung does not move with respiration. Sometimes the opening is valvular and allows air to enter but not to leave the pleural cavity with each breath ('tension' pneumothorax) and the patient may die in a few minutes or so.

Treatment: rest in bed, in the sitting position. Analgesic for pain. In a small pneumo-thorax the air is absorbed without treatment. In a large pneumothorax with

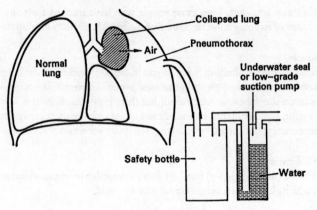

FIG. 7.17   Pneumothorax

moderate or severe dyspnoea a rubber catheter or needle is inserted into the pleural cavity through an intercostal space and the other end connected to an underwater seal (*Fig. 7.17*). Each time the patient coughs, air is expelled along the tube. Low-grade suction may be used. Surgery may be required in recurrent pneumothorax or pyopneumothorax.

Pleurisy

Pleurisy is inflammation of the pleura. The inflamed membrane becomes swollen and congested and serum exudes on to the surface and deposits fibrin which causes roughening of the surface. The two layers of pleura no longer move smoothly over each other but rub together causing pain, and a coarse crackling sound—a friction rub—is heard with the stethoscope. This is 'dry' pleurisy. If much fluid exudes (pleural effusion) the surfaces are pushed apart and pain disappears. The fluid is clear (serous). The fluid may become turbid due to infection and pus, and is then known as an empyema, or it may become blood-stained, as in tuberculosis and carcinoma. The exudate may be absorbed completely or the pleural surfaces may adhere and thicken (chronic or adherent pleurisy).

Causes:

1   Spread of infection from the lung: pneumonia, pulmonary tuberculosis, lung abscess, bronchiectasis.
2   Spread of infection through the diaphragm from an abdominal infection, e.g. peritonitis.
3   Septicaemia.
4   Carcinoma of the lung.
5   Pulmonary infarct.
6   Injury, e.g. stab wound, fractured rib penetrating the pleura.
7   Chronic nephritis.

Clinically: acute dry pleurisy causes sharp pain (a 'stitch') in the chest wall, worse on coughing and breathing, thus respirations are shallow. Movement of the chest wall, and therefore pain, is less on lying on the affected side. There is pyrexia, dry cough, and a friction rub. Diaphragmatic pleurisy is inflammation of the pleura lining the diaphragm and adjacent lung, and the pain may be felt in the epigastrium and be referred to the tip of the shoulder because the nerve supplying the diaphragm (the phrenic nerve) arises from the cervical nerve roots which also supply the shoulder. The affected side of the diaphragm is prevented from moving fully and there is 'guarding' by (contradiction of) the upper abdominal muscles, and hiccough.

Complications: (1) pleural effusion; (2) empyema; (3) chronic pleural thickening.

Treatment: rest in bed. Pain is reduced by strapping applied to the affected side during full expiration. The strapping should overlap the normal side by 10 cm (4 inches) front and back. A kaolin poultice, or warm pads also relieve pain. Warm pads have to be applied to the chest more frequently than a kaolin poultice but are less messy. An analgesic is also given, morphine 15 mg, pethidine 100 mg, or aspirin and a sedative. Antibiotic is given if there is infection.

Pleurisy with Effusion. Effusion separates the inflamed layers of pleura and pain disappears. As the amount of fluid increases the lung collapses and large effusions, e.g. 3 litres, cause dyspnoea and push the heart towards the opposite side. A moderate effusion is absorbed in about four weeks.

Complications: (1) empyema; (2) cardiac failure.

Investigations: (1) A little fluid is aspirated for examination for organisms, especially tubercle bacilli; (2) chest radiograph.

Treatment: rest in bed. Antibiotic for infection. Aspiration is not necessary unless there is dyspnoea. Treatment of the cause.

Pleural Effusion
Pleural effusion is the accumulation of fluid between the two layers of the pleura (*Fig. 7.18*).

Cause:
    A An Exudate is an effusion caused by inflammation and has a high content of protein. It may be cloudy from blood or pus and is due to:

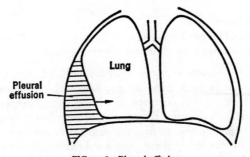

FIG. 7.18   Pleural effusion

1 Pneumonia.
2 Pulmonary tuberculosis.
3 Pulmonary infarct.
4 Carcinoma of the lung or breast.
5 Injury.

B   A Transudate (hydrothorax) is clear, sterile and low in protein and is due to:

1 Increased venous pressure, as in cardiac failure.
2 A low blood protein level (hypoproteinaemia) which causes a low osmotic pressure of the blood, hence fluid is not adequately reabsorbed into the blood capillaries from the tissues and body cavities, e.g. cirrhosis of the liver, nephrotic syndrome.
3 Fluid retention, as in renal failure.

Clinically: the fluid causes pressure on the lung which collapses and causes dyspnoea and cyanosis.

Treatment: fluid is aspirated (paracentesis thoracis) if it is causing dyspnoea. Following aspiration the pulse is checked half-hourly for several hours, and cyanosis and dyspnoea are watched for since acute pulmonary oedema may occur.

Empyema Thoracis

An empyema is a collection of pus in a cavity. Empyema thoracis is pus in the pleural cavity. Pus consists largely of leucocytes, mostly neutrophil polymorphs, but a few other cells and organisms, e.g. tubercle bacilli or staphylococci, are present depending on the cause.

Cause: spread to the pleura of adjacent infection in the lung, abdomen or chest wall.

Clinically: pyrexia due to the adjacent infection fails to respond to antibiotics and may increase; there is malaise, rigor, sweating, anorexia, weight loss, pleuritic pain in the early stages, and dyspnoea when the empyema is large and compressing the lung. The patient may die from toxaemia.

Complications:

1 The empyema may burst through the chest wall, the lung and bronchus, the pericardium, or the oesophagus, forming a fistula.
2 Collapse of lung, which may be permanent and cause scoliosis.

Investigations:

1 Chest X-ray.
2 The blood shows a leucocytosis.
3 Diagnostic aspiration and examination for organisms.

Treatment: The pus is aspirated on alternate days and antibiotic is injected into the empyema space, or the pus is drained using an intercostal tube attached to an underwater seal. If the pus is thick open operation (thoracotomy) may be needed and a wide bore open drain is inserted through a space made by removing a portion of a rib. In such cases the empyema and its surrounding sac may be excised complete (decortication) so that the lung can expand and function properly. Antibiotic is given orally. Breathing exercises help to re-expand the lung.

Respiratory Failure

Respiratory failure is the presence of hypoxaemia (a low level of oxygen in the arterial blood) and often hypercapnia (an increased level of carbon dioxide in the arterial blood).

Causes:

1. Depression of the respiratory centres in the brain by: (*a*) poisoning e.g. with barbiturates; (*b*) intracranial haemorrhage; (*c*) severe shock.
2. Restricted respiratory movements caused by : (*a*) pulmonary oedema or fibrosis; (*b*) pleural effusion; (*c*) pneumothorax; (*d*) paralysis due to poliomyelitis or neuropathy.
3. Obstruction of the airway with mucus, mucosal oedema, and/or bronchial muscle spasm, as in chronic bronchitis and in asthma.
4. Failure of alveolar function due to: (*a*) loss of alveoli caused by fibrosis or emphysema; (*b*) pneumonia.

Clinically: oxygen deficiency causes cyanosis and confusion; excess carbon dioxide causes tachycardia and dyspnoea. Other symptoms are of the cause.

Investigations:

1. Chest X-ray.
2. The forced expiratory volume in one second is reduced.
3. Blood oxygen (low) and carbon dioxide (high) content.

Treatment: treatment of the cause. Clear airway. Oxygen. Nikethamide (Coramine) 2–10 ml i.v. to stimulate the respiratory centres. Stop smoking. Tracheostomy and intermittent positive pressure ventilation (I.P.P.V.) if necessary.

8   THE DIGESTIVE SYSTEM

The Alimentary Tract

The alimentary tract is about 8·5 m (28 feet) in length, begins at the mouth; continues as the pharynx, oesophagus, stomach, small and large intestine; and ends at the anus.

Function. Nutritive substances taken into the alimentary tract (ingested) are complex materials which have to be broken down (digested) into simple substances which can then be transferred to the blood (absorbed). Food substances which cannot be absorbed, e.g. cellulose, are excreted from the bowel as faeces.

Digestion begins with the mechanical breakdown of food by chewing (mastication), followed by the chemical breakdown by digestive enzymes provided by the salivary glands, mucosa of the stomach and small intestine, and the pancreas, and aided in the stomach by hydrochloric acid and in the intestine by bile.

So that the food can be broken down fully it has to be thoroughly mixed with the digestive juices. The gastro-intestinal tract has a muscular layer which undergoes contractions (peristalsis and other movements) which aid mixing and the movement of food along the tract.

Ingested starch (one form of carbohydrate) is broken down into glucose, fat into fatty acids and glycerol, protein into amino acids, and at the same time the vitamins and minerals combined with the food substances are released ready for absorption.

Carbohydrates: starches are one form of polysaccharide ('many sugars') and consist of a chain of many glucose molecules joined together. Starch is present in peas, beans, potatoes and cereals and therefore in cereal products such as flour, bread, cakes and biscuits. Other carbohydrates are lactose in milk, fructose in fruit, and sucrose from sugar cane and sugar beet. The breakdown of starches begins in the mouth where salivary amylase (ptyalin) changes them into smaller carbohydrates (dextrins and maltose). The reaction continues in the stomach until it is prevented by hydrochloric acid mixing with the food, but continues again in the small intestine under the action of pancreatic amylase which converts polysaccharides such as starches and dextrins into the disaccharide maltose (two joined molecules of glucose.) The small intestine secretes enzymes (maltase, sucrase and lactase) which convert disaccharides (maltose, sucrose and lactose) into monosaccharides, e.g. glucose, which are absorbed.

Proteins consist of polypeptides. Polypeptides are amino acids joined together to form chains. Protein digestion begins in the stomach where pepsins (enzymes which act on polypeptides) and hydrochloric acid break parts of the protein molecules to form smaller polypeptides (peptones). In the small intestine trypsin and chymotrypsins, enzymes secreted by the pancreas, break down the polypeptides into still smaller polypeptides and dipeptides (a combination of two amino acids). These are then split into amino acids by peptidases (enzymes which act on peptides) secreted by the pancreas and intestinal mucosa. Cell nuclei are also proteins (nucleic acids) and are broken down by nucleases secreted by the pancreas. The amino acids are then absorbed from the small intestine. Undigested protein normally is not absorbed, but may be absorbed in certain diseases and cause the formation of antibodies against the protein, e.g. in ulcerative colitis the serum may contain antibodies to milk protein owing to the passage of protein through the ulcerated mucosa. The absorption of egg protein in infants causes allergy to eggs which is usually lost as the child grows older.

Fats (Lipids): the digestion of fats, e.g. triglycerides, begins in the duodenum where they are firstly emulsified by the detergent action of bile salts which are made in the liver and stored in bile in the gall bladder. After emulsification fats are broken down by lipase, an enzyme secreted by the pancreas. Triglycerides are broken into monoglycerides, glycerol and fatty acids. Bile salts, monoglycerides and fatty acids aggregate to form micelles ('organised grains') which are absorbed into the cells of the mucosa of the small intestine. From the mucosal cells small fatty acids enter the portal blood, but large fatty acids and other fats form small globules (chylomicrons) which enter the lymphatics. The bile salts pass back to the liver for re-use.

Vitamins and Minerals: the fat-soluble vitamins (A, D, E, and K) can be absorbed only along with fat, and their absorption is deficient if there is a lack of lipase, as in pancreatic disease, or a lack of bile, as in obstructive jaundice.

Water-soluble vitamins (the B group and C) are readily absorbed as are sodium and potassium.

Calcium is absorbed according to bodily needs and requires the influence of vitamin D. Its absorption is reduced by phosphate (in cereals) in the diet since this forms insoluble calcium phosphate.

THE MOUTH (ORAL CAVITY)

The mouth (*Figs. 7.1 and 8.1*) is lined with mucous membrane which is covered with squamous epithelium and contains mucous glands (glands which secrete mucus). The mouth is mostly surrounded with muscles (the muscles of the lips, cheeks, soft palate, pharynx and tongue). The mouth is separated from the nasal cavity by the palate which consists of an anterior bony portion (the hard palate) and a posterior muscular portion (the soft palate) from which hangs the uvula, a projection of muscle covered with mucous membrane.

Stomatitis is inflammation of the mucous membrane of the mouth. Inflammation may involve the gums (gingivitis), lips (cheilitis, cheilosis), angles of the mouth (angular stomatitis), or tongue (glossitis).

Acute Catarrhal Stomatitis is caused by measles, chemical irritation (smoking, excessive alcohol), carious teeth, or severe illness since infection is predisposed by a dry mouth due to dehydration and diminished salivation. Infection may spread up

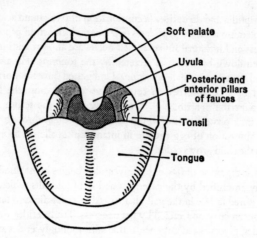

FIG. 8.1 The mouth

the parotid duct and produce suppurative parotitis. Stomatitis causes a red, painful and tender mouth, and a furred tongue; the breath may be offensive. It is prevented by oral hygiene, adequate hydration and the avoidance of irritants. Treatment is by rehydration of a dehydrated patient, stimulation of the flow of saliva with chewing gum or fruit juice, mouth washes with hydrogen peroxide solution (B.P.) 15 ml in half a tumblerful of warm water, and swabbing with glycerin and boric acid.

Thrush is an infection with the fungus *Candida* (*Monilia*) *albicans* which is predisposed by malnutrition in children, treatment with antibiotics (which suppresses the normal flora and allows fungi to grow) or corticosteroids, or by severe debility. White spots cover ulcers in the mucosa and may coalesce to give a 'thrush's breast' appearance.

Treatment is by painting with 1% gentian violet solution twice daily, swabbing with nystatin, or sucking nystatin tablets or amphotericin lozenges q.i.d.

Aphthous Stomatitis is due to a virus and consists of small painful ulcers in the mucosa. There is no specific treatment.

Benzocaine lozenges relieve pain in all types of stomatitis.

Non-specific Stomatitis is due to various micro-organisms and occurs in agranulocytosis and leukaemia.

Allergic Stomatitis may be due to toothpaste, dentures, antibiotics, or chemicals in sweets.

The Tongue
The tongue consists of muscle covered with mucous membrane which has numerous small projections (papillae) containing the nerve endings of the sense of taste (taste buds). Its muscle assists in chewing (mastication), swallowing (deglutition) and speech.

Glossitis is inflammation of the tongue and has the same causes as stomatitis. Ulceration of the tongue is due to broken teeth, ill-fitting dentures, tuberculosis, syphilis or carcinoma of the tongue.

The Teeth

The teeth are embedded in sockets in the upper and lower jaws (maxilla and mandible). Children have a temporary set of 20 deciduous teeth which are replaced by 32 permanent teeth between the ages of six and 24 years. In each half of the upper and lower jaws there are two incisors for cutting, one canine for tearing, two premolars and three molars for grinding and chewing food. Lack of teeth prevents proper mastication.

A tooth (*Fig. 8.2*) consists of a crown which protrudes from the gum, a root embedded in the bone with cement, and a neck between the crown and the root.

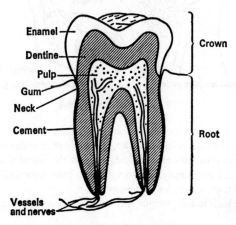

FIG. 8.2 A tooth, sectioned

The crown consists of very hard enamel beneath which is dentine. At the centre of the tooth is the pulp which contains blood vessels and nerves which enter via holes in the root.

Dental Caries (decay) is due to the growth of bacteria in food débris around the teeth and is reduced by regular cleaning of the teeth (brushed away from the gum) and by adequate vitamin C, vitamin D and calcium given to the growing child during the development of the teeth. The dentist should be visited regularly, e.g. every 6 months.

Pyorrhoea is purulent infection of the gum around the teeth, usually due to infection of food débris, and requires oral hygiene and hydrogen peroxide mouthwashes.

Haemorrhage from a tooth socket may follow the extraction of a tooth. The patient should bite on a rolled gauze swab for 15 continuous minutes. Prolonged haemorrhage may be due to blood disease, e.g. haemophilia.

Halitosis ('bad breath') is due to dental, sinus or tonsillar sepsis or poor oral hygiene.

The Salivary Glands (*Fig. 8.3*)

There are three pairs of salivary glands: the parotid, submandibular and sublingual. They consist of lobules of cells which secrete saliva which passes along the salivary ducts into the mouth. The flow of saliva is controlled by the autonomic nervous

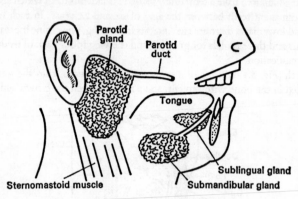

FIG. 8.3   The salivary glands

system as a reflex response to food in the mouth (unconditioned reflex) or to the sight or smell of food (conditioned reflex learned from previous experience). The function of saliva is to lubricate the food, to begin the digestion of cooked starch by the action of the enzyme ptyalin (α-amylase), to dissolve food in order to provide the sensation of taste, and to cleanse the mouth.

Dehydration leads to a dry tongue and mouth and predisposes to stomatitis and parotitis.

Parotitis is inflammation of the parotid glands and may be due to the mumps virus or to bacteria (septic parotitis). Septic parotitis is due to a dry mouth in an ill patient and is prevented by adequate hydration and proper care of the mouth. Treatment is with antibiotic, and surgical drainage if there is an abscess.

Parotid Tumours are usually benign but spread locally and require surgical excision.

A stone (calculus) in a salivary duct obstructs the duct and causes painful swelling of the gland during the secretion of saliva, i.e. when food is taken.

The Care of the Mouth

This is important in order to prevent stomatitis and parotitis, as well as for the patient's comfort. The mouth should be cleaned at least twice daily, and more often in fever, respiratory infection and coma, in which the mouth becomes dry.

Method: reassure the patient and explain the procedure. Screen the bed. The nurse's hands are washed and dried. A tissue is placed under the patient's chin, any dentures removed and placed in fresh water, adding whitener or antiseptic, e.g. 'Steradent', if required. First the lips, then the gums, tongue and teeth, are swabbed with gauze held in forceps and moistened with sodium bicarbonate solution, with particular attention to the space between the gums and teeth. The teeth are cleaned with an up and down movement. Gently remove any crusts. The procedure is repeated using glycothymoline. The mouth is rinsed with mouthwash such as glycothymoline. The dentures are cleaned and replaced, except in comatose patients, in whom dentures may slip into the larynx and cause asphyxia. A drink of water, lemonade, or fruit juice is given, if allowed. To prevent cracking, the lips are kept moist with glycerin, liquid paraffin, or petroleum jelly (Vaseline). Used swabs are placed in a disposable bag, which is sealed and burnt.

Swallowing (deglutition)
After mastication the bolus of food is pushed backwards into the pharynx by the tongue, the soft palate closes the nasopharynx, the larynx rises and is closed by the epiglottis and the muscles of the pharynx contract to push the bolus into the oesophagus where a wave of peristalsis is stimulated and carries the bolus into the stomach.

Dysphagia is difficulty in swallowing. It is caused by pain (glossitis, pharyngitis, tonsillitis, quinsy); paralysis of the muscles of deglutition (poliomyelitis, diphtheria, motor neuron disease); diseases of the oesophagus (oesophagitis, achalasia, carcinoma); pressure on the oesophagus (goitre, enlarged mediastinal glands); or hysteria.

The Plummer–Vinson Syndrome usually affects middle-aged women. It is dysphagia, glossitis, hypochlorhydria (low hydrochloric acid secretion by the stomach) and hypochromic anaemia, due to atrophy of the epithelium of the tongue, pharynx, oesophagus and stomach associated with deficiency of vitamin B and iron. It predisposes to carcinoma of the hypopharynx. *Treatment:* Vitamin B Co. and iron.

THE OESOPHAGUS

The oesophagus (gullet, *Fig. 8.4*) is 25 cm (10 inches) long and lies in front of the vertebral column and behind the trachea and heart. On passing through an opening in the diaphragm it joins the stomach. The oesophagus has four layers of tissue: the outer coat of fibroelastic tissue, a muscular layer of longitudinal and circular fibres, a submucosal layer containing blood and lymphatic vessels and autonomic nerves, and an inner lining of squamous epithelium and mucus-secreting glands.

Oesophageal Obstruction
Obstruction of the oesophagus (*Fig. 8.5*) may be due to the impaction (jamming) of a foreign body (swallowed toothplate, piece of bone), stricture of the oesophagus (which is due to the contraction of scar tissue following an injury to the wall by swallowed corrosives or reflux oesophagitis), cancer of the oesophagus or the upper

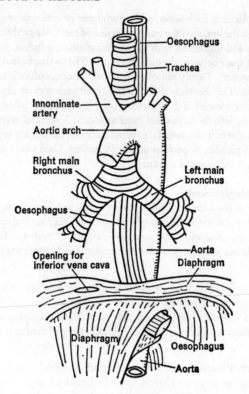

FIG. 8.4   The relations of the oesophagus

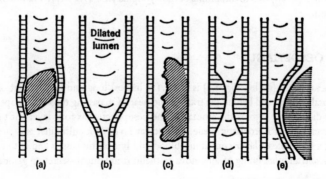

FIG. 8.5   Oesophageal obstruction: (a) foreign body; (b) achalasia; (c) carcinoma; (d) stricture (stenosis); (e) external pressure

end of the stomach, achalasia of the oesophagus (failure of relaxation of the muscle of the oesophageal 'sphincter'), pressure on the oesophagus by an aortic aneurysm or retrosternal goitre, or hysteria.

Clinically: there is dysphagia (difficulty in swallowing) and liquids and semi-solids are more easily swallowed than solids (except in hysteria). The patient may be able to indicate the level of the obstruction. Prolonged dysphagia causes malnutrition, emaciation and ketosis. Ketosis is due to the use of stored fat for energy and may cause ketonuria (ketones, e.g. acetone, in the urine).

Investigations: oesophagoscopy (the examination of the oesophagus through a tube, containing a light, passed into it) reveals tumour, stricture, inflammation or foreign body.
    Barium swallow—the patient is X-rayed on swallowing barium which outlines the oesophagus.

Treatment: treatment of the cause, e.g. removal of a foreign body or dilatation of a stricture with bougies. A semi-solid diet can be more easily swallowed than a solid one and includes milk, beaten eggs, custard, thickened soups, fruit juices and sugar. Small amounts are given frequently.

Achalasia of the Oesophagus ('Cardiospasm')
Achalasia is failure of relaxation of the oesophagogastric ('cardiac') sphincter associated with faulty peristalsis of the oesophagus due to a defective parasympathetic nerve supply to the oesophageal muscle.

Clinically: it usually affects middle-aged females. Retrosternal dysphagia is due to food being retained in the oesophagus, which dilates. If the food stagnates there is a foul odour. Undigested food regurgitates and may enter the trachea and lungs and cause aspiration pneumonitis (aspiration pneumonia). Weight is lost.

Investigations: oesophagoscopy after washing out the oesophagus. Barium swallow shows the dilated oesophagus and lack of peristalsis.

Treatment:
    1 Regular stretching of the sphincter by passing a bougie or dilator into the lower end of the oesophagus, e.g. Plummer's hydrostatic bag, Starke's dilator, or gum-elastic dilators.
    2 Heller's operation (oesophagomyotomy) is an incision through the muscle of the sphincter.

Carcinoma of the Oesophagus
Carcinoma of the oesophagus is a squamous carcinoma which spreads to the lymph nodes draining the oesophagus. Its development is predisposed by smoking and it mostly affects males.

Clinically: age over 50 years. There is dysphagia, at first for solids, later for liquids, including saliva. Dysphagia is due to obstruction of the oesophagus by the growth. Undigested food regurgitates (pseudovomiting), there is retrosternal discomfort, and weight is lost. Often the patient can point to the spot where food is held up. Pressure by the growth on the trachea causes cough, hoarseness and dyspnoea. The patient usually dies in six to 12 months.

Complications: perforation into the trachea, bronchi or lung causes broncho-pneumonia or gangrene of the lung, and these may be followed by empyema. Perforation into the mediastinum causes mediastinitis. Dysphagia leads to malnutrition.

Investigations: oesophagoscopy shows the growth, and biopsy is taken for histological examination to confirm the diagnosis. Barium swallow shows the site of obstruction and the dilated oesophagus above it.

Cytology, for malignant cells, on fluid aspirated from the oesophagus.

Treatment: the cure rate of any treatment is low.

Surgical: oesophagectomy (excision of the involved part of the oesophagus) and oesophago–gastrostomy (the joining of the remaining end of the oesophagus to an opening in the stomach).

Palliative treatment is used if the growth is inoperable, i.e. has spread outside the oesophagus: the insertion of a Souttar's tube past the growth allows feeding through the tube, as does dilatation of a stenosing carcinoma.

Gastrostomy, the making of a stoma (opening) into the stomach, is not justified since it does not affect the tumour and feeding through an intra-oesophageal tube avoids operation.

Radiotherapy: has poor results but reduces dysphagia for a few months.

The diet has to be in the form of fluids.

If saliva cannot be swallowed it must be aspirated or expectorated.

Hiatus Hernia

An hiatus hernia (*Fig. 8.6*) is the protrusion of part of the upper end (fundus) of the stomach into the chest through the oesophageal opening in the diaphragm. (Hiatus = gap, hernia = the protrusion of a part through an abnormal opening.) It is usually due to a widening of the opening or to weakening of the connective tissue holding the oesophagus to the hiatus. The condition is predisposed by obesity and pregnancy, both of which increase the intra-abdominal pressure.

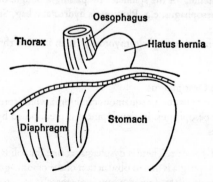

FIG. 8.6   Hiatus hernia

Clinically: age over 50 years. Hiatus hernia is often symptomless. It causes symptoms if the sphincter action at the lower end of the oesophagus is lost. This allows the regurgitation of acid gastric juice and causes reflux oesophagitis, i.e. the gastric juice begins to digest the oesophageal epithelium which cannot resist it.

The symptoms, investigations and treatment are the same as for reflux oesophagitis. The patient should sleep on the left side, which helps to prevent reflux.

Reflux (Peptic) Oesophagitis

Reflux oesophagitis is inflammation of the oesophagus due to regurgitation of gastric acid and pepsin into the oesophagus, caused by a hiatus hernia or repeated vomiting.

Clinically: burning pain ('heartburn') is felt behind the sternum and may be associated with the regurgitation of acid fluid into the mouth. The pain resembles that of angina pectoris but is not brought on by exertion. It follows large meals, stooping, lifting (which increases the intra-abdominal pressure), and lying down. It may be relieved by sitting up and by antacids. Chronic bleeding from the inflamed and ulcerated mucosa causes hypochromic anaemia.

Complications: stricture of the oesophagus due to fibrosis.

Investigations: oesophagoscopy reveals the inflammation. Barium meal shows an hiatus hernia.

Treatment: medical—reduction of weight if obese. Sleeping semi-upright at night, propped up on several pillows, with the foot end of the bed raised on blocks or on a chair to prevent the patient from sliding down the bed (*Fig. 8.7*). Avoidance of stooping and of tight clothes around the abdomen.

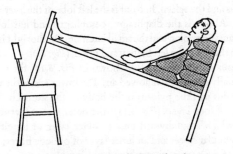

FIG. 8.7   Position for hiatus hernia

Diet: Small meals eaten slowly. An infant should be kept upright, its feeds thickened and a semi-solid diet given as soon as possible.

Peptic ulcer-type treatment for pain, i.e. antacids (magnesium trisilicate) hourly until pain ceases. Iron for anaemia.

Surgical: used if oesophagitis persists despite medical treatment. The operation closes the gap in the diaphragm and attaches the fundus of the stomach to the diaphragm. Dilatation of a stricture of the oesophagus.

THE STOMACH

Anatomy. The stomach is a **J**-shaped sac continuous with the oesophagus at the cardiac orifice which is at its upper end, and with the duodenum at the pyloric orifice which is at its lower end. It is situated in the epigastrium, but partly bulges into the umbilical region and left hypochondrium (*Fig. 8.8*).

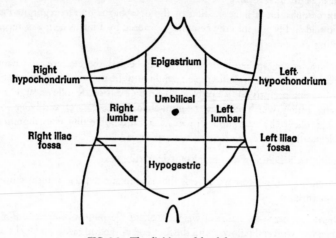

FIG. 8.8   The divisions of the abdomen

Behind the stomach lies the aorta, inferior vena cava, vertebral column, diaphragm, pancreas and the spleen. In front is the left lobe of the liver and the anterior abdominal wall. Above is the diaphragm, oesophagus and left lobe of the liver. Below lies the transverse colon and the small intestine. On the right is the duodenum and liver, and on the left is the left kidney and spleen (*Fig. 8.9*).

The subdivisions of the stomach are shown in *Fig. 8.10*; the upper part is the fundus and normally contains swallowed air. The lower end is the pyloric antrum. Between the fundus and the pylorus is the body of the stomach. The wall of the stomach consists of four layers (*Fig. 8.11*): the outer serous (peritoneal) coat; the muscular layer which is subdivided into an outer layer of longitudinal fibres, a middle layer of circular fibres and an inner layer of oblique fibres; the submucous layer consisting of connective tissue, blood and lymphatic vessels and autonomic nerves; and the inner lining of mucous membrane which has longitudinal folds (rugae) in it. The mucous membrane consists of columnar epithelium and goblet cells and contains numerous gastric glands.

Physiology. The functions of the stomach are:
1   To act as a temporary reservoir for food.
2   The secretion of gastric juice by the gastric glands. Gastric juice contains water, salts, hydrochloric acid (HCl), mucus and the enzymes pepsinogen, rennin and intrinsic factor. The water liquefies the food, the hydrochloric

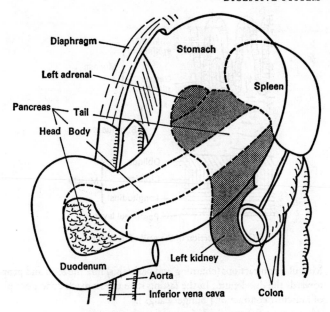

FIG. 8.9 The relations of the stomach

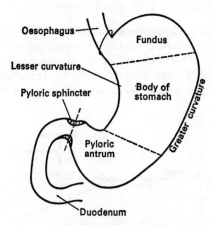

FIG. 8.10 The stomach

acid acidifies the gastric contents, killing many bacteria, making iron more soluble and converting the inactive pepsinogen into the active pepsin. Mucus protects the mucosa from acid and pepsin. Pepsin, assisted by strong acid (HCl) begins the breakdown of protein, converting it to peptones. Rennin clots milk in infants but is absent from adults. Intrinsic factor assists the release of vitamin B_{12} from protein.

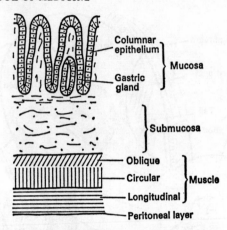

FIG. 8.11   Section of the wall of the stomach

3   Muscular contractions (churning and peristalsis) mix the food and propel it
    towards the duodenum. In the fasting state the stomach undergoes phases
    of muscular contraction ('hunger pangs').
4   Absorption of water, alcohol, glucose and some drugs.
5   The secretion of the hormone, gastrin, which is secreted directly into the
    blood and stimulates hydrochloric acid secretion.

The Control of Gastric Secretion and Motility is by the vagus nerves and
gastrin. The sight, odour or taste of food stimulates gastric secretion (cephalic phase)
by a reflex through the hypothalamus and the vagus nerves. Food entering the
stomach (gastric phase of secretion) stimulates the vagal reflex and also causes the
secretion, into the blood, of gastrin which stimulates the secretion of hydrochloric
acid (*Fig. 8.12*).

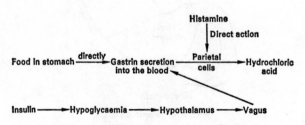

FIG. 8.12   The stimulation of gastric acid secretion

Vagotomy (cutting the vagus nerves) prevents the vagal stimulation of gastric
acid secretion and is used in the treatment of peptic ulcer. It also prevents gastric
motility and delays gastric emptying, and to prevent this pyloroplasty (division of
the pyloric muscle) must also be performed. The completeness of vagotomy can be
tested for by the insulin test described later.

SYMPTOMS AND SIGNS IN GASTRO-INTESTINAL DISEASE

Nausea is an unpleasant sensation in the epigastrium (feeling sick) due to changes in muscle tone and in peristalsis in the stomach. It may precede vomiting and has the same causes.

Vomiting (emesis) is the emptying of the stomach by the contraction of the abdominal wall and diaphragm with a relaxed cardiac sphincter and a closed glottis. It may be associated with reflex salivation (waterbrash), sweating and pallor, via the autonomic nervous system. In an unconscious patient the glottis may not close properly and vomit may be inhaled into the airway and cause asphyxia or pneumonia.

Causes:
1 Abdominal disease. Diseases of the stomach (gastric ulcer, pyloric stenosis, carcinoma, alcoholic gastritis); intestine (paralytic ileus, intestinal obstruction); gastro-enteritis; appendicitis; peritonitis; cholecystitis.
2 Sensitivity to food, e.g. mustard, fats, eggs.
3 Reflex vomiting due to pain, e.g. glaucoma, myocardial infarction, renal colic.
4 Diseases of the nervous system, e.g. increased intracranial pressure (meningitis, cerebral tumour or abscess); migraine; tabes dorsalis. Vomiting is not preceded by nausea.
5 Labyrinthine disturbance, e.g. travel sickness, vertigo.
6 Drugs and poisons, e.g. excessive intake of vitamin D, digitalis, morphine.
7 Endocrine disorders, e.g. Addison's disease, hyperparathyroidism, pregnancy (morning sickness, toxaemia), diabetic ketoacidosis.
8 Renal failure with uraemia.
9 Psychogenic, e.g. foul odour, unpleasant sight.

Vomiting may be induced as a first-aid measure by irritating the back of the throat with the fingers or by drinking warm salt solution.

Observations: the volume of vomit should be measured, its frequency, relation to food, and its appearance noted; i.e. the presence of bile, blood, undigested food, excess of mucus, and whether pain, if present, is relieved by vomiting.

Treatment:
1 Treat the cause.
2 Symptomatic treatment with antiemetics.
3 An unconscious patient who is vomiting must not be left on his own. The head should be turned to one side and vomitus removed from the mouth and pharynx by suction.

Flatulence ('wind', flatus) is the presence of air and other gases in the stomach and intestines. It is due to swallowed air, to carbon dioxide which is released from bicarbonate (in pancreatic secretions) by gastric acid, and to hydrogen and other gases caused by the fermentation of carbohydrates and the putrefaction of proteins by bacteria in the large intestine. Air may escape up the oesophagus (belching) or from the rectum. Borborygmi are sounds heard in the abdomen due to gas bubbling along the intestine.

Anorexia ('without appetite') may occur in many illnesses, or may be due to loss of the sense of smell, or to drugs such as amphetamines and cytotoxins.

Bulimia (increased appetite) may be due to habit; drugs such as oral contraceptives, corticosteroids and insulin; psychological compensation in frustration or loneliness; or giving up smoking.

Pain ('indigestion'). 'Heartburn' is a burning sensation behind the lower end of the sternum due to reflux of hydrochloric acid into an inflamed oesophagus, and is due to hiatus hernia, pregnancy or large meals. A burning pain in the epigastrium is due to gastric or duodenal ulcer. Colicky pain is due to increased peristalsis in the intestine because of intestinal irritation or obstruction. (Ureteric or biliary colic is due to obstruction of the ureter or biliary tract.) Continuous pain may be due to peritonitis or to the stretching of the capsule of an organ, e.g. the capsule of the liver in congestive cardiac failure. Pain may also be due to tabes dorsalis, aortic aneurysm, mesenteric embolism, pancreatitis, and many other conditions.

Pain sensation passes from the organ along the splanchnic sensory nerves to the posterior root ganglia of the spinal cord and then ascends in the spinal cord to the thalamus where it is relayed to the cerebral sensory cortex.

Hiccough is due to spasm of the diaphragm due to a reflex via the fourth and fifth segments of the cervical part of the spinal cord. It is caused by distension of the stomach, peritoneal irritation (e.g. peritonitis), uraemia, and encephalitis. Treatment is by taking a deep breath and holding it, or pressure on the epigastrium, e.g. by drawing the thighs up to the abdomen. Hiccough due to a serious disease may need chlorpromazine, the inhalation of amyl nitrite, or morphine.

Tenderness is pain felt on external pressure.

Rigidity is reflex spasm of muscle supplied by the same spinal segment which innervates the inflamed organ.

INVESTIGATIONS IN GASTRIC DISEASE

Endoscopy is the inspection of the interior of an organ using an illuminated hollow tube or a fibrescope, e.g. gastroscopy is the inspection of the stomach. The patient does not receive any food for eight hours before the examination. Local anaesthetic is used. A **biopsy** may be taken at the same time and examined microscopically.

The Investigation of Gastric Secretion

Fractional Test Meal (*Fig. 8.13*). After fasting overnight a Ryle's tube is passed via the nose into the stomach and the fasting juice is completely aspirated using a syringe attached to the Ryle's tube. In the original test meal 250 ml of porridge (gruel) was then eaten. In the alcohol test meal 100 ml of 7% alcohol is given in place of gruel. Samples of gastric contents are then aspirated every 15 minutes for $2\frac{1}{2}$ hours, completely emptying the stomach at $2\frac{1}{2}$ hours. Each sample is placed in a separate container labelled with the patient's name and the time it was taken. Each

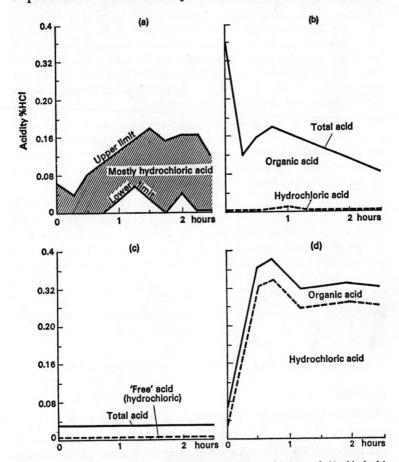

FIG. 8.13   Fractional test meal: (a) normal range; (b) carcinoma of the stomach; (c) achlorhydria; (d) hyperchlorhydria (e.g. duodenal ulcer)

sample is tested for 'free' acid, i.e. hydrochloric acid, and for organic acids, the two being 'total' acid. The samples are also examined for excess of mucus, bile and occult blood. In the gruel test the presence of starch is shown by a dark blue colour on adding iodine. The time of disappearance of the starch indicates the time taken for the stomach to empty.

The Augmented Histamine or Pentagastrin Test Meal. Histamine and penta-gastrin stimulate the secretion of hydrochloric acid when a gruel or alcohol test meal may show achlorhydria. The test has been described in Chapter 5, as has the 'tubeless' test using resin-dye.

Results: emptying of the stomach is delayed in pyloric stenosis and carcinoma of the stomach, thus there is an increased volume of fasting juice which contains organic acid (due to the fermentation of stagnant food by bacteria) but not free acid (*Fig. 8.13b*). Achlorhydria (absence of hydrochloric acid, *Fig. 8.13c*) occurs in chronic gastritis, carcinoma of the stomach, pernicious anaemia, and some patients with iron-deficiency anaemia. Hyperchlorhydria (increased secretion of hydrochloric acid, *Fig. 8.13d*) occurs in duodenal ulcer. Blood may be present in gastric juice due to bleeding from a carcinoma of the stomach or peptic ulcer, or may be due to trauma due to a roughly inserted Ryle's tube.

The Insulin Test Meal. This is used to determine whether vagotomy (cutting the vagus nerves) has been successful or not. Insulin causes hypoglycaemia (a low blood sugar) and a blood sugar below 2·5 mmol/l (45 mg%) stimulates the vagus nerves. If some vagal nerve fibres are intact hydrochloric acid will be secreted (*Fig. 8.12*) whereas if the vagus has been completely cut acid is not secreted.

Method: a Ryle's tube is passed into the stomach of the fasting patient, the stomach is emptied, and 20 units of soluble insulin are given intravenously. Gastric juice is aspirated every 15 minutes for 2½ hours. The blood sugar is checked 30 minutes after giving the insulin, and if it is above 2·5 mmol/l (45 mg%) more insulin is given to bring it below this level. A successful vagotomy will show an achlorhydria.

Detection of Bleeding

Faeces. Occult blood may be present in hiatus hernia, peptic ulcer or carcinoma of the stomach, and in diseases of the intestine such as carcinoma of the colon and ulcerative colitis.

The Blood Count may show a hypochromic anaemia if there is chronic bleeding.

Radiology

Plain Radiograph shows air under the diaphragm in perforated peptic ulcer.

Barium Meal shows a gastric ulcer crater, a filling defect due to carcinoma, the reflux of barium into the oesophagus in hiatus hernia, the rate of gastric emptying, and the shape, size, motility and position of the stomach.

Preparation for a Barium Meal: the patient is not allowed any medicines containing bismuth or calcium for three days before the X-ray since they cast shadows. Magnesium carbonate may be taken as an antacid. An aperient is given 24 hours beforehand. The patient fasts for at least six hours and is given neither solids nor fluids, and continues to fast until radiography is complete. In the evening a further aperient may be given to clear the barium from the intestines.

Cytology
Gastric cells obtained by lavage are examined for malignancy in suspected carcinoma.

DRUGS USED IN GASTRIC DISEASE

Antacids

Magnesium Salts. *Side-effects:* laxative in large doses. Magnesium trisilicate mixture B.P.C. 10 ml orally p.r.n. (contains sodium bicarbonate). Magnesium trisilicate powder 0·5–2 g orally in water p.r.n. Magnesium hydroxide mixture B.P 5–10 ml orally p.r.n. Magnesium oxide powder 250–500 mg p.r.n. is a powerful antacid (2–5 g as laxative). Magnesium trisilicate compound B.P.C. 1–2 tablets chewed before swallowing (contain aluminium hydroxide).

Magnesium carbonate liberates carbon dioxide and should not be used.

Aluminium Salts. *Side-effects:* constipation, reduced absorption of phosphate, tetracycline and vitamins. Aluminium hydroxide mixture 5–15 ml orally p.r.n.

Sodium Bicarbonate 1–5 g orally in water acts rapidly but liberates carbon dioxide which causes gastric distension and flatulence, and may cause alkalosis and renal damage if taken with milk (calcium) over prolonged periods (milk–alkali syndrome).

Proprietary Preparations are numerous and more costly but are usually no better than magnesium trisilicate.

Cimetidine (Tagamet) is not an antacid but it prevents the release of acid by blocking histamine H_2-receptors.

Antispasmodics

These are anticholinergic drugs (parasympatholytics) which prevent vagal nerve activity and therefore reduce gastric motility and vagal-stimulated, but not gastrin-stimulated, acidity. To be effective they have to be given in doses which paralyse cholinergic activity elsewhere, i.e. which cause side-effects such as blurring of vision, dry mouth, constipation and tachycardia.

Atropine sulphate 0·25–2 mg orally, s.c., i.m. or i.v. Belladonna tincture 0·5–2 ml orally. Propantheline (Probanthine) 15 mg orally six-hourly. Dicyclomine (Merbentyl) 10 mg six-hourly orally.

Liquorice Extracts

Carbenoxolone (Biogastrone) accelerates the healing of gastric ulcers. *Dose:* 50–100 mg t.d.s. *Side-effects:* sodium and water retention, oedema, hypertension and potassium deficiency. It may be given with a thiazide diuretic and potassium chloride. Spironolactone should not be used since it neutralises the healing effect of carbenoxolone. **Deglycyrrhizinised Liquorice** is ineffective. Each tablet of 'Caved-S' also contains 500 mg of antacid, the active agent.

Antiemetics

Hyoscine (scopolamine) hydrobromide 0·6 mg stat. then 0·3 mg six-hourly for travel sickness. *Side-effects:* dry mouth, blurred vision, constipation, difficulty in urination.

Antihistamines. *Side-effects:* drowsiness (danger if attempting to drive a vehicle), potentiation of hypnotics and alcohol.

Cyclizine (Valoid) 25–50 mg orally or i.m. p.r.n. Dimenhydrinate (Dramamine) 25–50 mg orally or i.m. p.r.n. (< 600 mg daily). Promethazine (Avomine, Phenergan) 25–50 mg daily orally or i.m. Mepyramine maleate (Anthisan) 25–50 mg orally, i.m. or i.v., p.r.n. Up to 600 mg daily may be given. Meclozine (Ancolan) 25–50 mg daily.

Phenothiazines. *Side-effects:* drowsiness, hypotension, Parkinsonism, agranulocytosis, rash, hypothermia.

Chlorpromazine (Largactil) 25–100 mg orally or i.m. Promazine (Sparine), perphenazine (Fentazin), prochlorperazine (Stemetil), and trifluoperazine (Stelazine) have a similar action.

GASTRIC DISORDERS

Acute Gastritis

Gastritis is inflammation of the mucous lining of the stomach.

Causes:
1. Badly chewed food due to bad eating habits or lack of teeth.
2. Excess of alcohol.
3. Irritants, e.g. excess of pickles, condiments, strong tea, tobacco chewing.
4. Drugs and chemicals, e.g. aspirin; swallowed corrosives such as lysol.
5. Swallowed infected material from the nose, sinuses or gums, or purulent sputum.
6. Reflux of bile into the stomach due to disturbed pyloric motility.
7. Food poisoning. Bacteria in food, e.g. salmonellae, or toxins produced by bacterial growth in food, e.g. staphylococci.
8. Viral gastritis or gastroenteritis ('gastric flu').

Clinically: anorexia, epigastric discomfort and tenderness, furred tongue, thirst, nausea, vomiting (which relieves pain), tachycardia, mild pyrexia.

Treatment: treat the cause, e.g. for poisons the stomach is washed out and the antidote given. Rest in bed. The diet is fluid at first (milk, jelly, custard), gradually adding solids as the patient improves.

Chronic Gastritis

Chronic gastritis has the same causes as those numbered one to six in acute gastritis, and also may be due to pyloric stenosis, smoking, or the habitual drinking of very hot liquids.

Clinically: anorexia and nausea, especially in the morning, flatulence due to swallowed air, vomiting, furred tongue, and dyspepsia.

Treatment: remove the cause, e.g. attention to teeth, tonsils, nasal infection. Smoking and alcohol are prohibited. Rough and fried food, pips and spices are avoided. Regular meals, chewed thoroughly. Regular exercise. Aperient for constipation.

Peptic Ulcer

Peptic ulcer is ulceration due to gastric acid and pepsin, and occurs in the lower end of the oesophagus in hiatus hernia (if there is reflux of acid), the stomach and duodenum, and at gastro-intestinal anastomoses (stomal or anastomotic ulcer). The normal stomach is protected from digestion by a layer of mucus.

Acute Peptic Ulcer

Acute peptic ulcers are often multiple (= acute erosive gastritis) and are due to:

1   Shock, e.g. burns. Shock reduces the blood supply to the gastric mucosa which produces less of the protective mucus. Local areas may have an especially poor blood supply and undergo ischaemic necrosis. Also, burns release histamine which increases gastric acid secretion, and this damages the poorly-protected mucosa.
2   Drugs, e.g. aspirin, phenylbutazone. Salicylates chemically alter the mucus which then loses its protective effect. Corticosteroids reduce the rate of healing of ulcers.
3   Heavy consumption of alcohol.
4   Uraemia.

Clinically: acute ulcers are symptomless unless they bleed. They heal rapidly.

Treatment: is of the cause, and a bland diet is given.

Chronic Gastric Ulcer

Cause: there is a familial tendency and it is slightly commoner in blood group O than A, B or AB. Males are slightly more often affected than females. It is commoner in the lower socio-economic groups and is caused by trauma by rough or poorly chewed food, alcohol, tobacco and drugs (e.g. aspirin), and by lack of mucosal resistance to hydrochloric acid due to a deficiency of mucus, as in atrophic gastritis.

Pathology: a chronic gastric ulcer is usually on or near the lesser curvature or antrum. Recurrent ulceration and healing causes fibrosis which may lead to stenosis.

Clinically: exacerbations of symptoms last for several days or weeks and remissions for months or years. Pain and tenderness is felt in the epigastrium. Pain is burning or gnawing in type and comes on shortly (20–30 minutes) after food, due to irritation of the ulcer by acid. Thus the patient is afraid to eat and loses weight. Appetite is not lost. Vomiting may occur and relieves the pain. Antacids relieve pain.

Complications:

1   Haemorrhage. Acute severe haemorrhage causes haematemesis (the vomiting of blood) and melaena (black stools). Chronic haemorrhage causes hypochromic anaemia due to iron deficiency.
2   Perforation, i.e. the ulcer extends through the mucosa and muscular layer

and finally penetrates the peritoneal layer. This releases the gastric contents into the peritoneal 'cavity' (*Fig. 8.14*) and the air from the fundus of the stomach rises to lie under the diaphragm. Immediate operation is required to close the perforation.

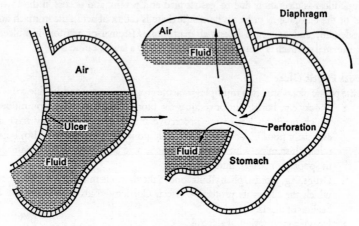

FIG. 8.14   Perforation of a gastric ulcer

3   Penetration of the pancreas. An ulcer in the lower part of the stomach or in the duodenum may erode the pancreas.
4   Stenosis, which may be pyloric, due to an ulcer in the duodenum or in the stomach near the pylorus, or 'hour-glass' due to an ulcer near the middle of the stomach (*Fig. 8.15*).

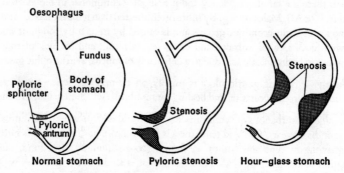

FIG. 8.15   Gastric stenosis due to peptic ulcer

5   Deficiencies. Iron deficiency due to chronic bleeding from the ulcer and to a poor diet. Deficiency of vitamin C due to 'milk and fish' diet.
6   Malignant change in a gastric ulcer, but never in a duodenal ulcer.

Investigations: gastroscopy shows the ulcer, and a biopsy is taken if carcinoma is suspected. Radiology (barium meal). Laboratory tests: blood count to detect anaemia, six consecutive faeces for occult blood (bleeding is often intermittent and blood may not be detected in only three or four specimens).

Treatment: Medical—physical and mental rest for two weeks, or more if symptoms persist. Rest in bed at home or in hospital. May get up to the lavatory. Mental rest away from sources of anxiety. Watching television and seeing visitors is not rest. Symptoms are usually relieved in a few days, but the healing of the ulcer takes two to 12 weeks. Smoking is prohibited since it delays healing, and drugs such as aspirin are avoided.

Diet: must consist of bland foods which do not damage the mucosa or stimulate gastric secretions. Milky foods are usually given for the first few days during acute symptoms, but it is probably immaterial whether the diet is of milk foods (milk, porridge, junket, milk pudding), starches (biscuits, bread, potatoes), egg or steamed fish, or a full diet which is finely minced, including minced meat. Food should be non-irritant, i.e. spices, pickles and rough foods (celery, radishes, cucumber, tough meat, chipped potatoes) should be avoided. Meals should be regular, small and frequent, with milk or antacids between them if pain persists, i.e. something should enter the stomach every two hours, or hourly at first if pain is severe. Adequate calories, protein and vitamins are needed to ensure good nutrition and promote the healing of the ulcer. The patient is advised to eat slowly and chew food properly. In intractable pain a milk drip, with added antacid, is given into the stomach at 40 drops a minute ($=$ 2·5 l in 24 hours). The Ryle's tube should be changed, cleaned and boiled every two days.

Drugs: antacid between meals to relieve pain and prevent further ulceration, e.g. magnesium trisilicate mixture B.P.C. 10 ml or tablets 1–2 orally p.r.n. Antispasmodic (anticholinergic) theoretically reduces gastric motility and secretions, but in practice their action is slight, e.g. belladonna given as magnesium trisilicate and belladonna mixture B.P.C. 10 ml orally between meals or at night. Liquorice preparations assist the healing of gastric ulcers, e.g. carbenoxolone (Biogastrone) 50 mg p.c. four- to six-hourly orally for five weeks. *Side-effects:* sodium and water retention, potassium depletion, hypertension. Vitamin C to improve the patient's general condition and to promote healing.

Surgical Treatment is used if exacerbations recur over several years, if medical treatment fails to cure, or if there are complications:

1 Partial gastrectomy is used in pyloric stenosis (whether due to gastric or duodenal ulcer) and carcinoma and is the best operation for chronic gastric ulcer. It may be used in recurrent haemorrhage or perforation. 60% of the stomach is removed either as a Billroth 1 or a Polya gastrectomy (*Figs. 8.16* and *8.17*). Partial gastrectomy has a low ulcer recurrence rate but a higher incidence of complications than vagotomy.

   Complications: (*a*) Loss of weight due to the small size of the remaining part of the stomach allowing only small meals to be taken; (*b*) iron deficiency anaemia due to deficient absorption of iron caused by the loss of hydrochloric acid or by the rapid passage of food through the jejunum; (*c*) dumping syndrome, of which there are two types: The early type comes on soon (30 mins.) after a meal and is due to the rapid entry of food into the

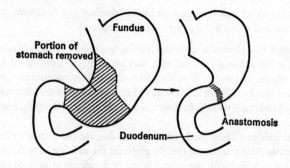

FIG. 8.16 Billroth I partial gastrectomy

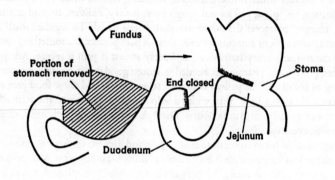

FIG. 8.17 Polya type partial gastrectomy

jejunum causing the outpouring of secretory juice into the jejunum. This results in a sudden reduction in blood volume which causes weakness, nausea and sweating, which is relieved by lying down and by taking meals 'dry', fluid being taken between meals. The later type occurs about 2 hours after food and is due to hypoglycaemia due to the rapid absorption of sugar being followed by the overproduction of insulin. Treatment is by taking sugar. Prevention is by taking carbohydrate in smaller amounts with each meal, and by taking meals more frequently.

2 Vagotomy and pyloroplasty (*Fig. 8.18*). Vagotomy reduces gastric acid secretion but also reduces gastric muscular contractibility and causes the post-vagotomy syndrome—discomfort and fullness after meals due to delayed emptying of the stomach. Pyloroplasty is widening of the pylorus which allows the stomach to empty. If emptying is too rapid 'dumping syndrome' may occur. Selective vagotomy is the cutting of the nerve fibres to the stomach, leaving intact those to the pancreas and liver. The various types of vagotomy are used especially in duodenal ulcer.

3 Vagotomy and antrectomy. Antrectomy (removal of the pyloric antrum) removes the gastrin-secreting part of the stomach.

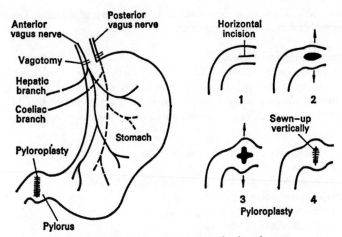

FIG. 8.18 Truncal vagotomy and pyloroplasty

Chronic Duodenal Ulcer

Cause: there is an hereditary tendency and an increased incidence in patients of blood group O. Excessive secretion of hydrochloric acid (hyperchlorhydria) and an increased serum gastrin is usual in duodenal ulcer, both during the day and at night, and is often associated with hypertrophy of the gastric mucosa. (Acid secretion is normal or low in gastric ulcer.) Duodenal ulcer is six to 12 times commoner in males than females. It is associated with long hours without food, business pressures, ambition and anxiety. It is as common in the lower as in the higher socio-economic groups (it was once thought to have a higher incidence in professional and executive classes).

Clinically: exacerbations and remissions occur as in gastric ulcer. Pain is epigastric, burning or gnawing in type, and comes on when the stomach is empty, i.e. when gastric acid is free to enter the duodenum without being neutralised by alkaline pancreatic juice. Pain therefore occurs 2–3 hours after meals (i.e. between meals) and at night. It is relieved by food and antacids and the patient 'eats anything'. Local epigastric tenderness may be present. Vomiting is rare unless pyloric stenosis is present.

Complications and Investigations are the same as for gastric ulcer except that carcinoma does not occur in duodenal ulcer.

Treatment is the same as for gastric ulcer except that carbenoxolone is ineffective. Cimetidine 200 mg t.d.s. and o.n. blocks acid secretion. In addition sedation may be needed for anxiety, e.g. phenobarbitone 30–60 mg t.d.s. orally, chlordiazepoxide (Librium) 5–10 mg t.d.s. orally or diazepam (Valium) 5–10 mg t.d.s. orally.

Zollinger–Ellison Syndrome

This is duodenal ulcer due to gastric hypersecretion due to a tumour of gastrin-secreting cells (gastrinoma) in the pancreas.

Note: Both the antrum of the stomach and the pancreas secrete gastrin. Treatment is removal of the tumour or gastrectomy.

Haematemesis and Melaena

Haematemesis is the vomiting of blood. Melaena is the passing of stools which are black and sticky, like tar, due to blood altered by enzymes and bacteria in the intestine. If bleeding is rapid, bright red blood may be vomited. If blood is retained in the stomach for a while it becomes brown and granular ('coffee-grounds').

Causes:
1 Duodenal ulcer is the commonest cause.
2 Gastric ulcer.
3 Acute erosive gastritis, e.g. due to aspirin, indomethacin.
These three causes account for 85% of all cases.
4 Hiatus hernia with reflux oesophagitis.
5 Carcinoma of the stomach.
6 Oesophageal varices (dilated varicose veins at the lower end of the oesophagus due to increased pressure and congestion in the portal venous system, i.e. portal hypertension, due to cirrhosis of the liver). The vein may rupture e.g. if abraded by rough food.
7 Swallowed blood from an epistaxis or tonsillectomy.
8 Blood disease, e.g. purpura, leukaemia, hypoprothrombinaemia (a low prothrombin level in the blood, due to vitamin K deficiency or oral anticoagulants).
9 Renal failure.

Clinically: nausea, vomiting of blood. Shock—the skin is pale and cold due to vaso-constriction, and clammy due to sweating. There is a fall in blood pressure, tachy-cardia, and weakness, and the patient is faint and anxious. Melaena may take 12–24 hours to appear, but frank blood may take only minutes.

Haematemesis must not be confused with haemoptysis: bright red frothy blood, alkaline in reaction, coughed up from the lungs.

Investigations:
1 Blood count. The haemoglobin does not alter until haemodilution occurs, i.e. the blood volume is replaced from tissue fluid or administered fluid, and takes some hours to begin and 24–36 hours for completion.
2 The blood urea rises due to the absorption of the breakdown products of blood protein from the intestines and to renal failure due to fall in blood pressure.
3 Blood group and serum for cross-matching taken before dextran (macrodex) is given since dextrans make grouping difficult by causing red cells to adhere to each other (rouleaux formation).
4 X-ray films of the patient's stomach and duodenum may be taken during the acute phase if Gastrografin is given. A barium meal should not be given until several days later.

Prognosis: the mortality rate is low below the age of 50 years but then rises.

Treatment: rest in bed. Sedation with morphine 15 mg to allay anxiety and restlessness, then phenobarbitone 30–60 mg six-hourly or diazepam 5 mg six-hourly orally. Raise the foot of the bed to combat shock. Treat the cause, e.g. vasopressin (Pitressin) 2·5–20 units i.m. for bleeding oesophageal varices (vasopressin causes splanchnic vasoconstriction and reduces portal blood flow).

Blood transfusion if more than two pints of blood are judged to have been lost or if shock is severe. Central venous pressure, C.V.P. (the pressure in the superior vena cava or right atrium), is measured so that transfusion can be given at a rate which will maintain a normal C.V.P. (5 cm of water, i.e. 500 Pa), circulatory overload can be prevented, and further bleeding detected by a fall in C.V.P. Pulse rate and volume and blood pressure are measured every 15–30 minutes at first, then hourly, and respirations and temperature are recorded. A falling blood pressure, weakening pulse or rising pulse rate, restlessness and sweating should be reported. Fluid balance chart. Stools and vomit are saved for inspection. Frequent mouth washes.

Diet: Water, half-strength saline or milk are given for a few hours and ice may be sucked, then an ulcer diet (normal, but bland, food) if the patient feels like it. NO starvation. Iron to restore any losses.

A soft rubber tube in the stomach aspirated hourly may detect further bleeding, but blood may not enter the stomach from the duodenum. Operation for recurrent bleeding, especially in the elderly since arteriosclerotic vessels cannot contract to stop bleeding.

Pyloric Obstruction

This is obstruction, at the pylorus, to the passage of food from the stomach into the duodenum.

Causes:

1 Chronic peptic ulcer near the pylorus, either duodenal or gastric.
2 Congenital hypertrophic pyloric stenosis in infants.
3 Carcinoma of the lower end of the stomach.

Pyloric Stenosis due to Chronic Peptic Ulcer

Chronic ulceration causes fibrotic scarring and muscular spasm. If it is near the pylorus it delays the emptying of the stomach.

Clinically: there is a history of peptic ulcer. Delay in emptying distends the stomach and causes anorexia, nausea, a feeling of fullness and vomiting. Vomiting relieves the discomfort but causes loss of water, electrolytes, vitamins and food, hence dehydration, constipation and wasting. Loss of hydrochloric acid causes alkalosis (*see* Chapter 3). The vomit may contain undigested food taken the previous day. Waves of gastric peristalsis may be visible in the epigastrium.

Investigations: aspirated fasting juice is of large volume, contains food, and is offensive due to fermentation. A barium meal shows the obstruction. Blood electrolytes (sodium, potassium, chloride) may show hypokalaemia and the blood urea may be increased due to dehydration.

Treatment: the stomach contents are aspirated via a Ryle's tube late each evening in order to relieve distension for the night. Dehydration and electrolyte disturbance are corrected. The diet is fluid at first (liquids may pass the obstruction) containing adequate calories, protein and vitamins, especially vitamin C. An i.v. drip is used if oral treatment is inadequate. When the patient's condition has improved operation is performed, e.g. partial gastrectomy.

Congenital Hypertrophic Pyloric Stenosis

This is hypertrophy of the muscle fibres of the pylorus which fails to relax properly.

Clinically: it affects mostly males, often the first-born. Vomiting usually begins at the age of three weeks, immediately after feeds at first; later delayed as the stomach dilates and hypertrophies. The vomit is ejected violently (projectile). Vomiting causes constipation, wasting, dehydration and alkalosis. There is a palpable pyloric thickening most easily felt immediately after a feed, and waves of peristalsis are visible in the epigastrium.

The condition cures spontaneously by the age of four months if the infant survives.

Treatment: dehydration is treated with i.v. saline. Atropine methonitrate (Eumydrin) 2–4 drops of 0·6% solution (0·4–0·8 mg) for infants, or hyoscine methonitrate, is given 20 minutes before feeds and the feeds should be small (30–60 ml) and given every two hours. If this is successful it is continued for several weeks. If it fails surgical treatment is necessary—Ramstedt's operation, which is an incision through the muscle of the pylorus.

Carcinoma of the Stomach

Carcinoma of the stomach (*Fig. 8.19*) is predisposed by atrophic gastritis, e.g pernicious anaemia (which shows five times the average incidence of carcinoma of the stomach), gastric polypi, and dietary pre-carcinogens such as cooking fat or nitrates. Some families show an hereditary tendency to it.

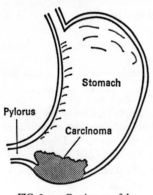

FIG. 8.19   Carcinoma of the stomach

Clinically: it most commonly affects the ages between 40 and 60 years, and is three times commoner in males than females. There is anorexia, especially for meat, nausea, fullness after small meals, vague dyspepsia, vomiting which does not relieve the discomfort, dysphagia if the growth is near the cardia, weight loss, a mass in the epigastrium, hypochromic anaemia causing tiredness and pallor, and there may be haematemesis and melaena. The growth spreads to lymph nodes, liver and peritoneum.

Investigations: barium meal demonstrates a 'filling defect'. Gastroscopy shows the growth and a biopsy may be taken for microscopical examination. Cytology on stomach washings. Gastric juice may contain blood and a high concentration of organic acid but the pentagastrin test shows hypochlorhydria or achlorhydria. The blood shows an hypochromic anaemia. Faeces may contain occult blood.

Treatment: correction of fluid and electrolyte imbalance and anaemia, improve nutrition, vitamins. Partial or total gastrectomy is performed if possible, as an attempt to cure. If the growth has spread outside the stomach it is 'inoperable', but a palliative gastrojejunostomy or oesophagojejunostomy will allow food to be taken.

Prognosis: 90% die in three to 12 months if untreated. A few survive five years if treated.

   Diet: Small frequent meals. Morphine or pethidine to relieve pain terminally.

Acute Dilatation of the Stomach
The stomach loses its muscular tone and dilates rapidly. It is a serious condition and may follow abdominal operation, childbirth or injury to the spine. It causes vomiting, dehydration and shock. The upper abdomen is distended.

Treatment: the foot of the bed is raised. The patient is on his side so that vomit is not aspirated into the lungs. Gastric contents, including gas, are aspirated, and fluid and electrolytes are given intravenously.

Perforation of a Peptic Ulcer
This is the penetration of a peptic ulcer through all the layers of the wall of the stomach.

Clinically: 95% are males, commonly aged 45 to 55 years. As the peritoneal layer ulcerates gastric contents are released into the peritoneal 'cavity' (*Fig. 8.14*) causing sudden agonising pain in the upper part of the abdomen, vomiting, board-like rigidity, tenderness, dullness to percussion, and the abdomen does not move with respiration, which is shallow and painful. Shock causes a subnormal temperature, tachycardia, low blood pressure and pallor. The patient lies quite still. After three to six hours fluid is secreted by the peritoneum and the patient appears to improve, but bowel sounds are absent (ileus) and bacterial peritonitis is beginning. The abdomen slowly distends, the pulse rate and temperature rise, and the condition of the patient deteriorates. The mortality is 15%.

Investigations: a plain X-ray of the abdomen shows air (gas) under the diaphragm.

Treatment: signed consent for operation then morphine 15 mg i.m. Gastric aspiration to keep the stomach empty, otherwise secretions continue to enter the peritoneal cavity. An i.v. drip, beginning with isotonic saline, replaces fluid losses, as indicated by the fluid balance chart. Antibiotic to prevent infection, e.g tetracycline into the i.v. drip.

   Surgical treatment is either simple closure of the perforation or one of the operations for peptic ulcer. Breathing exercises after operation help to expand the lungs and prevent hypostatic pneumonia.

THE PANCREAS

The pancreas (*Fig. 8.20*) is a gland in the epigastrium, extending into the left hypo-chondrium. It consists of a broad portion (the head), which lies in the curvature of the duodenum, narrowing to form the body, behind the stomach, and the tail

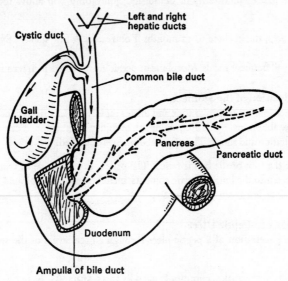

FIG. 8.20 The pancreas, gall bladder and bile ducts

which lies in front of the left kidney and just reaches the spleen. The aorta and the inferior vena cava lie behind the pancreas. The pancreas consists of lobules, each of which contains acini lined with cells which secrete pancreatic juice into the duodenum via the pancreatic duct. The duct, which runs through the whole length of the pancreas, enters the duodenum at the same point as the common bile duct, i.e. at the ampulla of the bile duct, which is controlled by the sphincter of Oddi.

Scattered throughout the pancreas are the islets of Langerhans which are collections of endocrine cells which secrete insulin, glucagon and pancreatic gastrin directly into the blood.

Physiology: pancreatic juice consists of water, salts (especially bicarbonate) and enzymes (trypsinogen, chymotrypsinogen, amylase, lipase, peptidases and nucleases). The bicarbonate makes the juice alkaline and this neutralises gastric acid and allows pancreatic enzymes to function. Trypsinogen is inactive (otherwise it would digest the pancreas) until it is activated to trypsin by enterokinase secreted by the duodenum. Inactive chymotrypsinogen is converted to active chymotrypsin in the duodenum. Trypsin and chymotrypsin convert peptones and other large polypeptides into small polypeptides. Amylase converts polysaccharides (starches) into disaccharides (sugars). Lipase converts fats into fatty acids and glycerol. To aid the action of lipase bile salts emulsify the fats, breaking the fat into smaller globules.

The secretion of pancreatic juice is stimulated by the vagus nerve and by two hormones, secretin and cholecystokinin–pancreozymin (C.C.K.), produced by the duodenal mucosa in response to gastric acid and partially digested food (chyme) in the duodenum. Secretin stimulates the secretion of juice rich in bicarbonate, C.C.K. stimulates pancreatic enzyme secretion and contraction of the gall bladder.

Investigations in Pancreatic disease

Duodenal Intubation. A tube is passed via the stomach (and its contents aspirated) into the duodenum. After the stimulation of the pancreas with intravenous secretin and pancreozymin, juice is aspirated from the duodenum, its volume measured (normally 2–5 ml a minute), and the bicarbonate concentration and enzyme activity (especially trypsin) measured. In severe pancreatic disease these levels are subnormal. Cytological examination is made for malignant cells. Secretin or Lundh test.

Lundh test meal: the patient is given a meal containing a known quantity of carbohydrate, protein and fat, and enzyme activity is measured in serial samples of duodenal contents.

Serum and Urine Enzymes. The serum and urine amylase are increased in acute pancreatitis, perforated peptic ulcer involving the pancreas, and cholecystitis. The normal serum amylase is 70–300 i.u. per litre.

Faecal Fat and Nitrogen Content are increased in pancreatic disease. Increase in fat (normal = up to 6 g daily) causes bulky, pale stools. Oil droplets and fatty acid crystals are seen microscopically, along with undigested meat fibres, but oily droplets, crystals, and meat fibres may be seen in any severe diarrhoea.

Sweat Electrolyte (sodium and chloride) concentration is increased in fibrocystic disease of the pancreas.

A Glucose Tolerance Test may show diabetes mellitus in chronic pancreatitis.

Radiography. A plain X-ray may show calcification in the pancreas in chronic pancreatitis. A barium meal may show an enlarged duodenal loop or displacement of the stomach in carcinoma of the head of the pancreas. Coeliac and mesenteric arteriography may demonstate a carcinoma.

Isotope scanning or **ultrasonogram** to detect cysts and tumours.

DISEASES OF THE PANCREAS

Acute Pancreatitis
This is acute inflammation of the pancreas with destruction of pancreatic tissue due to activation of pancreatic enzymes, which is caused by the regurgitation of duodenal

juice into the pancreatic duct. Trypsinogen is then activated and causes digestion of the pancreas, and the liberation of lipase causes fat necrosis.

Types: (1) oedematous: mortality 3% ; (2) haemorrhagic: mortality 40%.

Causes:

1   Gall bladder disease—gallstones and cholecystitis. The commonest cause. Oedema or spasm of the sphincter of Oddi may cause the reflux of bile along the pancreatic duct.
2   Alcoholism.
3   Virus infections, e.g. mumps.
4   Rarely, direct trauma to the pancreas, corticosteroid or cytotoxic therapy.

Clinically: the patient is often obese, with a history of gallstones. There is sudden severe pain in the upper part of the abdomen and across the back, which may radiate to the shoulder, with vomiting. Shock is due to the absorption of toxins and to hypovolaemia (loss of blood volume), the pulse is weak and rapid, the skin pale and clammy and slightly cyanosed. The temperature may be subnormal, normal or raised. Abdominal distension follows, with absent bowel sounds due to paralytic ileus, and there is tenderness and rigidity in the epigastrium.

Investigations: The blood shows a leucocytosis. The haemoglobin may be normal or increased at first, due to haemoconcentration, but later falls. The serum amylase is increased.

Complications: peritonitis. Acute renal failure. Haemorrhage from an eroded blood vessel. Retroperitoneal abscess. Hypocalcaemia. Diabetes mellitus.

Treatment: rest in bed. Nothing by mouth. Continuous gastric suction reduces the amount of acid entering the duodenum and thus reduces secretin output and pancreatic secretions. Fluid, e.g. saline, is given i.v. and the quantity is controlled by monitoring the central venous pressure. Plasma is given for severe shock, and blood is transfused if the haemoglobin falls below nine g/dl. A chart of fluid balance is kept. I.v. nutrition (amino acids, glucose) is given if ileus persists for more than two days.

Drugs: pethidine 100 mg, repeated, for pain. Chlorpromazine (Largactil) 50 mg for vomiting. Insulin for marked hyperglycaemia. Calcium chloride 2 g i.v. for hypocalcaemia. Antibiotic for infection. Anticholinergic drugs may be used to reduce pancreatic secretions, but they aggravate ileus, e.g. propantheline (Pro-Banthine) 15–30 mg six-hourly or atropine 0·5 mg four-hourly. Glucagon, 1 mg i.v. then 1 mg infused over five hours, may reduce the severity of the disease by inhibiting pancratic secretions. Aprotinin (Trasylol), a trypsin inhibitor, 200,000 units i.v. six-hourly for five days may reduce the mortality rate.

Surgical treatment for gallstones should be delayed until after recovery from the pancreatitis.

Chronic Pancreatitis
This is inflammation of the pancreas causing permanent damage and fibrosis.

Causes:
1 Idiopathic. Commonest.
2 Chronic alcoholism.
3 Repeated acute pancreatitis.
4 Obstruction of the pancreatic duct by stricture (fibrosis), ampullary papilloma or pancreatic stone.
5 Chronic biliary inflammation.

Clinically: there are attacks of pain in the epigastrium and back. Malabsorption causes loss of weight and steatorrhoea—pale, bulky stools which may be frothy and float on water. Diabetes mellitus occurs if the islets of Langerhans are involved.

Investigations: faecal fat is increased. The glucose tolerance curve may be diabetic. X-ray may show calcification of the pancreas. Radio-isotope scanning.

Treatment: avoidance of alcohol in alcohol-induced disease, cholecystectomy for gall bladder disease, insulin for diabetes mellitus. Low-fat diet to reduce steatorrhoea, with increased protein and carbohydrate for calories. Fat-soluble vitamins. Pancreatic enzymes (pancreatin) by mouth for steatorrhoea, either sprinkled on food or as tablets, taken with antacid to improve their action. Analgesic for pain, e.g. salicylate, paracetamol.

Mucoviscidosis (Fibrocystic Disease)
Cystic fibrosis is a recessively inherited disease which affects the pancreas, intestine and lungs. The mucus-secreting cells of these organs secrete viscid mucus which blocks ducts and bronchi. Pancreatic acini atrophy and are replaced with fibrous tissue. The islets of Langerhans are not affected. Obstruction to bronchi causes bronchopneumonia, bronchiectasis and pulmonary fibrosis.

Clinically: the infant may have meconium ileus (intestinal obstruction by viscid meconium). Failure to thrive is followed by emaciation but the appetite is good. The abdomen distends and there is diarrhoea with steatorrhoea (pale, bulky stools). Chronic cough is present. Death is from bronchopneumonia in childhood.

Investigations: sweat contains an increased concentration of salt (above 60 mmol/l, 60 mEq/l). Faecal fat is increased and trypsin is deficient in pancreatic juice.

Treatment: diet low in fat, high in carbohydrate, protein and vitamins. Pancreatin 2–6 g is given with each feed if the infant can take it. Antibiotic for respiratory infection.

Carcinoma of the Pancreas
This is an adenocarcinoma, commonly in the head of the pancreas. The prognosis is very poor; most patients die within six months.

Clinically: it is most frequent between the ages of 55 and 70 years. Epigastric pain radiates through to the back, is worse on lying supine and relieved by leaning forward. There is nausea, anorexia, weight loss, and there may be migrating thrombosis. A growth in the head of the pancreas presses on the common bile duct and causes obstructive jaundice, with pruritus and pale fatty stools. The gall bladder may dilate and become palpable.

Investigations: radio-isotope scanning. Coeliac and superior mesenteric arteriography. Duodenal cytology. Liver function tests.

Treatment is surgical. It is rarely possible to remove the growth. The usual operation is cholecystenterostomy—the gall bladder is drained into the small intestine.

THE SMALL INTESTINE

The small intestine (*Fig. 8.21*), which is about 6·4 m (21 feet) in length, begins as a continuation of the stomach at the pyloric sphincter and consists of duodenum,

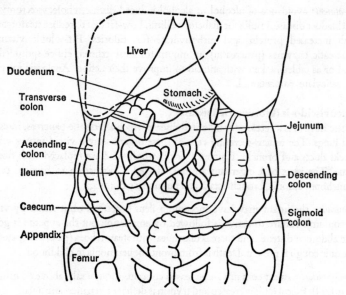

FIG. 8.21 The abdomen showing the intestines

jejunum and ileum. It ends by joining the large intestine at the ileocaecal valve, which controls the flow of material into the large intestine and prevents regurgitation into the ileum.

The duodenum is 25 cm (10 inches) in length and curves around the head of the pancreas. The pancreatic duct and the bile duct enter the duodenum together at the ampulla of the bile duct.

The wall of the small intestine consists of four layers (*Fig. 8.22*): the outer layer of peritoneum, continuous with the mesentery; the muscular layer of longitudinal and circular fibres; the submucous layer of loose connective tissue, blood vessels, lymph vessels and autonomic nerves; and the inner layer of mucous membrane. The

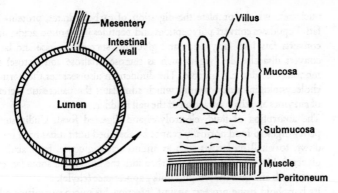

FIG. 8.22   The wall of the small intestines

surface area of mucous membrane is increased by circular folds and by villi. Villi (*Fig. 8.23*) are finger-like projections from the mucosal surface, lined with columnar epithelium. They contain a network of blood and lymph capillaries into which nutrients are absorbed from the lumen of the intestine. Lymph capillaries are called

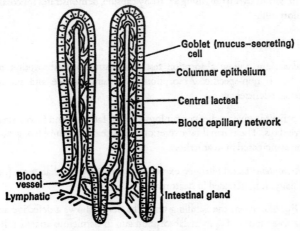

FIG. 8.23   Two villi in the small intestine

lacteals. Between the villi are the intestinal glands which secrete intestinal juice. In the mucous membrane there are numerous lymph nodes, the larger ones being called Peyer's patches.

Function:

1   Muscular activity. Segmental and pendular movements mix the chyme and intestinal secretions. Peristalsis propels the contents onwards.

2   The secretion of intestinal juice containing the enzymes enteropeptidase (formerly enterokinase), peptidases, lipase, sucrase, maltase, lactase and

nucleases, which complete the digestion of carbohydrates, proteins and fats. Peptidases convert polypeptides and peptides into amino acids; lipase converts fats into fatty acids and glycerol; sucrase, maltase and lactase convert disaccharides (sugars such as sucrose, maltose and lactose) into monosaccharides, e.g. glucose. The duodenum also secretes the hormone cholecystokinin–pancreozymin which stimulates the pancreatic secretion of enzymes and the contraction of the gall bladder.

3   The absorption of fluid, electrolytes and digested food. Undigested or partly digested food normally cannot be absorbed until it has been broken down to small molecules such as amino acids, glucose, fatty acids and glycerol. Most molecules are absorbed into the blood, but some fats enter the lacteals and give the lymph a milky appearance (chyle).

4   Its lymphoid tissue protects against infection by micro-organisms which have survived the action of hydrochloric acid in the stomach.

The Investigation of Small Intestinal Function

A Barium Meal and Follow-through shows gross defects such as Crohn's disease, fistulae and diverticulae.

Biopsy of Small Intestine, using a Crosby capsule, demonstrates mucosal changes such as short villi.

Tests of Absorption

Carbohydrate: the xylose absorption test demonstrates malabsorption of carbohydrate but is non-specific. Absorption tests using lactose and sucrose show disaccharidase deficiency.

Fat: the patient is given a diet containing 100 g of fat daily and faeces are collected over three days. The normal fat excretion is less than 21 mmol (six grams) daily. Excretion is increased in steatorrhoea.

Protein Absorption: faecal nitrogen excretion is normally less than 2·5 g ($\equiv$ 16 g of protein) daily. It is increased in steatorrhoea.

Vitamin B_{12} Absorption: the Schilling test (Chapter 5) shows a defective absorption of radioactive vitamin B_{12} in malabsorption and in pernicious anaemia. If intrinsic factor is given the absorption becomes normal in pernicious anaemia but remains poor in intestinal malabsorption.

Blood Count. Malabsorption may cause a megaloblastic anaemia due to folic acid or vitamin B_{12} deficiency, or hypochromic anaemia due to iron deficiency.

Acute Abdominal Pain (The 'Acute Abdomen')
The causes include:
Inflammation of abdominal organs: appendicitis, cholecystitis, pancreatitis, diverticulitis, salpingitis, peritonitis (perforated peptic ulcer, perforated colon, ruptured inflamed appendix), or mesenteric lymphadenitis.

Colic due to spasm of the smooth muscle in the wall of an organ which is obstructed, e.g. gallstones, renal calculi, intestinal obstruction (hernia), Crohn's disease, or from other causes, e.g. acute enteritis, lead poisoning, diabetic acidosis, Addison's disease, porphyria.

Vascular lesions, e.g. acute mesenteric embolism or thrombosis, dissecting or leaking aortic aneurysm.

Other causes are acute pyelonephritis, ruptured ectopic pregnancy, ruptured ovarian cyst, and tabetic crisis. Pneumonia and myocardial infarction may cause referred pain in the abdomen.

Intestinal Obstruction

Intestinal obstruction is any condition in which there is a delay in the onward passage of the contents of the gut, and may be due to mechanical narrowing of the lumen, thickening of the wall which interferes with peristalsis, or to paralysis of the muscle of the gut (paralytic ileus).

Causes:

Mechanical Obstruction—hernia, adhesions or bands of fibrous tissue due to previous operation or inflammation, volvulus, intussusception, Crohn's disease, stricture due to diverticulitis, neoplasm, or faecal impaction.

Mechanical Interference with Peristalsis—Crohn's disease, Hirschsprung's disease, amyloidosis, scleroderma.

Paralytic Ileus—post-operative (drugs, anaesthetics, handling of gut), peritonitis, uraemia due to renal failure, fractured spine (interference with the autonomic nerve supply), hypokalaemia, retroperitoneal haemorrhage.

Clinically: vigorous peristalsis above a mechanical obstruction is an attempt to overcome the obstruction and causes attacks of colicky pain and increased bowel sounds. Pain and bowel sounds are absent in paralytic ileus since the bowel is paralysed. Vomiting is early in disease of the small intestine; late in colonic obstruction. Dehydration is due to loss of fluid and electrolytes by vomiting and by stagnation of intestinal secretions in loops of dilated intestine, the secretions are not being absorbed and are lost to the circulation. Normally eight to 10 litres of fluid are secreted into the gut every 24 hours and all except 100 ml are reabsorbed. Both gastric acid and alkaline pancreatic juice are lost, therefore there is no tendency to acidosis or alkalosis. The abdomen distends, there is constipation, and the urine is concentrated and of low volume with a low chloride content.

Investigations: a plain radiograph shows distended loops of gut with fluid levels in the loops. A barium meal should not be used since barium increases the obstruction, but x-ray following gastrografin, which is absorbable, shows the site of the obstruction. Serum electrolytes. Blood count.

Treatment is surgical in mechanical obstruction, usually medical in paralytic ileus. In both types, fluid and electrolytes are given i.v. Losses and intake of fluid must be recorded. The stomach, and preferably also the intestinal, contents should be aspirated (decompression). Enemata, or manual removal if necessary, of impacted faeces.

Malabsorption

Malabsorption is the defective absorption of protein, fat, carbohydrate, or vitamins. It may involve a single substance, e.g. lactose, a group of substances, e.g. fats (causing steatorrhoea), or a wide range of substances.

Causes:

1 Deficiency of pancreatic enzyme action occurs in pancreatic disease (chronic pancreatitis, mucoviscidosis, carcinoma of the pancreas), inadequate mixing of enzymes with food in gastro-intestinal anastamoses, e.g. gastro-enterostomy, or inactivation of enzymes by an excess of hydrochloric acid in the Zollinger–Ellison syndrome.

2 Deficiency of bile salts due to biliary obstruction, or to bacterial destruction of bile salts which occurs in blind (stagnant) loops of bowel (diverticulae, gastro–intestinal operations, *Fig. 8.24*).

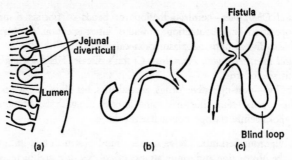

FIG. 8.24 Blind loops: (*a*) jejunal diverticuli; (*b*) polya gastrectomy; (*c*) ilial fistula with a blind loop

3 Diseases of the small intestine, e.g. fistulae, regional ileitis, tuberculous enteritis, gluten enteropathy, mesenteric thrombosis; lymphatic obstruction, e.g. Hodgkin's disease; systemic sclerosis; or intestinal parasites, e.g. *Giardia lamblia*.

4 Drugs such as neomycin, kanamycin or colchicine.

Clinically: there may be general malnutrition with loss of weight and, in a child, failure of growth. Abdominal distension and diarrhoea, often with steatorrhoea, is common. Anaemia is due to deficiency of iron, folic acid or vitamin B_{12}; haemorrhages may be due to vitamin K deficiency, tetany to hypocalcaemia, osteomalacia to vitamin D deficiency, oedema to hypoalbuminaemia or scurvy, and glossitis and dermatitis to vitamin B deficiency. Steatorrhoea causes the stools to become bulky, pale, offensive, and greasy, and to float on water.

Investigations include faecal fat and nitrogen, blood count to detect anaemia, absorption tests, barium meal and follow-through, and biopsy of the small intestine.

Treatment is of the cause, the correction of deficiencies, and symptomatic, e.g. a low-fat diet, drugs to prevent diarrhoea.

Drugs: Codeine phosphate 30–60 mg t.d.s. or q.i.d. or chalk for diarrhoea. Antispasmodic, e.g. propantheline 15 mg once to three times daily, or belladonna for colic (belladonna also reduces diarrhoea). Antibiotic for sepsis or malabsorption due to the blind-loop syndrome.

Steatorrhoea

Steatorrhoea is the presence of excess fat in the stools. The faeces become bulky, pale, offensive, and float on water and are not easily flushed down the lavatory. The causes and investigations have been given under malabsorption. The treatment is of the cause, a low-fat diet if the cause cannot be treated, adequate protein, vitamins especially the fat-soluble A, D and K, and calcium.

Gluten Enteropathy (Coeliac Disease, Non-tropical Sprue)

Coeliac disease may be due to an immunological defect or to a genetic deficiency of an enzyme (a peptidase) which normally digests a peptide present in gluten (a mixture of proteins found in wheat and rye). The undigested peptide damages the mucosa of the jejunum, the villi of which become short and may disappear. This reduces the absorptive surface area of the intestine and causes malnutrition. There is a familial tendency.

Clinically: it usually affects children under the age of 5 years, but may present at any age. Symptoms begin when the child starts to eat solid food (wheat or rye). The child is irritable and miserable, and has anorexia, loose stools which are bulky, pale and offensive, float on water and are not easily flushed down the lavatory (i.e. steatorrhoea), abdominal distension, and a proneness to infections. Nutritional deficiencies cause failure of growth (protein and calorie deficiency), anaemia (folate, iron and vitamin B_{12} deficiency) and rickets (calcium deficiency).

Investigations: jejunal biopsy shows flattened villi. A barium meal and follow-through shows an abnormal mucosal pattern of the jejunum.

Treatment: a gluten-free diet cures. A relapse indicates that the patient is not keeping to the diet. A gluten-free diet excludes all food containing wheat and rye, i.e. wheat (ordinary) flour, bread, cakes, biscuits, soups thickened with flour. The patient may take rice flour, cornflour, soya flour, maize and oatmeal.

Vitamins, iron, folic acid and calcium are needed until there is recovery from these deficiencies.

Regional Ileitis (Crohn's Disease)

Regional ileitis is a chronic inflammation of areas of the small intestine, particularly the terminal ileum, but may occasionally affect the colon, and rarely the rectum, stomach and oesophagus. The cause is unknown, but is probably an infection. The ileal wall is thickened by fibrosis, oedema and inflammatory cells, including giant cells, and may be ulcerated. Inflamed loops of bowel adhere to adjacent structures and fistulae (channels joining two epithelial surfaces) may form.

Clinically: the patients are usually young adults with anaemia, fever, anorexia, weight loss and diarrhoea. There are attacks of colicky pain in the right lower quadrant of the abdomen due to increased peristalsis attempting to overcome the partial obstruction caused by the thickened segment of ileum, adherent loops of which may be palpable as a tender mass. A few have steatorrhoea and malabsorption, due to involvement of the jejunum.

Complications:
1   Fistulae may involve the bladder, vagina and abdominal wall (especially through an operative suture-line), or may be perianal.
2   Strictures, which may cause intestinal obstruction.
3   Abscess.

Prognosis: the disease is one of relapses and remissions over years.

Investigations: a barium meal and follow-through shows segmental narrowing of the ileal lumen. Sigmoidoscopy and biopsy demonstrate any colonic involvement. The blood shows anaemia and an increased erythrocyte sedimentation rate.

Treatment: there is no specific treatment. Medical treatment is advisable, since local resection of intestine is followed by recurrence. Surgery is used only for complications, e.g. intestinal obstruction, for which a short-circuit operation is preferable to excision. Rest in bed during relapse. Diet of low residue during attacks, high in energy, e.g. 12·6 MJ (3000 kcal.) a day, adequate in protein. Low in fat if there is steatorrhoea. Correct anaemia with iron and folic acid.

Acute Enteritis and Gastroenteritis
Acute enteritis is inflammation of the intestine. Often the stomach is also inflamed.

Causes:
1   Food poisoning is due to pathogenic bacteria, bacterial toxins, or chemicals taken in food or drink. Bacteria multiply readily in food, even at room temperature, but especially in food kept warm for a length of time, as in canteens and restaurants. Common pathogens are salmonellae, *Cl. welchii*, and pathogenic *E. coli* (both in infants and in adults) e.g. *E. coli* number 0148K causes traveller's diarrhoea. Typhoid, paratyphoid, cholera and dysentery are also spread via contaminated food or water. Sometimes food poisoning is due, not to the bacteria themselves, but to toxins which they produce, e.g. toxins produced by staphylococcus pyogenes or by *Cl. botulinum*.
     Allergies to food or symptoms due to overeating are not food poisoning.
2   Viruses, e.g. ECHO viruses.
3   Chemical poisons accidentally contaminating food or drink.

Clinically: several people may be affected at the same time. The mucosa of the stomach and small intestine, and sometimes the colon, is inflamed. There is nausea, vomiting, abdominal pain (colic due to spasms of the small intestine) and diarrhoea, which may cause dehydration. Vomiting within half an hour of taking food suggests chemical poisoning; within six hours suggests a bacterial toxin; and between 12 and

48 hours (the time taken for the multiplication of organisms) suggests bacterial infection, e.g. salmonella.

Investigations: vomit, faeces and suspected food should be sent to the laboratory since salmonellae, typhoid, dysentery and cholera are notifiable to the area medical officer of health.

Treatment: rest in bed, at home for mild disease, in hospital if dehydrated. The stomach is washed out with saline in chemical poisoning or if the 'death-cap' fungus has been eaten (in mistake for the edible mushroom), and the appropriate antidote is given. Fluid and electrolyte losses are replaced. A semi-solid, then a normal, diet is given as soon as the patient feels like it. Diarrhoea is controlled with codeine phosphate. In infectious diseases (Chapter 4) the patient is barrier-nursed and the stools are treated with 5% carbolic acid. Antibiotic for dysentery.

THE LARGE INTESTINE

Anatomy. The large bowel (*Fig. 8.21*) is about 1·5 m (5 feet) in length. It consists of the colon and rectum. The colon begins as the caecum at the ileo-caecal valve in the right iliac fossa. The caecum is a pouch from which the appendix opens. From the caecum the colon ascends in the right side of the abdomen (ascending colon) to the lower surface of the liver where it bends (right colic flexure, hepatic flexure) to continue across the abdomen as the transverse colon, in front of the duodenum and stomach. On reaching the spleen in the left side of the abdomen it turns downwards (splenic flexure) to continue as the descending colon which becomes the sigmoid (S-shaped) colon as it curves into the pelvis to join the rectum. The rectum is 13 cm (5 inches) long, lies in the pelvis in front of the sacrum, and ends at the anal canal. The anal canal is closed by the anal sphincter, a thickening of the circular muscle fibres of the bowel.

The transverse and sigmoid colon are mobile, being held in a fold of peritoneum.

The large intestine has four layers: an outer peritoneal layer; a muscular layer of longitudinal and circular fibres; a submucous layer containing blood vessels, lymphatics and autonomic nerve fibres; and the inner lining of mucous membrane of columnar epithelium containing goblet cells which secrete mucus. The anus is lined with squamous epithelium continuous with that of the skin. The longitudinal fibres of the muscular layer of the colon do not cover the colon completely but form three narrow bands (taeniae coli) running down the colon.

Functions. Absorption of water: the intestinal contents are fluid at the caecum and semi-solid at the rectum. Salt, glucose and corticosteroids can also be absorbed. Bacterial action: bacteria in the colon synthesise vitamin B, B_{12} and K_2 but only vitamin K_2 is absorbed.

Defaecation: the entry of food into the stomach causes a reflex contraction of the colon (gastrocolic reflex) forcing material into the rectum, which is normally empty. Stretching of the rectal wall causes impulses to pass to the spinal cord and on to the brain where the conscious desire to defaecate is aroused. The pressure in the abdomen is increased by fixing the diaphragm (holding the breath) and contracting the muscles of the abdominal wall and pelvic floor. This compresses the rectum, which also contracts, and the anus relaxes. The anal sphincter is under the control of autonomic nerves as part of the defaecation reflex, but is also under voluntary control. The gastrocolic reflex is important in the management of constipation and of a colostomy.

Investigation of the Large Bowel

Faeces consists of unabsorbed food residue, water and bacteria. Its quantity, frequency, consistency, colour, odour, and the presence of abnormal material should be noted.

The quantity is normally 80–200 g daily, depending on the diet. Fruit and vegetables provide 'roughage' which increases faecal bulk. Bulk is increased in steatorrhoea and diarrhoea. The consistency is normally semi-solid and formed into a cylinder. Stools are soft if the diet is high in roughage, hard lumps (scybala) in constipation, and abnormally liquid in diarrhoea, e.g. dysentery, ulcerative colitis. The colour is normally dark brown due to altered bile pigments. The stools are pale in obstructive jaundice and coeliac disease, black and sticky from melaena (blood from the stomach or duodenum altered by digestion), dull black with iron or bismuth, bright red blood comes from the large intestine or anal canal (ulcerative colitis, dysentery, haemorrhoids). The odour is offensive if excess of protein is present, due to small intestinal hurry and putrefaction of protein in the large bowel. The presence of mucus (constipation, inflammation, tumours), blood, worms, pus, or coins and buttons swallowed by children and passed in the stools should be recorded. Laboratory examination for pathogenic organisms (shigella, salmonella, pathogenic E. coli, amoebae, tubercle bacilli), fat droplets, and muscle (meat) fibres.

Endoscopy is visual examination of the organ with an illuminated instrument, e.g. the rectum (proctoscopy), sigmoid part of the colon (sigmoidoscopy), or the whole of the colon using a fibrescope (colonoscopy). Inflammation, tumours and the motility of the wall can be seen.

Radiology. A barium meal and follow-through may show abnormalities but a barium enema is preferable and demonstrates ulcerations, tumours and diverticulae. A *Barium Enema* is the injection, into the rectum and colon, of 2 l of radio-opaque material followed by radiography. Careful preparation to empty the bowel is essential.

Preparation: a low-residue diet is given for three days beforehand, and fluids only on the day before. The day before the examination an aperient is given in the morning and an evacuant enema in the evening. On the morning of the X-ray another enema or a Dulcolax suppository is given and the bowel is washed out twice with tepid water to remove débris.

Constipation

Constipation is infrequent passage of faeces, residues being excreted more than three days after the food was taken. Some people are healthy if the bowels are emptied only twice weekly, others are normal on defaecating thrice daily.

Causes:

1 Persistent neglect of the call to empty the rectum (dyschezia), the rectum becoming distended with faeces and relatively insensitive.
2 Lack of opportunity to open the bowels at a convenient time.
3 Weakness of the abdominal muscles, e.g. the elderly and the ill.
4 Mechanical obstruction in the large bowel.
5 Defective peristalsis of the colon. Paralytic ileus causes acute constipation. A spastic colon absorbs more water from the faeces. Hypothyroidism.
6 Small faecal bulk. Low food intake (depression, anorexia nervosa, dementia), low roughage, dehydration (fevers).
7 Painful defaecation due to an anal fissure.

Symptoms are of the cause, and also headache, abdominal discomfort, and lassitude.

Complications: faecal impaction.

Prevention: training to empty the bowel after meals at a regular time each day. Adequate fluids. Roughage, e.g. fruit (prunes, apples), green vegetables, wholemeal bread. Regular exercise. Treatment of haemorrhoids and anal fissure.

Treatment is of the cause. For dyschezia the patient must be trained to answer the call to defaecation, assisted with liquid paraffin or agar, and a high residue diet. Normal bowel physiology should be explained to the patient. Abdominal exercises for weak muscles. Enema if necessary. Purgatives and laxatives: magnesium sulphate 4–15 g orally, taken in the morning, followed by a hot drink, acts by osmosis. Cascara 1–2 tabs. (20–40 mg), senna 1–4 tabs. (7·5–30 mg), or rhubarb Co. mixture 10 ml taken at night, act by stimulating the muscle of the large bowel. Bisacodyl (Dulcolax) 5–10 mg orally or as a suppository. Liquid paraffin emulsion 10–30 ml orally, acts as a lubricant but interferes with the absorption of fat-soluble vitamins and may leak out of the anus. Agar 4 g or methylcellulose granules 1·5–6 g orally provide bulk. Digital removal of impacted faeces, if necessary.

Enemas are liquids injected into the rectum. They may be evacuant or purgative for emptying the bowel, or retention enemas for absorption from the bowel.

The sodium phosphate enema, or the less-often-used soap and water enema (15 ml green soap in 500 ml of warm water at 38°C), is used to evacuate the bowel and should be retained for 10 minutes. It is used if Dulcolax suppositories are ineffective in constipation, and prior to a barium enema or surgery to the large bowel. Retention enemas may contain drugs, e.g. corticosteroids (used in ulcerative colitis), and should be retained as long as possible. The bowel and bladder should be emptied beforehand.

Method of Administration of Enemas: the bed is screened, the procedure explained to the patient, the bedclothes (except the sheet) turned back, and a blanket laid across the trunk. The patient lies on his left side with the hips flexed, and a plastic sheet or paper towel is placed beneath the buttocks, which are near the edge of the bed. The foot of the bed is raised so that the enema flows into the colon. A rectal tube or catheter is lubricated with a swab wiped in KY or petroleum jelly, solution is run into it to expel air, and the tube is nipped with the fingers. It is passed 10 cm into the rectum and the enema-container raised so that the solution runs slowly into the rectum over five minutes. The enema must be at 38°C, otherwise it may be expelled. The tube is gently withdrawn and the patient covered with the bedclothes. The buttocks are held together to help to prevent the enema from being expelled prematurely. A bedpan, kept nearby, is placed under the patient when requested. The result should be inspected and the findings recorded.

A sodium phosphate enema is simple to use and is given directly from a disposable pack and its attached tube. The pack is warmed before use and the tube lubricated.

A Flatus Tube is passed to remove gas from the lower part of the bowel, usually after abdominal operations. The patient is positioned as for an enema and the bed protected with a plastic cover. The tube is warmed in water, lubricated with petroleum jelly and gently passed into the bowel for 10–40 cm, the free end being kept under water. It is removed after 10 minutes.

Diarrhoea
Diarrhoea is the passing of unformed or frequent stools.

Causes:
1 Psychogenic. Nervousness, anxiety, fear.
2 Inflammation. Enteritis (tuberculous, staphylococcal, food poisoning, viruses, dysentery, salmonellae, pathogenic *E. coli*), ulcerative colitis, diverticulitis, Crohn's disease.
3 Parasites. Amoebic dysentery, *Giardia lamblia* (in small intestine).
4 Irritation of the bowel. Purgatives, dietary indiscretion, irritant poisons (mercury, arsenic).
5 Malabsorption. Pancreatic disease, gluten enteropathy, ileal resection.
6 Gastric disorders. Achlorhydria, carcinoma, vagotomy or gastrectomy.
7 Others. Thyrotoxicosis, food allergies, excess roughage in the diet, oral antibiotics, constipation with overflow (pseudodiarrhoea).

Complications: dehydration, producing a rapid pulse and fall in blood pressure. Loss of electrolytes, especially potassium, which may cause coma and death. Loss of blood proteins, causing oedema.

Investigations: stools for organisms, parasites, ova, fat, poisons. Record of the appearance and number of stools. Rectal examination and sigmoidoscopy. Barium enema.

Treatment of the cause, rest in bed, barrier nursing for infectious disease. Replacement of fluid and electrolyte losses orally, or i.v. if dehydration does not respond to oral fluids. Diet free from roughage. Local barrier cream or silicone spray to perineum.

   Drugs: kaolin to absorb poisons, atropine to relieve spasm, codeine phosphate or morphine, e.g. kaolin and morphine, to relieve pain.
Bedpans may be:
   1 Disposable papier mâché which are used once, macerated in a destructor, and

flushed into the sewage system. Drains may be blocked by inadequately macerated bedpans.

2 A non-disposable plastic carrier for each patient, with a polyethylene liner which is removed with its contents and incinerated.

3 Metal bedpans disinfected and heated to at least 80°C for one minute to destroy vegetative bacteria, then washed with water jets. They should be warmed with hot water before use.

4 Polypropylene pans do not conduct heat and therefore may not be adequately sterilised.

Appendicitis

Appendicitis is inflammation of the appendix. It may be acute, subacute or recurrent ('chronic'). It is due to bacteria or viruses, bacterial infection being predisposed by obstruction of the lumen of the appendix by hard faeces (faecoliths).

Clinically: it is commonest between the ages of five and 25 years. It begins with generalised abdominal colicky pain, nausea, anorexia, and maybe vomiting. After a few hours pain localises to the right iliac fossa and there is tenderness, guarding and rigidity over the appendix, associated with pyrexia, tachycardia and a furred tongue.

Investigations: the white blood cell count is increased ($10,000-15,000 \times 10^6/l$). The urine is normal, which distinguishes appendicitis from pyelonephritis, since in pyelonephritis the urine contains albumin, pus, blood and organisms.

Complications: abscess. Rupture (perforation) and peritonitis. Fistulae. Intestinal obstruction later due to adhesions.

Treatment is appendicectomy unless there is an abscess. The pulse is recorded half- to two-hourly and the temperature and any vomiting noted. Nothing is given by mouth for 24 hours. Laxatives must be avoided since they increase peristalsis and may cause perforation of the appendix. An abscess is drained and an antibiotic given, appendicectomy being performed three months later, i.e. after recovery, to prevent recurrence.

Colitis

Colitis is inflammation of the colon. It may be due to amoebic or bacillary dysentery (Chapter 4), Crohn's disease, ulcerative colitis, diverticulitis, tuberculosis, or ischaemia of the colon.

Ulcerative Colitis

Ulcerative colitis is inflammation of the colon and rectum with ulceration of the mucosa. The cause is unknown, with the result that many causes have been suggested such as auto-immune disease, food allergy, infection, reduced blood flow to the colon, genetic abnormality, and psychological disorder.

Clinically: age 20–40 years. The condition varies from mild diarrhoea to fatal acute fulminating disease. It begins in the sigmoid colon and rectum and spreads along the entire colon. There are attacks of diarrhoea with blood and mucus in the stools, abdominal discomfort, and a tender colon, and there may be tenesmus (painful straining) due to proctitis. There is depression, fever, loss of weight, anaemia and vitamin deficiency, e.g. deficiency of vitamin B causing glossitis. Emotional stress is not the cause of the condition but may predispose to an attack (emotional stress may cause diarrhoea in normal people).

Complications:

Intestinal—massive haemorrhage, perforation into the peritoneal cavity due to acute dilatation of the colon, fistulae due to adherence of the inflamed colon to nearby structures e.g. bladder, pseudopolypi (islands of mucosa remaining in an area of ulceration), carcinoma of the colon after 10 years of colitis.

Systemic—skin rash due to drug therapy, arthropathy, liver damage (fatty degeneration, portal tract inflammation). In acute fulminating ulcerative colitis there is severe diarrhoea, pyrexia, toxaemia, tachycardia and exhaustion.

Investigations: sigmoidoscopy and biopsy. Barium enema (not in the acute phase owing to the risk of perforation) annually to detect carcinoma. Stools for blood and mucus; pus indicates secondary infection; examination for pathogenic organisms to exclude infective colitis. The blood count shows anaemia, and the E.S.R. is increased. The serum protein level may be low.

Treatment: rest in bed in the acute phase until diarrhoea ceases. Mild disease may be treated at home, more severe disease in hospital. Diet should be varied and full, with a low residue (residues irritate the inflamed bowel), high energy (10·5–12·6 MJ, 2,500–3,000 kcal. daily), high protein, e.g. 120 g daily since protein (blood, exudate and mucosa) is being lost from the bowel into the stool. Protein is given as eggs, fish, meat, cheese and milk, but milk is avoided if there is sensitivity to it. Plasma transfusion may be needed if there is severe hypoalbuminaemia. Vitamin B and C are given, and also vitamin K if there is bleeding due to a low prothrombin level in the blood.

Dehydration is corrected with i.v. fluids if oral fluids are inadequate, and fluid losses and intake are recorded. Hypokalaemia is corrected by giving potassium citrate 10–15 g daily orally, potassium chloride 1 g t.d.s. orally, or Darrow's solution i.v. Iron for anaemia, blood transfusion for severe haemorrhage. Temperature, pulse and respirations are recorded four-hourly. The daily number of stools is recorded and one is saved for inspection.

Local Treatment of Colon: colon washout with saline, perineal cleanliness and a barrier cream applied to the perianal skin. General care of the skin and changes of position to prevent bedsores.

Psychological: encouragement and reassurance are required and the patient is encouraged to talk to relieve his anxiety. Occupational therapy is provided.

Drugs: sedation with phenobarbitone 30–60 mg t.d.s. orally or chlordiazepoxide (Librium) 5–30 mg t.d.s. orally. To relieve diarrhoea and pain, codeine phosphate 15–60 mg t.d.s. is given orally, or tincture of opium 0·5–1 ml orally for severe diarrhoea, but there is the risk of addiction. Antispasmodic, e.g. propantheline (Pro-Banthine) 15–30 mg orally or atropine 0·6 mg orally. Treatment of the colitis itself is with:

1 Sulphasalazine (Salazopyrin) 0·5–2 g q.i.d. orally. Side-effects are rash, nausea, vomiting, anorexia, neutropenia, haemolytic anaemia, headache.

2 Retention enema; or better, an intrarectal drip at 1–2 drops a second, of prednisolone-21-phosphate 40 mg in 70 ml of tap water, or hydrocortisone hemisuccinate 100 mg in 100 ml of warm saline, held as long as possible, given nightly, or morning and night, for three weeks.

3 In severe colitis either prednisolone 10–20 mg t.d.s. orally, or corticotrophin (Acthargel) 20–60 units i.m. b.d. is given in addition to intrarectal corticosteroid.

Surgical treatment for intestinal complications, i.e. perforation of the colon, fistula, carcinoma, and if intensive medical treatment fails in severe colitis. Total proctocolectomy with ileostomy cures. A ring with a bag is attached to the abdominal wall. The efflux from the ileostomy contains digestive enzymes and must not come into contact with the skin which will be digested and become ulcerated. The efflux is fluid and appears every hour or two and always follows a meal. It causes loss of fluid, and a high fluid intake may be needed to prevent dehydration. An ileostomy does not prevent active sports, e.g. swimming. Help can be obtained from the ileostomy association.

Diverticulosis and Diverticulitis

Diverticulosis is the presence of diverticuli. These are pouches of mucosa projecting outwards from the lumen of a hollow organ. Diverticulitis is inflammation of diverticuli. Inflammation causes fibrous thickening.

Cause: diverticulosis of the colon (*Fig. 8.25*) is due to increased pressure in the lumen of the colon, often due to constipation, gradually producing pouches of mucosa at sites of weakness in the wall (e.g. at the entrance of blood vessels).

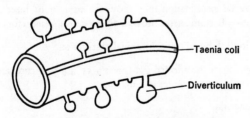

FIG. 8.25   Diverticulosis of the colon

Clinically: age over 50 years. Diverticuli are symptomless until they become inflamed, e.g. after obstruction by a faecolith. Diverticulitis causes discomfort and tenderness in the left iliac fossa, and thickened bowel may be palpable. There is constipation with attacks of diarrhoea, and blood is passed per rectum if haemorrhage occurs. Tenesmus occurs if inflammation involves the rectum.

Complications: recurrent inflammation causes fibrosis and stenosis of the bowel which may cause intestinal obstruction. Fistulae form, e.g. between the bladder and the colon (vesico-colic fistula). An abscess may form around an infected diverticulum. Hypochromic anaemia from recurrent bleeding.

Investigations: barium enema shows the sacs and any stenosis. Faeces may contain blood, mucus and pus, and there is a polymorph leucocytosis during acute attacks.

Treatment is usually medical: Rest in bed during an acute attack, relieve pain and spasm of the colon with an antispasmodic, e.g. propantheline, inhibit infection with a broad spectrum antibiotic. During remissions constipation must be prevented with a high-residue diet (a low-residue diet is likely to worsen the condition), but substances producing gas in the colon (turnip, swede, peas) should be avoided. Surgical treatment for complications, e.g. intestinal obstruction, when a temporary colostomy or partial colectomy may be needed.

Carcinoma of the Colon and Rectum

The cause is unknown but it is associated with a diet low in roughage. Bacterial breakdown of colonic contents forms chemical carcinogens which are concentrated unless diluted by faecal bulk (roughage) and are retained for a longer time in constipation. Carcinoma of the colon is also associated with ulcerative colitis, and polypi.

Carcinomas of the colon and rectum are slowly growing adenocarcinomas which spread locally, into the lymphatics, and via the portal blood to the liver.

Clinically: age over 50 years. Change in bowel habit (constipation, diarrhoea, or alternation of both) and anaemia are common. In the ascending colon, where the contents are liquid, a carcinoma causes toxaemia due to absorption through the ulcerated tumour, anorexia, and weight loss, and a mass may be palpable. In the descending colon and rectum, where the contents are semi-solid, a tumour may cause intestinal obstruction with constipation and colicky pain, or haemorrhoids. A tumour in the rectum may cause tenesmus.

Investigations: rectal examination may show the tumour or bleeding. Sigmoid-oscopy and biopsy. Barium enema shows a 'filling defect'. Faeces for occult blood.

Complications: local abscess. Fistula. Intestinal obstruction.

Treatment: resection of the affected gut (gives a 55% 5-year cure) after correcting dehydration, electrolyte imbalance and anaemia.

Intestinal Ischaemia

A deficient blood supply to the gut is caused by obstruction to the mesenteric arteries by atheroma, embolism, aortic aneurysm, thrombosis (e.g. oral contraceptive), or arteritis (e.g. collagen disease). Treatment is of the cause, e.g. embolectomy, and resection of bowel if it is gangrenous.

Megacolon

Megacolon is dilatation, elongation and hypertrophy of the colon which may be idiopathic or due to Hirschsprung's disease.

Idiopathic Megacolon. Both the colon and the rectum are dilated and there is constipation. Treatment is with a diet high in roughage, and laxatives. Colon washouts with saline may be necessary.

Hirschsprung's Disease. This is due to a congenital absence of autonomic nerve cells in a segment of the wall of the colon causing a block in peristalsis and the part of the colon above the obstruction dilates.

Clinically: symptoms begin at birth with chronic constipation and abdominal enlargement. The rectum is empty.

Investigations: sigmoidoscopy or barium enema shows the narrow segment of colon and rectum with dilatation above. Biopsy shows the absence of nerve cells.

Treatment is resection of the narrow abnormal segment, which cures. Colon wash-outs may be necessary.

Spastic Colon ('Mucous Colitis')

This is spasm of the colon causing pain in the left iliac fossa, and chronic constipation which causes the production of an excess of mucus.

Treatment is with an antispasmodic.

THE PERITONEUM

The peritoneum (*Fig. 8.26*) is a serous membrane having two layers, the parietal layer lining the abdominal wall, and the visceral layer covering the organs (viscera) in the abdomen and pelvis. The two layers are in contact, but between them is a potential cavity (the peritoneal cavity) containing lubricating serous fluid secreted by the cells of the membrane.

The mesentery is a double layer of peritoneum which encloses the jejunum and ileum, attaching them to the posterior abdominal wall and containing the arteries, veins, nerves and lymphatics to the intestines.

The lesser omentum is a fold of peritoneum hanging from the lower surface of the liver and supporting the stomach.

The greater omentum (*Fig. 8.27*) is a loose fold of peritoneum hanging like an apron from the greater curve of the stomach, with its posterior layer attached to the posterior abdominal wall behind the stomach, and supporting the transverse colon. It contains arteries, veins, nerves, lymphatic vessels, lymph nodes and fat. It surrounds areas of inflammation in the peritoneal 'cavity' e.g. in appendicitis it may surround the appendix.

The pocket of peritoneum behind the stomach is the lesser sac. The rest of the peritoneal cavity is the greater sac.

Functions. The peritoneum supports the abdominal organs, secretes serous fluid to permit the organs to slide over each other without causing friction, and protects against infection. The greater omentum also protects the abdominal organs and acts as a store for fat.

Peritonitis

Peritonitis is inflammation of the peritoneum.

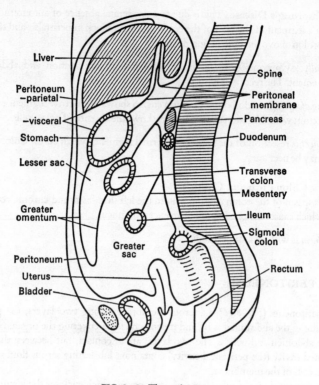

FIG. 8.26   The peritoneum

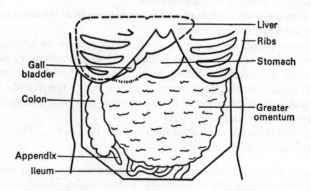

FIG. 8.27   Abdomen showing the greater omentum

Causes: acute peritonitis is due to perforation of a peptic ulcer, the colon or the appendix, to pancreatitis, septicaemia, abdominal operation, septic abortion, extension from local infection, e.g. appendicitis, cholecystitis, salpingitis or diverticulitis, or through the gut wall, as in unrelieved intestinal obstruction. In all these the infecting bacteria are, e.g., *E. coli*, streptococci and bacteroides. Primary peritonitis is due to gonococci or pneumococci.

Clinically: in acute peritonitis there is pyrexia, tachycardia, flushed face, repeated bile-stained vomiting, abdominal pain, rigidity and tenderness and the abdomen does not move with respiration (movement causes pain). The knees are flexed, which slightly relieves pain. The tongue becomes dry due to dehydration. By the third day paralytic ileus is present and causes an absence of bowel sounds, abdominal distension and a very tender abdomen. By the fourth day the skin is cold and clammy, the pulse rapid and thready, and the eyes sunken but bright.

Complications: abscess. Paralytic ileus. Acute intestinal obstruction due to adhesions.

Treatment: rest in bed in the semi-sitting position. Gastro-intestinal aspiration and an i.v. drip. 30 ml of water hourly is put into the stomach (probably aspirated later). Fluid balance chart. Correction of electrolyte imbalance, especially potassium, since hypokalaemia delays the return of peristalsis. Measurement of abdominal girth. A flatus tube is passed and the presence or absence of flatus noted. Blood transfusion is given for a low haemoglobin, e.g. below 8·8 per g/dl (60%). Sedation with morphine 10–15 mg four-hourly. Vitamins B and C. Antibiotic, e.g. penicillin plus streptomycin, or tetracycline 0·5 g in 1 l dextrose-saline drip every 12 hours. Frequent changes of position.

Treatment is of the cause, e.g. operation for perforated peptic ulcer.

Chronic peritonitis is due to tuberculosis from an infected mesenteric lymph node or pyosalpinx, or to malignancy. There is ascites (peritoneal effusion), weight loss, diarrhoea or constipation, weakness, pyrexia and abdominal discomfort.

Ascites
Ascites is the collection of fluid in the peritoneal sac. The mechanism of its formation is the same as for oedema (Chapter 3).

Causes: raised venous pressure (cardiac failure, constrictive pericarditis), hepatic cirrhosis, nephrotic syndrome, tuberculous peritonitis, carcinoma invading the peritoneum.

Clinically: massive ascites causes discomfort and restricts breathing.

Treatment is of the cause, a low sodium diet, a diuretic, and a high protein intake. It may be necessary to remove fluid from the peritoneal cavity (paracentesis abdominis).

Paracentesis Abdominis. The procedure is explained to the patient. The bladder must be emptied. A many-tailed bandage or abdominal binder is placed in position. The appropriate area of abdominal skin in the iliac fossa or in the midline of the abdomen between the umbilicus and pubis is sterilised with iodine and local anaesthetic injected. Avoiding old operation scars (since organs may adhere to the abdominal wall and thus be liable to injury), a trocar (needle) and cannula (tube) is inserted, the trocar is removed and a plastic tube attached to the cannula to drain the ascitic fluid into a container through a drip chamber so that the rate of flow can be controlled. The binder is kept tight while fluid is draining and for 24 hours afterwards, otherwise removal of fluid, which reduces the pressure in the abdomen, may cause shock.

Enlargement of the Abdomen

This may be due to fat (obesity), fluid (ascites), gas (fermentation of carbohydrates, putrefaction of proteins, swallowed air), both fluid and gas (intestinal obstruction), pregnancy, enlargement of the liver and spleen (e.g. myeloid leukaemia, malaria), or tumours of the ovary, kidney or liver.

9 THE LIVER AND BILIARY SYSTEM

THE LIVER

The liver is a gland weighing about 1·5 kg (3 lb) and is situated in the upper part of the abdomen (*Fig. 8.21*) in the right hypochondrium and epigastrium and extends into the left hypochondrium. Above is the diaphragm, below is the stomach, duodenum, colon, right kidney and adrenal, behind is the oesophagus, inferior vena cava, aorta, vertebral column and diaphragm. Laterally are the ribs and diaphragm, and in front is the anterior abdominal wall.

The liver is enclosed in a capsule and covered by peritoneum attaching it to the diaphragm. It has four lobes: the large right lobe, the left lobe, and the quadrate and caudate lobes. On the posterior surface of the liver is the gall bladder. Entering the liver at the portal fissure are the portal vein (carrying blood from the stomach, spleen, pancreas and intestines), the hepatic artery (carrying arterial blood), and autonomic nerve fibres, and leaving it are the right and left hepatic bile ducts carrying bile to the gall bladder, and lymph vessels (*Fig. 9.1*).

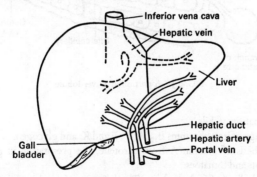

FIG. 9.1   Diagram of the vessels of the liver

The liver consists of numerous tiny hexagonal lobules. Each lobule contains columns of cubical cells (*Fig. 9.2*) radiating from a central vein. Between the columns of cells there are sinusoids which receive blood from branches of the portal vein and hepatic artery (*Fig. 9.3*). The sinusoids are lined with Kupffer cells which belong to the reticuloendothelial system and are phagocytic, taking up foreign particles from the blood, for example bacteria which enter the portal blood from the intestine. Blood flows through the sinusoids into the central vein which drains into the hepatic veins. The hepatic veins enter the inferior vena cava.

Bile formed by the liver cells enters the bile capillaries, and from these drains into the bile ducts which join to form the right and left hepatic ducts.

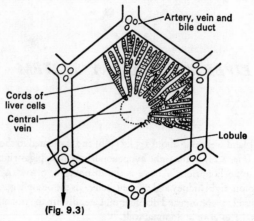

FIG. 9.2 A liver lobule

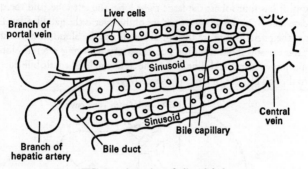

FIG. 9.3 A portion of a liver lobule

Function.

1 Formation of bile.

2 Storage of iron, vitamins B_{12}, A, D, E and K, and glycogen.

3 Synthesis of vitamin A from carotene, the provitamin in green leaves, carrots and tomatoes.

4 Metabolism of carbohydrate. The liver converts glucose into glycogen, then releases glucose from glycogen, as required.

5 Metabolism of protein. Formation of plasma proteins (albumin, fibrinogen, prothrombin and other blood clotting factors). The deamination of (removal of amino groups from) proteins to form urea. The conversion of unwanted nucleoprotein to uric acid. The conversion of excess protein into glucose (gluconeogenesis). The synthesis of non-essential amino acids.

6 Metabolism of fat.

7 Heat production, due to the energy used by the liver in its metabolism.

8 Inactivation of hormones, e.g. aldosterone and oestrogens.

9 Detoxification of drugs, e.g. morphine and atropine, and of poisons, e.g. ammonia.

INVESTIGATIONS IN LIVER DISEASE

Liver Function Tests

Serum Bilirubin: the normal is 5–14 μmol/l (0·3–0·8 mg%). In the Van den Bergh test bilirubin may be direct-reacting (conjugated bilirubin, cholebilirubin) or indirect-reacting (unconjugated bilirubin, haemobilirubin). Increased cholebilirubin is due to obstruction to the secretion of bile (obstructive jaundice). Increased haemobilirubin is due to increased haemolysis of red cells or failure of the liver to convert it to cholebilirubin.

Serum Alkaline Phosphatase is an enzyme formed in bone and liver and excreted by the liver. The normal is 20–90 iu/l (3–13 KA units%). It is increased in obstructive jaundice, hepatocellular damage and in bone diseases.

Serum Transaminases (aminotransferases) are enzymes present in many tissues, especially liver and heart. They are released from damaged cells, increasing the serum level. The normal serum level of both glutamic–pyruvic transaminase (S.G.P.T., alanine aminotransferase) and glutamic–oxaloacetic transaminase (S.G.O.T., aspartate aminotransferase) is 4–17 i.u./l (= 11–40 Wu/ml).

Serum Thymol Turbidity is increased in liver damage. The normal is up to 4 units. The zinc sulphate turbidity and cephalin flocculation tests are similar. Positive tests are due to changes in the serum proteins.

Serum Proteins: the serum albumin (normal = 50 g/l) is low in liver disease and the serum globulin (normal = 25 g/l.) is raised.

Plasma Prothrombin Level is low in vitamin K deficiency, liver damage or treatment with vitamin K antagonists, e.g. Dindevan.

Urine: bilirubin is present in obstructive jaundice. Urobilinogen is increased in haemolytic anaemia and absent in obstructive jaundice.

Bromsulphalein (B.S.P.) Test. The liver handles B.S.P. in the same way as bilirubin. 95% of a dose of 350 mg i.v. should be removed from the serum in 45 minutes and 98% in 60 minutes. It is retained in the serum in diseases affecting hepatic blood flow, liver function and biliary excretion.

Liver Biopsy demonstrates cirrhosis and other disorders.

Liver Scanning, after giving a radio-isotope, demonstrates tumours and excretory function. **Ultrasonic scanning** shows cysts.

Barium Swallow or **Fibreoptic Oesophagoscopy** shows oesophageal varices in cirrhosis of the liver.

Splenic Venography. Contrast medium is injected into the spleen and X-rays are taken to show the splenic and portal veins.

JAUNDICE, AND DISORDERS OF THE LIVER

Jaundice is yellow pigmentation due to accumulation of bile pigments in the blood and tissues. It is most easily seen in the conjunctivae.

Physiology. Old red blood cells are broken down by the reticuloendothelial system, especially the spleen. The haemoglobin is broken into globin, which is fragmented into amino acids to be used again, iron which is also re-used, and haemobilirubin (unconjugated bilirubin). These are released into the blood and the bilirubin attaches to albumin, from which it is detached by the liver and conjugated with (joined to) glucuronic acid to become cholebilirubin (conjugated bilirubin) which is excreted into the bile to reach the intestine. Here, bacteria change bilirubin into stercobilinogen, some of which is absorbed and excreted in the urine where it is called urobilinogen (*Fig. 5.4*). Urobilinogen oxidises in air to urobilin.

Types. Jaundice may be haemolytic, hepatocellular, or obstructive in origin (*Table 9.1*).

TABLE 9.1 *The features of the different types of jaundice*

	Type of jaundice		
	Haemolytic	*Hepatocellular*	*Obstructive*
Appetite	Normal	Poor	Normal or poor
Skin			
jaundice	Pale lemon	Usually moderate	Often pronounced and greenish
bruising	None	May be present	Common
pruritus	No	No	Common
Urine			
urobilinogen	Increased	Slightly increased	Decreased
bilirubin	Absent	Present	Present
bile salts	Absent	Absent	Present
Faeces, colour	Dark	Normal unless obstruction	Pale and bulky
Blood			
Anaemia	Always present	May be present	None
Van den Bergh (bilirubin)	Indirect+	Direct and indirect+	Direct+
alkaline phosphatase	Normal	Slightly increased	Increased
turbidity tests	Normal	++	Normal
transaminase	Normal	Increased in acute damage	Normal
albumin	Normal	Decreased	Normal
prothrombin concentration	Normal	Low	Low

Haemolytic (Pre-hepatic) Jaundice

Excessive destruction of red blood cells increases bilirubin formation. Haemobilirubin in the blood is bound to albumin and cannot enter the urine (acholuric jaundice), but the urine contains an excess of urobilinogen.

Causes:

1 Congenital abnormalities of the red blood cells such as an abnormal haemoglobin i.e. haemoglobinopathy (sickle-cell anaemia, thalassaemia), spherocytosis (spherical cells which rupture easily), or defective enzymes in the red cells.
2 Toxins. Drugs such as quinine, sulphonamides, nitrofurantoin, phenylhydrazine, phenacetin, methyldopa. Poisons.
3 Infections, e.g. malaria (Chapter 4).
4 Antibodies to red cells, e.g incompatible blood transfusion, 'rhesus' baby (erythroblastosis fetalis), acquired acholuric jaundice (Chapter 5).

Clinically: the skin is a lemon (pale) yellow due to the combination of anaemia and jaundice. There is anaemia and splenomegaly due to the destruction of red cells. The stools are a normal colour.

Investigations: the blood count shows a normochromic anaemia. The reticulocyte count is increased owing to regeneration of blood. Serum bilirubin (indirect, i.e. unconjugated) is increased. The Coombs test is positive in anaemia due to red cell antibodies. The red cell fragility may be increased. Fresh urine is of normal colour but contains an excess of urobilinogen, and darkens on standing due to the oxidation of urobilinogen (colourless) to urobilin (brown).

Treatment: see anaemia, Chapter 5.

Hepatocellular Jaundice
Damaged liver cells are less able to convert haemobilirubin into cholebilirubin, thus increasing the serum haemobilirubin. They also have difficulty in secreting bile. Swelling of cells compresses bile canaliculi and causes intrahepatic cholestasis, thus increasing the serum cholebilirubin (*Fig. 9.4*).

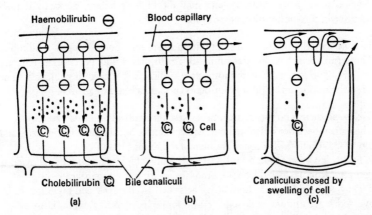

FIG. 9.4   Mechanism of the high serum bilirubin in hepatocellular damage: (*a*) normal liver cell; (*b*) moderately damaged cell; (*c*) severely damaged cell

Causes:

1 Infections: virus hepatitis, leptospirosis, yellow fever, glandular fever, septicaemia.
2 Drugs: pyrazinamide, ethionamide, chlorpropamide, iproniazid, oestrogens, tetrachloroethane, halothane sensitivity, cytotoxins used in malignant diseases, paracetamol overdose (15 g).
3 Other toxins: toluene, carbon tetrachloride, alcohol, selenium, mycotoxins, (toxins from fungi).
4 Congenital deficiencies of enzymes in liver cells, e.g. Gilberts disease (glucuronyl transferase deficiency).
5 Others: Hepatic cirrhosis, carcinoma of the liver.

Viral Hepatitis

Viral hepatitis is usually due to infective hepatis or to serum hepatitis, or hepatitis virus C, but is ocassionally due to other viruses such as glandular fever.

Acute Infective Hepatitis

This is due to hepatitis virus A which is spread via faecally-contaminated food, water or shellfish or by direct contact. It is predisposed by alcohol and a poor diet.

Clinically: the incubation period is two to six weeks. It is commonest in children and young adults. Anorexia is the first symptom, followed by headache, nausea, vomiting, constipation, pyrexia and jaundice.

Swelling of liver cells enlarges the liver and stretches its capsule, causing tenderness in the right hypochondrium and epigastrium. The stools are a normal colour at first, but severe infection obstructs bile canaliculi and the stools become pale and the urine darkens.

Complications: most patients recover completely within three months. A few develop acute yellow atrophy (and may die of liver failure, especially if malnourished), chronic hepatitis, or cirrhosis.

Investigations: the urine contains albumin and an excess of urobilinogen or bilirubin. The serum bilirubin and transaminases are increased and flocculation tests are positive. The serum alkaline phosphatase is increased if there is cholestasis. The faeces are normal unless biliary obstruction occurs, when they are pale.

Treatment: there is no specific treatment. Rest in bed usually for two to three weeks. The patient need not be isolated but requires barrier nursing since faeces, urine and blood are infectious. Thorough washing of the hands.
Diet: high energy (3000 kcal., 13·3 MJ daily), high protein, fat is allowed if desired. Alcohol is forbidden for six months since it is toxic to the liver.
Drugs: many drugs are normally inactivated by the liver and these should be avoided, e.g. barbiturates. If jaundice is prolonged corticosteroids may be given.
Severe disease is treated as for liver failure.
Convalescence may be slow owing to tiredness and depression.

Prevention: γ-globulin given before the incubation period attenuates the disease and limits epidemics in schools and institutions.

Note: Briefly boiling syringes does not destroy the virus, but autoclaving does.

Serum Hepatitis (Homologous Serum Jaundice)

This is due to hepatitis B virus which is spread by plasma or blood transfusion, inoculations using contaminated needles (drug addicts, tattooing) or contaminated vaccine (yellow fever vaccine), or by mosquito bites. Those handling blood may become infected, e.g. workers in pathology laboratories, haemodialysis or organ transplant units. It may also be spread orally, sexually or by dental instruments. The incubation period is two to 14 weeks (average three months). Symptoms and signs are similar to infective hepatitis but the mortality is higher and hepatitis B antigen (Australia antigen) is present in the serum.

Leptospirosis

Leptospira are spirochaetes. *Leptospira icterohaemorrhagica* causes Weil's disease and is spread by drinking or immersion (e.g. swimming) in water or taking food contaminated by urine of small animals which carry the disease, e.g. rats, mice, hedgehogs, sometimes dogs, cats, pigs and cattle. Another Leptospira is *L. canicola*, spread by dogs, and causing meningitis. The portals of entry are by ingestion, through damaged skin or the nasal, genital and buccal mucosa or conjunctiva.

Weil's Disease is an occupational hazard in farmers, coal miners, abattoir and sewage workers, fish cutters and veterinary surgeons.

Clinically: it is a generalised disease but particularly attacks the liver and kidneys. The incubation period is four to 21 (average 10) days. It begins with headache, pyrexia, pains in the muscles, anorexia, nausea, vomiting and conjunctival congestion, then jaundice, pain and tenderness in the right hypochondrium due to hepatitis, dark urine and haemorrhages, e.g. purpura, epistaxis. Renal damage causes albuminuria, haematuria and uraemia. Myocarditis leads to tachycardia and cardiac failure, and meningitis causes headache and neck stiffness.

Investigations: the blood shows a polymorph leucocytosis and an increased bilirubin. Urine contains red cells, protein and an increased urobilinogen.

Treatment: benzylpenicillin 300 mg 6-hourly i.m. for seven to 14 days, or tetracycline. Barrier nursing. Disinfection of urine.

Acute Liver Necrosis (Acute Yellow Atrophy)

Acute necrosis of the liver may be a complication of viral hepatitis, drugs, toxins such as phosphorus, benzene, carbon tetrachloride, and chloroform, or toxaemia of pregnancy. Symptoms are the same as for infective hepatitis but progress to deep jaundice, severe headache, vomiting, haemorrhages, confusion, delirium, and perhaps coma and death due to hepatic failure.

Treatment is the correction of fluid and electrolyte imbalance, and glucose orally or i.v.

Cirrhosis of the Liver

Hepatic cirrhosis is hardening of the liver by fibrous tissue.

Causes:

1   Portal cirrhosis is due to excessive alcohol, the commonest cause (which is associated with a poor diet owing to anorexia from chronic gastritis), poor diet (deficiency of protein and vitamin B), and rarely virus hepatitis.
2   Biliary cirrhosis may be primary, due to autoimmunity, or secondary, due to cholangio-hepatitis caused by gallstones or by bile-duct stricture.
3   Chronic cardiac failure causes venous congestion in the liver and finally cirrhosis.
4   Haemochromatosis, an excessive deposition of iron in the body.
5   Hepatolenticular degeneration, an excessive deposition of copper.

Clinically: the onset is insidious. In portal cirrhosis the liver is enlarged at first, but shrinks and becomes small as it is gradually destroyed. Hepatocellular failure causes malaise, vague dyspepsia, flatulence, anorexia, nausea, vomiting, furred tongue, mild fever, weight loss and spider naevi (tiny vessels in the skin). A diminished production of prothrombin causes bleeding, whilst diminished albumin production leads to oedema and ascites. The liver fails to metabolise aldosterone, causing sodium and water retention, which contributes to oedema and ascites.

Obstruction to the portal circulation by the damage in the liver leads to portal hypertension which contributes to ascites and causes splenomegaly, distension of veins around the umbilicus, haemorrhoids, and oesophageal varices. Oesophageal varices may bleed and cause haematemesis and anaemia.

Eventually there is jaundice, foetor hepaticus (an offensive smell), and encephalopathy.

Complications: haematemesis; infection, e.g. bronchopneumonia; primary carcinoma of the liver; and hepatic coma.

Investigations: liver function tests. Liver biopsy to show the type of cirrhosis. Barium swallow to demonstrate oesophageal varices.

Treatment: avoidance of alcohol. Normal fluid intake e.g. 2 l daily.

Diet: normal fat (80 g daily), high protein (80–120 g daily) if there is hypo-albuminaemia, but low protein (20 g daily or less) if there is encephalopathy. Salt restriction if there is ascites. Vitamins B and C. Iron or folic acid for anaemia.

Drugs: diuretic, e.g. bendrofluazide (Aprinox) 10 mg daily orally for oedema, plus potassium chloride 0·5 g q.i.d. Spironolactone (Aldactone-A) 100 mg daily orally. Vitamin K_1, 10 mg i.m. daily if the prothrombin level is low.

If there is ascites and a low urinary output paracentesis abdominis (tapping of ascites) is performed, assisted with a many-tailed bandage applied from above downwards and gently tightened to maintain pressure as fluid drains from the peritoneal cavity.

Treatment of complications, e.g. vasopressin 1 ml (20 units) i.v. in 100 ml 5% dextrose over 10 minutes and surgery for bleeding oesophageal varices.

Surgical: anastomosis of the portal vein to the inferior vena cava (porto-caval anastomosis) to relieve portal hypertension.

Hepatic Coma and Pre-coma (Hepatic Encephalopathy)

This is abnormality of brain function due to liver failure. It may occur in cirrhosis, acute liver necrosis, or severe viral hepatitis. It is due to failure of the liver to detoxicate toxins, e.g. ammonia, produced in the intestine by the action of bacteria on proteins. In cirrhosis, coma may be precipitated by haemorrhage into the gastro-intestinal tract, alcohol, general infection, or the rapid tapping of ascites. It causes a flapping tremor of the outstretched hands, abnormal behaviour, delirium and coma in addition to the signs of hepatocellular damage and portal hypertension described under hepatic cirrhosis.

Treatment: correction of water and electrolyte imbalance, and especially potassium depletion.

Diet: high carbohydrate (at least 400 g daily) to minimise protein catabolism, no protein in severe encephalopathy. Glucose i.v. if the patient is unable to swallow (coma). Prevent the formation of toxins by killing bacteria in the gut with neomycin 1 g six-hourly orally, assisted with enemas or purgation. Lactulose (Duphalac) may help by promoting the growth of starch-splitting bacteria which reduces the number of protein-splitting bacteria and releases lactic acid into the gut which traps the toxic ammonia.

Drugs should be avoided, since many are normally detoxicated by the liver, but small doses of sodium phenobarbitone i.m. may be needed if there is restlessness and noisiness.

Portal Hypertension

Portal hypertension is a high pressure with congestion in the portal venous system (*Fig. 9.5*). It is due to cirrhosis of the liver, back pressure from congestive cardiac failure or pressure by a tumour on the portal vein. Jaundice is often absent, owing to adequate liver function. The organs which drain into the portal vein (stomach, small and large intestine, spleen and pancreas) become congested since their venous return is impaired. This is particularly seen in the veins of the oesophagus, which become varicose (oesophageal varices) and may rupture and cause haematemesis. Veins of the rectum also become varicose (haemorrhoids, piles).

The high pressure in the veins increases the hydrostatic pressure in the blood capillaries and causes ascites (the accumulation of fluid in the peritoneal cavity).

Treatment is of the cause where possible, and of symptoms where necessary, e.g. salt-low albumin for oedema due to hypoalbuminaemia, or porto-caval anastomosis may be performed for bleeding oesophageal varices.

Carcinoma of the Liver

Primary carcinoma of the liver is rare but occurs particularly in hepatic cirrhosis.

Secondary deposits of malignant growth are common and are due to spread from primary carcinoma in the stomach, colon, rectum, pancreas, breast and lung.

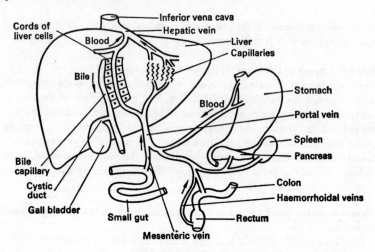

FIG. 9.5   Diagram of the portal venous system

The liver enlarges and causes discomfort in the upper part of the abdomen, and nodules may be palpable. Nodules often have a central depression due to necrosis. Jaundice is common and is due to pressure by the growth on bile ducts. The patient soon dies.

Treatment consists of analgesics for pain, and the removal of ascitic fluid. A single nodule may be removed by hemihepatectomy if the primary is also treatable.

Obstructive Jaundice

Obstructive jaundice is jaundice due to obstruction of the outflow of bile from the liver cells into the duodenum. Bile accumulates in the liver and is reabsorbed into the blood.

Causes: intrahepatic cholestasis is due to obstruction of the small bile ducts in the liver, often due to swelling of liver cells which compresses bile canaliculi. It is caused by oral contraceptives, methyl testosterone, phenothiazines, chlorpropamide, cholangitis, primary biliary cirrhosis, or severe hepatitis.

Extrahepatic obstructive (post-hepatic) jaundice is due to obstruction of the main bile ducts, usually the common bile duct, by gallstones, carcinoma of the head of the pancreas, carcinoma or stricture of the bile duct, or malignant lymph nodes in the porta hepatis *(Fig. 9.6).*

Clinically: symptoms are of the cause, e.g. pain in the back from carcinoma of the pancreas, and also jaundice which may be greenish, malaise, anorexia, and pruritus (itching, due to bile salt retention). Lack of bile salts in the intestine prevent the absorption of fat, so the stools contain excess of fat and are pale (no bilirubin), bulky and offensive smelling. Haemorrhages, e.g. into the skin, are due to a low plasma prothrombin level caused by deficiency of vitamin K which is fat-soluble and therefore is not absorbed.

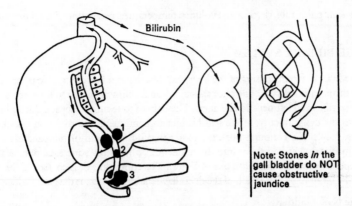

FIG. 9.6   Causes of obstructive jaundice: (1) glands in the porta hepatis; (2) gall stone in the common bile duct; (3) carcinoma of the head of the pancreas

Investigations: liver function tests show a raised direct-reacting bilirubin and an increased alkaline phosphatase in the serum. The urine is dark due to cholebilirubin, but the urobilinogen concentration is low.

Treatment is of the cause, and a high-protein, fat-free diet is administered.

Nursing Observations in a Jaundiced Patient

History of taking drugs, injections or contact with infective hepatitis. Symptoms, e.g. pain (colic).

Jaundice: degree (pale yellow in haemolytic anaemia, often marked and greenish-yellow in obstructive jaundice), whether there is variation in its degree (jaundice may vary from day to day if it is due to gallstones, but is gradually increasing in carcinoma of the head of the pancreas or liver).

The State of the Skin: the presence of rashes (drugs, certain liver diseases), pallor (anaemia), scratch marks (pruritus, i.e. obstructive jaundice), bruising (prothrombin deficiency).

Haemorrhages: haematemesis (oesophageal varices, vitamin K deficiency), bruises or petechiae in the skin.

Vomitus: description (the presence of bile excludes obstruction of the common bile duct), volume (for fluid balance), presence or absence of blood (oesophageal varices, vitamin K deficiency).

Faeces: colour, quantity, odour (pale, bulky and offensive in obstructive jaundice, dark in haemolytic anaemia).

Food intake: appetite, type of food, e.g. dislike of fat especially in gall-bladder disease, anorexia early in hepatitis.

Fluid Intake and Output so that fluid and electrolyte balance can be maintained.

General: pulse, rate, rhythm and volume, temperature, respirations, blood pressure.

THE BILIARY SYSTEM

The biliary system consists of the liver, gall bladder and bile ducts. Bile is secreted by the hepatic cells into fine bile capillaries (canaliculi) which join to leave the liver as the right and left hepatic bile ducts. These unite to form the hepatic duct which joins the cystic duct from the gall-bladder to continue as the common bile duct (*Fig. 8.20*). The common bile duct passes through the head of the pancreas and immediately before its exit into the duodenum it joins the pancreatic duct at the ampulla of the bile duct (ampulla of Vater). The common exit is controlled by the sphincter of Oddi. The walls of the ducts have the same layers as the gall-bladder.

The Gall-bladder

This is a pear-shaped sac attached to the undersurface of the liver. It has a fundus, a body, and a neck which continues into the cystic duct. The wall of the gall-bladder has three layers. An outer layer of peritoneum (except over that part in contact with the liver), a middle layer of smooth muscle consisting of longitudinal, circular and oblique fibres, and an inner lining of mucous membrane.

Function: the gall-bladder acts as a reservoir for bile, its mucosa secretes mucus into the bile and concentrates the bile by absorbing water from it, and the muscular wall contracts to expel bile via the bile ducts into the duodenum.

Bile secreted by the liver cannot enter the duodenum when the sphincter of Oddi is closed, so it passes into the relaxed gall-bladder where it is concentrated and stored. When food containing fat enters the duodenum the duodenum secretes the hormone cholecystokinin–pancreozymin which causes the contraction of the gall-bladder (in addition to stimulating pancreatic enzyme secretion).

Bile. Bile is composed of water, mineral and bile salts, mucus, cholesterol, lecithin and bile pigments. The bile salts emulsify fats in the duodenum. The bile pigments are waste products from the breakdown of red blood cells and the bile is their route of excretion into the faeces. Bile has an aperient action, colours the faeces, and is necessary for the absorption of fat and the fat-soluble vitamins A, D, E, and K.

Emulsification of fat is the reduction of large globules to the tiny globules essential for its absorption. Tiny globules provide a large surface area (*Fig. 9.7*) for the action of pancreatic lipase.

INVESTIGATIONS IN GALL-BLADDER DISEASE

1 *Plain X-ray:* most gallstones (90%) are radiotranslucent and do not show on a plain radiograph.

2 *Cholecystography:* an aperient is given two days before the test since a loaded colon obscures the gall-bladder on X-ray. A fatty meal is taken at 6 p.m. on the day before the test to empty the gall-bladder so that later the 'dye' will fill it.

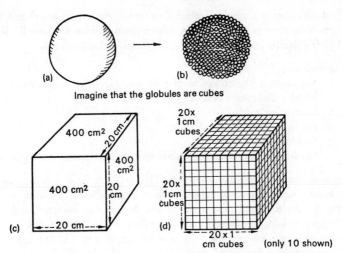

FIG. 9.7 Increase in surface area due to emulsification: (a) single large globule surface area 25 cm²; (b) the same volume but as small globules, surface area 25,000 cm²; (c) one cube with six faces each 20 × 20 cm = 6 × 400 = 2400 cm²; (d) 20 × 20 × 20 (= 8000) cubes with six faces, each 1 × 1 cm, total surface area = 6 × 8000 = 48,000 cm²

Graham–Cole test: a substance ('dye') which is excreted into the bile and which is opaque to X-rays is given orally (six tablets of 'telepaque') in the evening (10 p.m.) and no food or fluid is allowed by mouth until radiographs have been taken on the following morning, then the patient is given a meal with a high fat content (eggs, bacon, heavily buttered toast, and milk or cream) and one hour later further radiographs are taken.

Intravenous Test: biligrafin (sodium iodipamide) is injected i.v. and radiographs are taken at intervals afterwards. A fatty meal is given as with the oral test.

If the gall-bladder is functioning normally it will concentrate the 'dye', which will outline any stones. The fatty meal causes a normal gall-bladder to contract and empty. A cholecystogram should not be performed within three days of an attack of biliary colic or if the bilirubin is above 50 μmol/l (3 mg%) since the function of the liver is depressed and the 'dye' will not be excreted into the biliary system.

DISEASES OF THE BILIARY SYSTEM

Cholecystitis

Cholecystitis is inflammation of the gall-bladder (chole = bile, cyst = sac, itis = inflammation). It may be acute, subacute or chronic and is due to infection with *E. coli*, streptococci, staphylococci or rarely by salmonellae. Gallstones may obstruct the neck of the gall-bladder and cause biliary stasis which predisposes to infection.

Clinically: in acute cholecystitis there is pyrexia, polymorph leucocytosis, tachycardia; pain and tenderness in the right hypochondrium, the pain radiating to the right shoulder; nausea, vomiting which does not relieve the pain, and there may be rigors. The patient is usually female, fat-intolerant (dislikes fatty food), 'fertile' (has several children), aged forty to fifty, fat (obese) and has flatulence.

Complications:

1 Suppuration (the collection of pus), forming an empyema of the gall-bladder. The patient becomes very ill.
2 Perforation, rarely.
3 Fistula, e.g. with the duodenum.
4 Gallstones.
5 Cholangitis, due to spread of infection along the bile ducts, causing jaundice.

Treatment: conservative—the patient should rest in bed in the semi-sitting position. Fluids are given orally when there is no vomiting. If there is vomiting an intra-gastric or intraduodenal tube is passed and the contents aspirated; and fluids, electrolytes and dextrose given i.v. Pethidine (Demerol) 100 mg s.c. or i.m. and an antispasmodic, e.g. atropine 0·4–2 mg s.c. or i.m. or propantheline 15 mg, are given to relieve pain. Antibiotic for infection, e.g. sulphadimidine 3 g then 1–1·5 g six-hourly i.m., ampicillin 250 mg six-hourly, or cotrimoxazole 2–3 tablets b.d. A fat-free diet is given when vomiting stops and is continued during convalescence. Increase in pyrexia, pulse rate or vomiting should be reported since suppuration or perforation may be developing.

Surgical: cholecystectomy is sometimes performed within 3 days of the onset of an acute attack, otherwise it is performed 2 months later since recurrences are common.

Gallstones (Cholelithiasis, Biliary Calculi)

Gallstones are formed by the deposition from solution of substances in the bile. The gall-bladder concentrates bile, thus favouring deposition. The presence of bacteria in stagnant bile forms a nucleus on which cholesterol and bile pigment is deposited to form stones. Gallstones may consist of cholesterol, bile pigment (as in haemolytic anaemia), or a mixture of cholesterol and bile pigment, sometimes with calcium also.

Clinically: many stones are 'silent' and there are not any symptoms if they remain in the gall-bladder, or there may be flatulence, a feeling of fullness after meals, and discomfort after fatty food. If a stone enters the bile duct it causes colic. The patient is usually a middle-aged female who has had several children.

Complications: obstruction of the common bile duct, cholecystitis, acute pancreatitis, mucocele, cholangitis, and carcinoma of the gall-bladder.

Investigations: cholecystogram.

Treatment: diet low in fat and calories if obese; chenic (chenodeoxycholic) acid 15. mg/kg/day to dissolve cholesterol stones, or cholecystectomy.

A Stone in the Common Bile Duct. This condition causes obstructive jaundice and biliary colic—severe colicky pain in the right hypochondrium and epigastrium, which may make the patient roll about in agony. The pain radiates to the right shoulder and is associated with sweating, tachycardia and vomiting. A small stone may enter the duodenum and be passed in the faeces. A larger one may obstruct the common bile duct and after 24 hours causes jaundice which may fluctuate in intensity.

Investigations: i.v. cholecystogram and cholangiogram.

Treatment: rest in bed. Diet low in fat, and low in calories in obese subjects. Antispasmodic, e.g. atropine; analgesic, e.g. pethidine (a side-effect is mild contraction of smooth muscle. Morphine cannot be used since it causes more marked spasm). Sedation with phenobarbitone. Vitamin K (menaphthone) 10 mg b.d., i.m. Cholecystectomy and choledochotomy (opening the bile duct) to remove the stone(s).

Mucocele of the Gall-bladder. This is distension of the gall-bladder with mucus, usually due to obstruction of its neck with a gallstone. The treatment is cholecystectomy.

10 THE URINARY SYSTEM

The urinary system is one of the excretory systems of the body. The other excretory systems include the skin, hair, and lungs, and the biliary-intestinal-faecal system.

The urinary system consists of two kidneys which filter the blood to form urine, their ureters which propel the urine to the bladder, and the urinary bladder where urine is temporarily stored until it is discharged via the urethra.

THE KIDNEYS

Anatomy. The kidneys are situated behind the peritoneum on the posterior part of the abdomen, one on each side of the vertebral column. Each is surrounded by a fibrous capsule and outside this is the protective perirenal fat. The fat is surrounded by a sheath of fibroelastic tissue, the renal fascia, which holds the kidney in place. On the upper pole of each kidney is an adrenal (suprarenal) gland, behind are the muscles of the posterior abdominal wall and the diaphragm, in front of the right kidney is the duodenum, the right flexure of the colon and part of the liver. In front of the left kidney is the spleen, stomach, pancreas, jejunum and left colic flexure (*Figs. 10.1 and 10.2*).

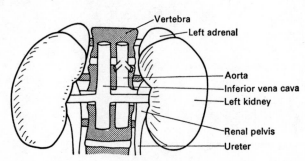

FIG. 10.1 The kidneys

The kidney consists of an outer part, the cortex, surrounded by the renal capsule; and an inner part, the medulla, which is attached to the calyces. The calyces are branches of the pelvis of the kidney. The renal pelvis narrows to become the ureter. The medulla forms conical projections called the renal pyramids which project into the renal pelvis (*Fig. 10.3*).

The renal artery and nerves enter, and the renal vein and lymphatics leave, the kidney at the hilum of the kidney adjacent to the pelvis.

Each kidney contains one million nephrons. A nephron is the functional unit of

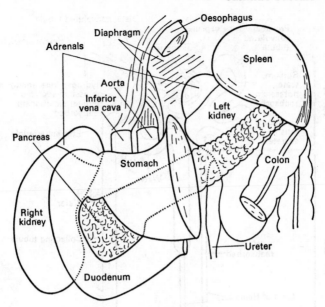

FIG. 10.2 The relations of the kidneys

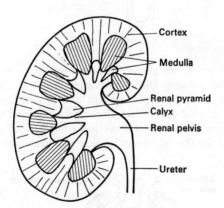

FIG. 10.3 A section of the kidney

the kidney and consists of a tubule and its glomerulus. The tubule is closed at one end. This end is indented by, and surrounds, a mesh of blood capillaries, the glomerulus. The indented end of the tubule thus forms a capsule around the glomerulus. The tubule is a single layer of cells forming a tube consisting of five parts: the glomerular capsule, the proximal convoluted tubule, the loop of Henle, the distal convoluted tubule and the collecting tubule. The collecting tubule drains into a renal calyx (*Fig. 10.4*).

The renal artery divides into small arteries then arterioles. One arteriole, the

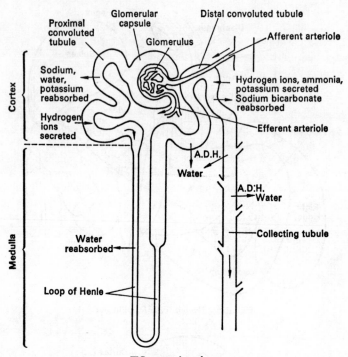

FIG. 10.4   A nephron

afferent arteriole, enters each glomerular capsule where it divides to form the glomerular capillary network. Unlike other tissues, in which the capillaries join to form venules, the glomerular capillaries join to form a second arteriole, the efferent arteriole (*Fig. 10.5*), which then redivides into capillaries around the tubules before ending in venules which lead blood to the renal vein. The renal vein empties into the inferior vena cava. The arterioles are supplied with autonomic nerves.

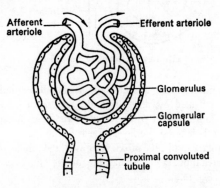

FIG. 10.5   A glomerulus

Physiology. Chapter 3 should be revised at this point. The function of the kidneys is to maintain water balance, electrolyte balance, the normal pH of the blood (Chapter 3), and to dispose of waste materials in the urine.

Urine is formed by simple filtration through the semi-permeable walls of the glomerular capillaries and glomerular capsule, and by selective reabsorption and secretion by the tubular epithelium. Filtration is brought about by the blood pressure which forces water and small molecules, such as salt, glucose and urea, out of the capillary into the glomerular capsule; but cells and large molecules such as protein remain in the capillary blood. An increase in blood pressure increases the amount of glomerular filtrate. A decrease in blood pressure, as in haemorrhage or burns, reduces glomerular filtration thus retaining fluid in the body and helping to combat shock. Substances which are essential to the body (e.g. water, some salts, glucose, amino acids and fatty acids) are then reabsorbed by the tubular cells as the filtrate passes along the tubule, and these substances do not appear in the urine. The ability of the tubules to reabsorb these substances is limited, thus glucose is completely reabsorbed at normal levels (80–120 mg%, 4·4–6·7 mmol/l, in the blood and glomerular filtrate), but if the blood glucose level rises above 10 mmol/l (180 mg%), as in diabetes mellitus, it cannot be reabsorbed completely and some is lost in the urine. This level is the renal threshold. The renal threshold is sometimes lower than normal; for example glucose may appear in the urine when the blood level is 8·9 mmol/l (160 mg%) and this is called a low renal threshold. The tubular cells secrete some substances from the blood into the tubule, for example corticosteroids and penicillin.

Control of Water Balance: normally 180 l of fluid are filtered from the glomeruli daily. The urine volume is 1·5 l, thus 178·5 l are reabsorbed. The minimum urinary output required to remove waste substances from the body is 500 ml in 24 hours. Water reabsorption by the tubule is partly controlled by the antidiuretic hormone (A.D.H., vasopressin). A.D.H. is made in neurons in the hypothalamus and passes down their axons to be stored in the posterior pituitary. Release of A.D.H. into the blood is controlled by cells in the hypothalamus (osmoreceptors) which are sensitive to changes in the osmotic pressure of the blood. If the osmotic pressure of the blood rises, as in dehydration, the osmoreceptors are stimulated and cause the release of A.D.H. If the osmotic pressure of the blood falls the amount of A.D.H. released into the blood is reduced. A.D.H. increases the permeability of the distal and collecting tubules and thus increases the reabsorption of water into the blood (*Fig. 10.6*).

If the tubules contain an abnormally high concentration of dissolved substances the A.D.H. is overpowered and water is excreted (osmotic diuresis). In diabetes mellitus the blood glucose concentration is high. If it exceeds the renal threshold for glucose it passes into the glomerular filtrate, thus increasing the osmotic pressure of the filtrate and preventing water from being absorbed into the blood. This increases urinary volume and the patient becomes dehydrated unless the fluid intake is increased (by thirst) to compensate for the extra water lost.

Control of Electrolyte Balance is by the adrenocorticosteroids (steroids secreted by the adrenal cortex, Chapter 12), hydrocortisone and aldosterone. Both of these act on

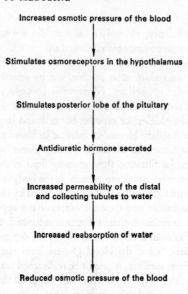

Increased osmotic pressure of the blood

Stimulates osmoreceptors in the hypothalamus

Stimulates posterior lobe of the pituitary

Antidiuretic hormone secreted

Increased permeability of the distal
and collecting tubules to water

Increased reabsorption of water

Reduced osmotic pressure of the blood

FIG. 10.6   Control of antidiuretic hormone secretion

the cells of the convoluted tubules to cause the reabsorption of sodium from the glomerular filtrate, but aldosterone has the more powerful action. An increased reabsorption of sodium causes a decreased reabsorption of potassium, thus more potassium is excreted in the urine. The reabsorption of sodium is automatically followed by the reabsorption of water.

Specialised cells are present in the wall of the afferent arteriole as it enters the glomerulus in contact with the distal convoluted tubule. A fall in the blood pressure in the renal artery (for example due to a fall in blood volume caused by haemorrhage, burns, or dehydration from vomiting) stimulates these juxta-glomerular cells to secrete renin into the blood. Renin converts angiotensinogen in the plasma into angiotensin, and angiotensin has two actions: it is a vasoconstrictor and it stimulates the adrenal cortex to release aldosterone. Aldosterone causes the kidney to retain sodium, and hence water, by an action on the convoluted tubular cells, and helps to restore the blood volume and blood pressure (*Fig. 3.4*). A reduced sodium intake also stimulates the secretion of aldosterone. Deficiency of aldosterone occurs in Addison's disease (hypoadrenocorticism) and causes the retention of potassium and the loss of sodium and water; hence dehydration and hypotension.

Control of Acid–Base Balance: the kidneys help to maintain the normal slightly alkaline blood pH by excreting acids such as phosphoric and sulphuric acids which are produced by the catabolism (breakdown) of protein. The tubular cells make carbonic acid from water and carbon dioxide. From the carbonic acid they secrete hydrogen ions (H^+) which are acid, and retain the bicarbonate ions (HCO_3^-) which are alkaline. If a positive ion such as hydrogen is secreted it must be replaced by another positive ion, so sodium (Na^+) is reabsorbed from the glomerular filtrate.

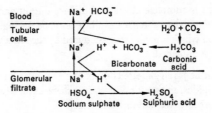

FIG. 10.7   Effects of hydrogen ion secretion

In this way sodium and bicarbonate are retained while hydrogen ions, sulphate and phosphate (= sulphuric and phosphoric acids) are excreted (*Fig. 10.7*). The tubular cells also make ammonia which can be secreted along with a hydrogen ion, forming an ammonium ion (NH_4^+) and this can also be exchanged for sodium or potassium. In renal failure acids accumulate in the blood (metabolic acidosis).

Hormonal Functions: the juxta-glomerular complex secretes renin which maintains the blood pressure by the two mechanisms described above. The kidney makes erythropoietin which is required by the bone marrow for red cell production (erythropoiesis); thus chronic renal disease causes anaemia. The kidney metabolises vitamin D into a more active form.

Mechanisms of Action of Diuretics
Diuretics act on the kidney to increase the excretion of water and certain electrolytes, especially sodium.
1   Inhibition of the secretion of antidiuretic hormone, such as by water or alcohol.
2   Osmotic action. Substances which pass into the glomerular filtrate and are not reabsorbed by the tubules provide a high osmotic pressure (*see* Chapter 3) in the tubules so that water is prevented from being reabsorbed and is excreted; for example by mannitol (250 ml of 20% solution i.v.).
3   Inhibition of sodium reabsorption by the tubules, for example by mercurials, thiazides, frusemide, or ethacrynic acid. If sodium is excreted water is automatically excreted with it.
4   Inhibition of aldosterone by spironolactone (Aldactone), thus preventing the sodium-reabsorptive action of aldosterone.
5   Decreased hydrogen ion secretion has a weak diuretic action by slightly reducing sodium reabsorption from the tubules; for example carbonic anhydrase inhibitors such as acetazolamide (Diamox).

SYMPTOMS AND SIGNS IN RENAL DISEASE

Oliguria ('less urine') is a urinary volume below the amount needed to excrete waste products. It may be due to a reduced renal blood flow caused by hypotension (shock, vomiting, diarrhoea) or cardiac failure, or to renal disease such as acute nephritis.

Anuria ('no urine') is complete absence of urinary output and occurs in severe shock, crush injury or bilateral renal calculi. It must be distinguished from acute retention of urine in which urine is being produced by the kidney but is retained in the bladder, which is distended.

Polyuria ('much urine') is an increased output of urine and is due to excessive fluid intake, diabetes insipidus, an osmotic diuresis as in diabetes mellitus, or chronic renal disease in which the tubules cannot reabsorb water.

Haematuria is blood in the urine and is due to haemorrhage from the urinary tract.

Causes:

1 Blood disorders. Anticoagulant therapy, thrombocytopenia, bacterial endocarditis.
2 Renal injury, tumour, infarct, tuberculosis, calculus, polycystic kidneys, acute pyelonephritis, polyarteritis nodosa.
3 Bladder papilloma, carcinoma, calculus, cystitis.
4 Prostatic carcinoma, benign hypertrophy with venous congestion, prostatitis.
5 Urethral injury, urethritis.
6 Others: malignant hypertension, contamination by menstruation. A reddish or brownish colour may be due to dyes in food or sweets, beetroot, or drugs such as senna.

Urine may be collected in three portions. Blood is present mostly at the beginning of micturition in urethral disease, at the end of micturition in bladder disease, and throughout in renal disease.

Proteinuria (protein in the urine). Normally the urine does not contain detectable amounts of protein. Albuminuria may follow severe exertion or be due to venous congestion as in congestive cardiac failure, or to poisons such as phenacetin and mercury, but albuminuria is usually due to urinary tract disease (for example nephritis, nephrotic syndrome or cystitis.)

Bence-Jones protein is often present in the urine in myelomatosis.

Glycosuria (glucose in the urine). Normally the urine does not contain detectable amounts of sugar, but glucose may be present if there is a low renal threshold for glucose (renal glycosuria) or in diabetes mellitus.

Ketonuria (ketones in the urine) may be present if fat is being used for energy, as in starvation, vomiting, or diabetes mellitus.

Pyuria (pus in the urine) occurs in pyelonephritis, renal tuberculosis, cystitis, prostatitis, and urethritis.

INVESTIGATIONS OF THE RENAL TRACT

Urine. The nurse tests the urine of the newly admitted patient for pH ('reaction'), albumin, sugar, blood and ketones.

For microscopy and culture a sterile early morning specimen is obtained by collecting a midstream specimen or by suprapubic aspiration. Passing a catheter is unnecessary and dangerous since it may cause urinary tract infection.

Method: in females vaginal contamination is prevented with a gauze tampon. In both sexes the external genitals are cleaned e.g. with 'Hibitane'. The first part of the specimen is collected into a receiver and discarded. The second part (midstream specimen) is collected in a sterile screw-capped bottle, kept cool, and sent to the laboratory while fresh, i.e. within one hour.

For a 24-hour specimen, urine is collected in a large vessel containing a few drops of toluol or hydrochloric acid as a preservative, labelled with the patient's name, and kept in a cool place. After discarding the first morning specimen, urine is collected at the same time the next morning, and includes the fresh early morning specimen.

The **volume** is normally 1–1·6 l in 24 hours but depends on water intake, and water losses by the skin (depending on climate) and faeces. It is recorded on the fluid balance chart. The **colour** is amber, but is pale if dilute, or dark if concentrated or containing bile or coloured drugs. The appearance is hazy (smoky) with small amounts of blood, or red to brown with larger amounts.

The **specific gravity** (S.G.) is an indication of the quantity of substances dissolved in it. The S.G. of water is 1·000 and of normal urine varies between 1·010 and 1·030 (300–1000 mosmol/kg). It is low in polyuria due to renal disease or excessive fluid intake, but is high if there is glycosuria or oliguria.

The **reaction** is normally slightly acid (pH 6·0), but is alkaline (pH above 7·0) after vomiting, alkaline drugs (potassium citrate, sodium bicarbonate), or if left standing because certain bacteria transform urea into ammonia, which is alkaline (the fact that bacteria grow while urine is left standing is one reason why urine should be tested when fresh).

The **deposit** may contain crystals of phosphate, which are white and dissolve in acid; oxalate; or urates which are light pink in colour. It may contain casts, which are cylinders of coagulated protein formed in the tubules, red blood cells, pus or organisms. In a fresh specimen 100,000 or more organisms per ml or over 200,000 white (pus) cells an hour indicate infection somewhere in the urinary tract.

Bile salts, bile pigments and urobilinogen may be tested for.

Urine Concentration and Dilution Test. At 6 p.m. the patient is given a meal with a good protein content but no more than 200 ml of fluid. No more fluid is allowed after this meal. Any urine passed during the night is discarded. On the following morning at 8, 9 and 10 a.m. urine is collected in separate containers labelled with the time; the bladder being emptied completely. These specimens should be concentrated; one should have a specific gravity of over 1·022 (= 800 mosmol/l). The patient is then given 1 l of water to drink within the next 30 minutes and the urine is collected hourly in separate containers for four hours. These should become dilute and at least one should have a specific gravity below 1·004. In severe chronic renal disease the specific gravity stays around 1·010 (= 300 mosmol/kg) throughout, since the kidney can neither concentrate the urine nor rapidly excrete a water load. Impaired concentration indicates tubular dysfunction or lack of antidiuretic hormone.

Urea Clearance Test. The urea clearance is the amount of blood theoretically completely cleared of urea in one minute. It is low if there is a low glomerular filtration rate. No fasting is necessary. The patient has breakfast and at 9 a.m. is given 200 ml of water; the bladder is emptied completely and the urine discarded. At 10 a.m. the bladder is completely emptied and the urine labelled with the exact time and its volume. Blood is taken between 10 and 11 a.m. and at 11 a.m. the bladder is again emptied and the urine collected and labelled with the exact time it was actually passed (e.g. 11·02 hours) and volume. The urea content of the blood and urines is measured. The normal urea clearance is 54 ml per minute if the urine flow is less than 2 ml per minute, or 75 ml per minute if the urine flow is above 2 ml per minute. These two levels are used because, although urea is filtered into the glomerular filtrate, it is partly reabsorbed from the tubule by diffusion, and less urea diffuses out of the tubule if the urine flow is increased.

The Creatinine Clearance is independent of urine flow and is measured on a 24-hour urine and a blood sample. Normal = 85–140 ml/min.

Blood Urea is normally 3·3–6·7 mmol/l (20–40 mg%); **Electrolytes** (Chapter 3).

Percutaneous Renal Biopsy. A fragment of kidney is taken, using a hollow needle, and is examined microscopically. Urine should be examined afterwards for blood, since renal bleeding is a complication.

Radiology. Plain X-ray shows the size and shape of the kidneys and calcification due to calculi or tuberculosis.

Intravenous Urogram (Pyelogram, I.V.P.): into a vein is injected material which is excreted in the urine and opaque to X-rays, causing the urine to cast a shadow. X-rays are taken at intervals and show the function, size, and any distortion, of the kidneys, ureters and bladder.

Preparation: minerals (e.g. bismuth or calcium) and food containing pips are avoided for three days before the X-ray. An aperient is given the preceding evening and a Dulcolax suppository one hour before the test, so as to remove faecal shadows. The patient has nothing to drink for six hours before the X-ray so that the urine will be concentrated. On completion of the test, fluid is given to relieve thirst.

Retrograde Pyelogram: radio-opaque material is injected into the pelvis and calyces of the kidney via the bladder and ureter and radiographs are taken.

Isotope Renogram: radioactive hippuran is given i.v. and the radioactivity over the urinary tract is measured.

Renal angiogram: radio-opaque material is injected into the renal artery, via a catheter passed into the femoral artery, and radiographs taken.

Ureteric Catheterisation. A special catheter is passed via the bladder into the ureter and urine can be collected separately from each kidney or a retrograde pyelogram performed.

DISEASES OF THE KIDNEY

Nephritis
Nephritis is inflammation of the kidney.

Types:
1 Pyelonephritis is bacterial infection of the kidney, particularly of the renal pelvis and medulla. It may be acute or chronic.
2 Glomerulonephritis is inflammation of the glomeruli of the kidney. There is no bacterial infection in the kidney: (*a*) acute glomerulonephritis; (*b*) chronic glomerulonephritis; (*c*) focal and other types of glomerulonephritis.
3 Nephrotic syndrome.

Pyelonephritis
Pyelonephritis is infection of the kidney (especially the medulla) and renal pelvis.

Acute Pyelonephritis (Acute 'Pyelitis'). This is common and should be treated early and thoroughly since, if it becomes chronic, renal damage occurs and may lead to renal failure. It is usually due to infection by *E. coli*, *Strept. faecalis*, *Proteus*, or *Pseudomonas*, ascending from the bladder. It is predisposed by catheterisation, by urinary tract obstruction such as prostatic enlargement, tumours, calculi, urethral stricture, or the pressure of a pregnant uterus (during pregnancy there is also relaxation of the ureter by hormones which contributes to stasis and infection), by diabetes mellitus, and by analgesic (e.g. phenacetin) abuse.

Clinically: the patient feels ill, has pain and tenderness in the loins, pyrexia, vomiting and rigors. Children may have convulsions, often without other symptoms. Associated cystitis causes suprapubic pain, dysuria (difficult or painful micturition), strangury (a painful desire to pass urine although the bladder is empty), and the frequent passage of small amounts of 'scalding' urine.

The blood shows a leucocytosis and the urine contains protein, numerous pus cells (pyuria), organisms and some blood. An intravenous pyelogram shows any obstruction.

Prognosis: the urine becomes sterile within a few days of treatment but organisms are still present in renal tissue for several more days; thus treatment should be given for a minimum of three weeks, otherwise mild infection may remain and cause chronic pyelonephritis.

Complications are acute renal failure, and chronic pyelonephritis.

Treatment: treatment of the predisposing cause. Rest in bed. A midstream specimen of urine is examined while fresh (within two hours of voiding) for organisms and their sensitivity to antibacterial drugs, and the appropriate drug is given, such as: sulphadimidine 2 g then 1 g orally four- to eight-hourly, or sulphamethizole (Urolucosil) 200 mg then 100 mg orally four-hourly. Co-trimoxazole (trimethoprim with sulphamethoxazole; Septrin) 2–6 tablets orally daily. *Side-effects* are nausea, vomiting, headache, rash, agranulocytosis.

Nalidixic acid (Negram) 0·5–1 g six-hourly. Resistance easily develops. It gives a positive Clinitest. Side-effects: nausea, vomiting, rash.

Nitrofurantoin (Furadantin) 50–150 mg orally p.c. six-hourly. Side-effects are peripheral neuropathy, pulmonary damage, arthralgia, nausea, and diarrhoea.

Gentamicin (Genticin) 80 mg 8-hourly i.m. or Kanamycin (Kantrex) 1 g i.m. daily. Side-effects are vestibular nerve damage (ataxia, vertigo) and rash. Since they are normally excreted via the urine, toxic levels are likely if there is renal failure.

Ampicillin (Penbritin) 0·5–1·5 g (or amoxycillin 250 mg) eight-hourly, orally. Side-effects: rash, hypersensitivity.

Tetracycline 250 mg orally six-hourly. It should not be used in pregnancy since it stains fetal teeth and bone.

Sulphonamides and kanamycin act best in alkaline urine and are given with sodium bicarbonate 3 g orally two-hourly or sodium citrate 3–6 g orally six-hourly until the urine is alkaline, then just enough to keep it alkaline.

Penicillins (e.g. ampicillin), tetracyclines, and usually nitrofurantoin, act best in acid urine, for example with ascorbic acid 1 g orally six-hourly.

Fluid intake should be normal, since if it is increased it dilutes the effect of the drug.

Chronic Pyelonephritis. This may be due to acute pyelonephritis, urinary tract obstruction, chronic cystitis (associated with, for example, multiple sclerosis or paraplegia), diabetes mellitus, or abuse (excessive intake) of analgesics.

There is vague ill-health and lassitude and there may be frequency of micturition. The urine is sometimes normal but may contain pus and show slight proteinuria. The infection is difficult to eradicate and requires prolonged treatment. Complications are hypertension and renal failure.

Acute Glomerulonephritis

This is also known as acute nephritis, acute diffuse glomerulonephritis, acute proliferative glomerulonephritis and Ellis type 1 nephritis. It is an acute diffuse inflammation of the glomeruli of both kidneys due to hypersensitivity to microbial toxins. The toxins cause the formation of immunoglobulins (antibodies and anti-toxins) which are deposited in the glomeruli and damage them. It is, therefore, an autoimmune disease. The causative microbes include bacteria and viruses, the commonest being the ß-haemolytic streptococcus. The streptococcus itself does not infect the kidney but remains confined to the throat.

Clinically: the disease usually affects children and adolescents. Acute tonsillitis or scarlet fever is followed, one to three weeks later, by renal inflammation which causes fever, malaise, anorexia, aching in the loins, and blood, albumin, casts and a few leucocytes in the urine. Damage to glomeruli reduces glomerular filtration and causes fluid and salt retention, hence oliguria and oedema. Oedema causes puffiness of the face (unlike the oedema of heart failure since the patients with heart failure are dyspnoeic and do not lie flat but sit up, thus fluid gravitates to the limbs and lower part of the trunk), and swelling of the hands and legs. If there is marked fluid retention effusions occur in the peritoneal cavity (ascites) and pleural cavities (hydrothorax). Oedema of the lungs causes breathlessness.

Oliguria leads to retention of waste products (uraemia) which causes tachycardia, headache, nausea, vomiting, and perhaps coma.

Hypertension is due to increased secretion of renin caused by the poor glomerular blood flow.

Investigations: the urine is smoky due to haematuria and contains up to 10 g/l of albumin. The blood shows a mild normochromic anaemia, increased blood urea, and an increased erythrocyte sedimentation rate (E.S.R.). The serum shows an increased antistreptolysin O (A.S.O.) level. Antistreptolysin O is an antibody to streptolysin O, a toxin produced by the β-haemolytic streptococcus. The serum electrolytes show potassium retention. The serum cholesterol is normal.

Prognosis: most patients improve after a few days and 90% recover completely in a few weeks. A few die of acute complications or go on to chronic glomerulonephritis.

Complications:

1 Acute heart failure.
2 Infection.
3 Uraemia due to renal failure.
4 Hypertensive encephalopathy.
5 Convulsions or coma due to uraemia or hypertensive encephalopathy.
6 Chronic glomerulonephritis.

Treatment: rest in bed, kept warm until symptoms disappear and the E.S.R. is normal. Mild proteinuria may persist for months but the patient is not kept in bed if proteinuria is the only abnormality. The urine volume and protein content, and the blood pressure, are measured daily, the temperature, pulse and respirations four-hourly at first, and the E.S.R. weekly.

Diet: fluid, salt and protein are limited. Water excretion is impaired, so the fluid intake is limited to 500 ml daily plus the volume of the previous day's urinary output. Salt is not added to food or used in cooking, since it leads to fluid retention. Protein is restricted to nil, 20 or 40 g daily if there is uraemia, since protein is broken down to urea and other waste products which cannot be excreted, and collect in the blood. To prevent muscle wasting, calories are given as carbohydrate and fat.

A child may begin with sweetened fruit juice 500 ml daily for a few days. When improvement in oedema and uraemia begin to occur, salt-free bread, salt-free butter and 20 g of protein are added. The diuresis due to recovery should be watched for so that excessive loss of fluid and electrolytes can be replaced. A normal diet is given as soon as oedema and uraemia have subsided.

Penicillin is given to clear the throat infection, if it is still present, e.g. procaine penicillin 600 mg daily i.m., or benzyl penicillin 300 mg b.d., i.m. for 5 days. For recurrent streptococcal infection prophylactic phenoxymethylpenicillin 250 mg orally daily is used, or tonsillectomy is performed during remission.

Immunosuppressive drugs such as azathioprine and corticosteroids are ineffective. A diuretic is not usually necessary since the oedema is frequently mild. If uraemia is severe peritoneal dialysis or haemodialysis may be needed.

Chronic Glomerulonephritis

Chronic glomerulonephritis may follow acute glomerulonephritis, membranous glomerulonephritis or sometimes the nephrotic syndrome. Symptoms, signs and treatment are as described under 'Chronic Renal Failure'. Hypertension is always present.

Other Types of Glomerulonephritis

Focal glomerulonephritis is due to bacterial endocarditis, Henoch–Schönlein syndrome, or polyarteritis nodosa. These cause proteinuria and haematuria.

Minimal-change Glomerulonephritis and **Membranous Glomerulonephritis** are abnormal immune disorders of the kidney which cause proteinuria and oedema, sometimes severe enough to cause the nephrotic syndrome.

Nephrotic Syndrome

A syndrome is a group of symptoms and signs which have more than one cause. The nephrotic syndrome is any condition in which proteinuria is severe enough to lower the plasma albumin levels, and therefore plasma osmotic pressure, sufficiently to cause oedema. Other plasma proteins may also be lost.

Causes:

1 Glomerulonephritis, especially minimal lesion glomerulonephritis (also called subacute nephritis, Ellis type 11 nephritis, or lipoid nephrosis) and membranous glomerulonephritis. The commonest causes in the United Kingdom and U.S.A.

2 Quartan malaria. The commonest cause in the tropics.

3 Occasional causes are: diabetes mellitus, systemic lupus erythematosus, thrombosis of the renal vein or inferior vena cava, amyloidosis, hypersensitivity to pollen, and poisons (mercury, gold, troxidone). The mechanism of oedema is shown in *Fig. 10.8.*

Clinically: any age is affected. The patient may rest in bed although this is not essential. Albuminuria is present before the oedema. Oedema is severe and generalised, its site depending on posture. It is worse in the legs in adults (or sacral region

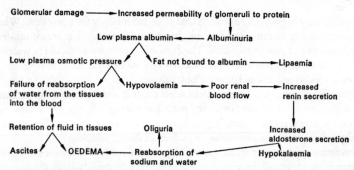

FIG. 10.8 The mechanism of oedema in the nephrotic syndrome

if in bed), but is more obvious in the face in children. In men the genitals may be swollen. The skin is pale ('a pale swollen patient with a pale swollen kidney'). In subacute nephritis haematuria, hypertension and uraemia are absent at first. Most children under 10 years of age recover, but the outlook in adults is uaually poor and many develop chronic nephritis with renal failure, or die from infection.

Complications:
1   Protein malnutrition, which causes muscular wasting.
2   Increased coagulability of the blood, causing venous and arterial thromboses.
3   Infection due to a low serum γ-globulin and malnutrition, for example pneumonia, cellulitis, or peritonitis.
4   Progression to chronic nephritis and renal failure.

Investigations: urine daily for albumin estimation. The serum albumin is low (below 36 g/l), the serum potassium may be low due to excessive aldosterone, and the blood cholesterol is above 6·5 mmol/l (250 mg%). The blood urea is normal (3·3–6·7 mmol/l; 20–40 mg%) at first, but rises if renal failure occurs. Renal function tests and renal biopsy, in those patients not responding to prednisolone, show the type of disease.

Treatment: rest in bed. The diet should be high in protein (80–110 g daily) and low in salt (no salt added to food on the plate or in the cooking; salt-free bread). The high protein diet is safe since the blood urea is normal. The patient may need encouragement to persevere with the tasteless low-salt diet.

Drugs: diuretic such as bendrofluazide (Neo-naclex, Aprinox) 5–15 mg orally daily. Spironolactone (Aldactone-A) 100–200 mg orally daily is added if the diuretic is inadequate. If oedema persists salt-free albumin may be given i.v. to raise the osmotic pressure of the plasma.

Prednisolone 60–80 mg daily for one to four weeks produces a rapid remission in subacute ('minimal change') nephritis but not in most of the other types. The dose is then reduced gradually to a maintenance level (e.g. 20 mg daily). Side-effects include growth retardation in children. Potassium chloride 14 mmol (1 g) t.d.s. orally to replace the potassium lost by the diuretic and prednisolone. For repeated attacks of subacute nephritis an immunosuppressive drug such as cyclophosphamide (Endoxan) 3 mg/kg daily is given for eight weeks; a weekly white cell count being done since leucopenia may develop. Prophylactic penicillin to prevent infection. Infection, e.g. of the upper respiratory tract, may precipitate relapse. Ascites may need aspirating if diuretics fail. Record of fluid balance and daily weight to observe progress.

Acute Renal Failure (Suppression of Urine)
This is sudden failure of the function of the kidneys due to poor glomerular filtration.

Causes:
Pre-renal—fall in blood pressure sufficient to severely reduce glomerular filtration, as in severe shock due to haemorrhage, burns, crush injury with extensive tissue damage, acute pancreatitis, incompatible blood transfusion (shock and obstruction

of tubules by haemoglobin), septicaemia due to Gram-negative organisms (bacter-aemic shock), dehydration due to severe vomiting, diarrhoea, diabetes mellitus, Addison's disease, heat stroke, intestinal obstruction, myocardial infarction, or toxaemia of pregnancy.

Renal disease: acute glomerulonephritis, acute pyelonephritis, malignant hyper-tension, polyarteritis nodosa, toxins (mercury, gold, lead, pesticides, kanamycin, gentamicin, methicillin), hypersensitivity, obstruction of the renal tubules by crystals such as poorly-soluble sulphonamides or uric acid.

Post-renal: obstruction of the lower urinary tract by bilateral renal calculi, prostatic hypertrophy, or tumours, causes acute retention of urine and may also cause acute renal failure.

Clinically: there is sudden oliguria (small urinary volume) or anuria (absent urine) but the bladder is not distended, which distinguishes anuria from acute retention of urine. The levels of waste products in the blood rise ('uraemia') rapidly, for example the blood urea rises by 4·2 mmol/l (25 mg%) daily, if untreated. Retention of acids which are normally excreted in the urine produces metabolic acidosis which causes hissing (Kussmaul) respiration, anorexia, nausea, vomiting, headache and apathy. Twitchings or convulsions are due to uraemia or to hypertension. Hiccough, drowsiness and stupor are present by the sixth day and coma by the tenth day. With recovery a marked diuresis occurs and water and electrolytes are lost.

Complications: infection, haemorrhage, convulsions. Cardiac arrest due to hyper-kalaemia.

Investigations: daily urine volume, daily blood urea and electrolytes.

Prevention: regular recording of the pulse and blood pressure after operation or injury, adequate blood transfusion for haemorrhage, plasma for burns and saline i.v. for dehydration. Careful checking before blood transfusion. The use of soluble sulphonamides in place of those causing crystaluria.

Treatment: the cause is treated. Acute renal failure is usually reversible if the patient can be kept alive for three weeks. Fluid is restricted to 500 ml daily (water lost via the lungs and skin) plus the volume of the previous day's urine, vomit and diarrhoea and an allowance made for fever, if present. A fluid balance chart and daily weight record help to judge therapy. A patient can expect to lose 0·3 kg of flesh daily by catabolism.

Diet: protein is restricted to 14–20 g daily. In order to reduce the breakdown of tissue protein 8·4–10·5 MJ (2000–2500 kcal.) are needed daily as fat and carbo-hydrate. Lactose 300 g in 500 ml water may be given orally. If vomiting prevents oral feeding 500 ml 40% glucose or 15% fructose or sorbitol is given i.v. Glucose is irritant to veins and tends to cause thrombosis, so has to be given via a catheter passed through a superficial vein into the superior or inferior vena cava where blood flow is rapid and prevents thrombosis. Fructose is less irritant. Electrolytes are not given since they are not being lost. Acidosis is treated with isotonic sodium bicarbonate i.v. or 3–10 g orally daily. Multivitamins are given.

Barrier nursing is preferable, to avoid infection. Careful mouth toilet, prevention of constipation.

Haemodialysis (artificial kidney) or peritoneal dialysis may be necessary.

In the diuretic phase (recovery) salt 3 g and sodium bicarbonate 2 g is needed for each litre of urine passed. Fruit is given to provide potassium, and dietary protein is gradually increased.

Patients with uraemia are unduly sensitive to many drugs, such as digoxin or warfarin.

Chronic Renal Failure

Causes: chronic glomerulonephritis, chronic pyelonephritis, malignant hypertension, polycystic kidneys, bilateral renal calculi, bilateral hydronephrosis, carcinoma of the bladder, involvement of the ureters by spread from carcinoma of the cervix, irradiation of the kidneys, diabetes mellitus, hyperparathyroidism, gout, amyloidosis, myelomatosis, systemic lupus erythematosus, and toxins such as phenacetin (analgesic nephropathy) and mercury. 60% of renal function has to be lost before uraemia begins.

Clinically: the onset of uraemia is gradual. Destruction of nephrons causes a greater filtration per glomerulus, thus there is an increased quantity of dissolved substances passing through the tubules and this causes an osmotic diuresis; i.e. polyuria and nocturia (unlike acute renal failure), which causes thirst. A high fluid intake delays the onset of uraemia but when polyuria exceeds fluid intake dehydration, constipation, uraemia, oliguria and hiccough occur. Polyuria causes loss of electrolytes such as sodium and bicarbonate, and loss of bicarbonate (plus retention of acid) leads to metabolic acidosis.

The tongue is dry and furred and there is anorexia, nausea, and vomiting (increasing the tendency to dehydration and uraemia). The skin is sallow due to anaemia and to the retention of urinary pigments, and may itch. Anaemia is due to deficiency of erythropoietin and to the toxic effect of uraemia on the bone marrow.

Complications: osteodystrophy (bone disease, due to defective metabolism of vitamin D), pericarditis, convulsions, cardiac arrhythmias, and anaemia.

Investigations: urine for S.G., pus, blood and organisms, urine dilution test, and blood creatinine or urea.

Treatment: treat the cause, e.g. malignant hypertension, stop analgesic abuse.

Diet: at least 8·4 MJ (2,000 kcal.) daily to reduce tissue catabolism. In severe uraemia carbohydrate may be given as lactose 300 g (5·2 MJ, 1,230 kcal.) daily, with fat 65 g (2·5 MJ, 604 kcal.) daily. Since protein contains a high concentration of potassium, and is metabolised into waste products such as urea and phosphate, less than 40 g (0·7 MJ, 164 kcal.) should be taken if the blood urea is above 33 mmol/l (200 mg%). Vitamins B Co. and C should be given, and vitamin D if there is bone disease.

The mouth is dry and requires care. A bed bath is performed at least daily since waste products are secreted into the sweat. Calcium resonium reduces hyperkalaemia by taking up potassium in the gut. Chlorpromazine may prevent hiccough and vomiting. Antacid (aluminium hydroxide, which is not absorbed) for dyspepsia.

'Renal' function is provided by using repeated dialysis (artificial kidney) if the blood urea is over 50 mmol/l (300 mg%) or serum potassium above 7 mmol/l (7 mEq/l). Waste products diffuse from the blood into the solution.

(a) *Peritoneal dialysis* is simple but often causes complications, such as peritonitis. The bladder is emptied. 1–2 l of fluid is run into the peritoneal cavity through a cannula, retained for 30 minutes so that electrolytes and urea diffuse into it, and is then drained off and the volume measured. This is repeated several times daily.

(b) *Haemodialysis*. The patient's blood from an artery, usually at the wrist, is passed through a coiled tube of semi-permeable membrane or a double plate of membrane which is immersed in dialysing fluid, then returned to the patient into a vein near the cannulated artery. The patient receives heparin during haemodialysis in order to prevent clotting in the apparatus. A permanent arteriovenous shunt may be attached at the wrist or ankle (*Fig. 10.9*). Complications of haemodialysis are

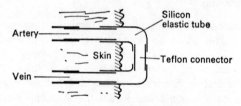

FIG. 10.9   Arteriovenous shunt for haemodialysis

clotting and infection of the shunt, and haemorrhage. Staff in a dialysis unit have an increased risk of virus hepatitis from hepatitis-contaminated blood.

(c) *Diafiltration*. This is purification of the patient's plasma after it has been separated from the cells; then the cells and reconstituted plasma are returned to the patient.

A Renal Transplant tends to be rejected since it is a foreign tissue. Donor kidneys from close relatives are best since they have a closer tissue typing. The patient's immune system produces antibodies and cellular immunity against the kidney, thus immunosuppressive drugs have to be given to prevent this, e.g. prednisolone 15 mg daily and azathioprine 2·5 mg/kg body weight orally daily maintenance, higher doses, e.g. prednisolone 200 mg daily, being used initially and during an acute rejection crisis.

After a transplant operation the patient is barrier-nursed in a cubicle owing to the danger of infection due to the immunosuppressive drugs. Staff enter the cubicle only when essential, and wear cap, gown, gloves and overshoes. Daily haemoglobin, white cell and platelet counts are performed to detect overdose of azathioprine. Complications of azathioprine are alopecia, megaloblastic anaemia, leucopenia, thrombocytopenia, liver damage, and lymphoma (tumour of the lympho-reticulo-endothelial system). Renal function is also measured daily at first.

Calculi (Stones) in the Urinary Tract
Calculi are aggregates of crystals formed by the precipitation of dissolved substances out of solution.

Causes:

1 An increased concentration of the urine precipitates poorly soluble material from solution, e.g. chronic dehydration due to a hot climate or an occupation involving excessive sweating.

2 A high concentration of calcium in the urine (hypercalciuria) precipitates calcium oxalate or calcium phosphate and occurs in prolonged immobilisation (calcium is withdrawn from the bones), hyperparathyroidism, Cushing's syndrome, sarcoidosis and an excessive intake of vitamin D. Calcium oxalate stones form if there is a high content of oxalate in the diet, e.g. rhubarb.

3 Urinary infection and stasis. Epithelium damaged by infection or by vitamin A deficiency acts as a nidus (nest) on which salts are deposited. Calcium phosphate and magnesium ammonium phosphate are insoluble in alkaline urine. They form stones if there is infection with alkali-producing organisms such as *B. proteus,*which split urea to form ammonia.

4 Similar calculi form if there is an excessive intake of milk (calcium) and alkali, as in peptic ulcer (the milk–alkali syndrome).

5 Gout and leukaemia predispose to uric acid calculi. Uric acid is precipitated from acid urine.

6 Cystinuria is a rare congenital abnormality due to failure of the renal tubules to reabsorb cystine, producing cystine stones.

Clinically: calculi are commonest at age 30–50 years and may be symptomless or may cause tenderness and a dull ache in the loin or back; worse on movement and relieved by lying down. A small stone may pass into the ureter and cause ureteric ('renal') colic, a sudden severe colicky pain in the loin or groin due to violent peristaltic contractions of the ureter attempting to push the stone onwards, associated with restlessness, sweating, pallor and vomiting. A small stone may be passed in the urine. A large stone remains fixed in the renal pelvis and calyces, e.g. a 'staghorn' calculus (*Fig. 10.10*).

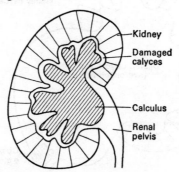

FIG. 10.10   A 'staghorn' calculus

Complications: renal infection (pyelonephritis, pyonephrosis), hydronephrosis, impaction (jamming) of the stone in the ureter, renal atrophy, or retention of a stone in the bladder.

Investigations: urine may contain crystals, pus, protein or blood. Blood count and urea, serum calcium and phosphate. Cystoscopy. Plain radiograph after a vegetable laxative (not a mineral laxative which casts a shadow). Pyelogram. Analysis of the stone.

Prevention: a high fluid intake is necessary in a patient who is immobilised for a length of time and for people going to tropical areas or working near furnaces.

Treatment: rest in bed, local warmth, a liberal fluid intake (minimum 4 l daily) to help to wash a small stone down the ureter, keep dissolved substances in solution and prevent further calculous deposition. A reduced dietary intake of predisposing substances. A low-calcium diet if there is idiopathic hypercalciuria; avoidance of rhubarb, spinach, tomatoes, celery and cocoa if there are oxalate calculi; and of liver, kidney, sweetbreads and fish roe if there are urate or uric acid stones.

Drugs: analgesic such as pethidine 100 mg i.m. with an antispasmodic such as atropine sulphate 1–2 mg i.m. four-hourly if necessary, to relax the ureteric muscle. Ammonium chloride 450 mg to 13 g daily, in divided doses, to make the urine acid if there are calcium phosphate calculi. In the body ammonium chloride is broken into hydrochloric acid, which is excreted into the urine and acidifies it, and ammonia which is metabolised to urea. All urine should be collected and examined for the presence of a small stone if there is colic.

Surgical removal of larger stones.

Hydronephrosis
Hydronephrosis is dilatation of the renal pelvis and calyces due to partial obstruction to urinary outflow (*Fig. 10.11*).

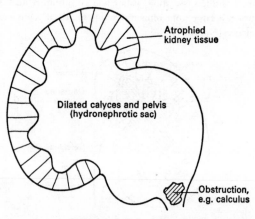

Atrophied kidney tissue

Dilated calyces and pelvis (hydronephrotic sac)

Obstruction, e.g. calculus

FIG. 10.11   Hydronephrosis

Causes include calculi, tumours of the renal pelvis or bladder, pressure on the ureter from outside by, e.g. carcinoma of the cervix or rectum, stricture of the ureter or urethra, kinking of the ureter, and an enlarged prostate.

Clinically: there are symptoms of the cause, e.g. haematuria due to tumour; of the hydronephrosis, which may cause a dull ache in the loin brought on by an excessive fluid intake, and swelling in the loin; and of complications.

Complications: (1) renal atrophy. If this is bilateral there is chronic renal failure. (2) Pyonephrosis, which is infection of a hydronephrosis.

Treatment is of the cause. The ureter may be re-implanted, or a nephrectomy performed if the kidney is functionless.

Renal Tuberculosis
Tuberculosis of the kidney is due to blood-borne infection from tuberculosis elsewhere in the body, usually in the lungs. It spreads to the bladder. The changes are the same as in pulmonary tuberculosis (Chapter 4), with necrosis (caseation) and abscess cavity formation.

Clinically: there is aching and tenderness in the loin, pyrexia, and frequency of micturition. The urine often contains a little albumin, blood and pus. The patient loses weight.

Investigations: the 24-hour urine is acid and contains tubercle bacilli. T.B. require special culture and grow slowly, ordinary culture being sterile. The E.S.R. is increased. Cystoscopy may show tuberculosis of the ureteric orifices and a small bladder. Pyelography shows ulceration of the calyces and renal calcification.

Treatment: anti-tuberculous drugs, good nutrition, vitamins and fresh air (*see* Chapter 4).

Polycystic Disease of the Kidneys
This is the formation of multiple cysts throughout both kidneys due to a genetic abnormality. Both kidneys are enlarged and there is haematuria, hypertension, anaemia and chronic renal failure with death in childhood or middle age. Cysts may be present in the liver. Treatment is as for chronic nephritis.

Tumours of the Kidney

Renal Carcinoma ('hypernephroma') arises from tubular epithelium. It causes fever and haematuria; clots in the ureter cause colic. It spreads to the lungs, liver and bones. Treatment is nephrectomy.

Papilloma and Carcinoma of the renal pelvis, ureter or bladder arise from transitional epithelium and cause haematuria, and obstruction and infection of the urinary tract.

Treatment is by diathermy, excision of the affected part, or radiotherapy.

Wilm's Tumour is a malignant tumour of the kidney which affects children.

Hypertension in Renal Disease

Hypertension may be caused by renal disease such as stenosis of the renal artery (by atheroma), renal injury, chronic nephritis and hydronephrosis, and is due to an excessive production of renin.

Investigations: urine is collected separately from each kidney by ureteric catheterisation. Aortography shows an obstruction in the renal artery. Pyelography shows, e.g. hydronephrosis.

Treatment: arterial graft for arterial stenosis. Nephrectomy for unilateral renal disease cures the hypertension. Antihypertensive drugs for symptomatic treatment.

Note: Severe hypertension may damage the renal arteries and cause renal failure. This is malignant ('accelerated') hypertension. Papilloedema (oedema of the optic disc) is also present.

THE URETERS, BLADDER AND URETHRA

The Ureters. These are narrow tubes 28 cm (11 inches) in length, which convey urine from the renal pelvis to the bladder by peristaltic action. The ureters pass obliquely through the wall of the bladder so that when the bladder contracts the ureters are closed, thus preventing reflux of urine into the ureters. The ureters have three layers, an outer fibrous coat, a middle muscular layer, and an inner mucous membrane of transitional epithelium.

The Urinary Bladder. This is a reservoir for urine. It lies in the cavity of the bony pelvis but its fundus can rise into the abdomen when distended. In front is the symphysis pubis; above is small intestine. In the male behind the bladder is the rectum and the seminal vesicles, below is the prostate and urethra (*Fig. 10.12*). In the female the uterus and vagina are behind the bladder, and the muscles of the pelvic floor and the urethra are situated below it (*Fig. 10.13*).

The bladder consists of four layers: the outer peritoneal layer covering its superior surface, a muscular layer of longitudinal and circular fibres, a submucous

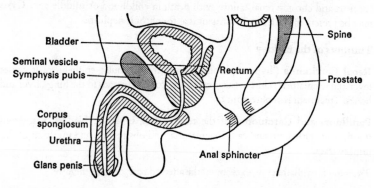

FIG. 10.12 The urinary bladder and its relations in the male

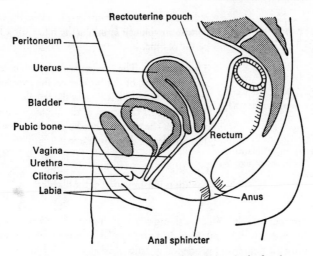

FIG. 10.13 The urinary bladder and its relations in the female

layer containing blood vessels, lymphatics and autonomic nerves, and an inner mucous membrane consisting of transitional epithelium which is folded when the bladder is empty but the folds disappear as the bladder fills with urine. The wall is pierced by the ureters (*Figs. 10.14 and 10.15*). A third orifice in the bladder is the origin of the urethra. The area between the three orifices is the trigone of the bladder.

Function: when sufficient urine has accumulated (about 300 ml in adults) the tension in the bladder wall stimulates the autonomic nerve endings in the wall. This causes

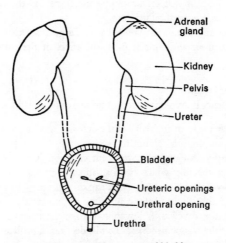

FIG. 10.14 The ureters and bladder

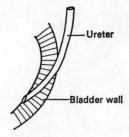

FIG. 10.15 The oblique entry of the ureter into the bladder

reflex micturition in infants, but in adults the cerebral cortex can voluntarily inhibit the reflex for a limited period of time.

The Urethra. The urethra is a tube which extends from the neck of the bladder to the exterior. The length of the urethra is 4 cm in the female and 20 cm in the male. At the origin of the urethra is a muscular sphincter. The urethra is lined by mucous membrane. The ejaculatory duct opens into it.

Cystitis
Cystitis is inflammation of the bladder.

Causes:

1 Infection of the bladder with organisms such as *E. coli*, *Strept. faecalis* and *B. proteus,* is the usual cause. It is predisposed by urinary obstruction, e.g. prostatic hypertrophy, urethral infection, catheterisation, and neurological lesions such as paraplegia and multiple sclerosis.
2 Sterile inflammation is due to radiation therapy to the lower part of the abdomen for carcinoma of the cervix, or to cytotoxic drugs such as cyclophosphamide.

Clinically: inflammation increases the sensory stimulation of the micturition reflex causing urgency, frequent painful (scalding) micturition and strangury (the desire to pass more urine, and spasm of the detrusor muscle, although the bladder is empty). There is perineal and retropubic pain and tenderness. The urine contains albumin, pus, blood and organisms. A bacterial count of 100,000 or more per ml indicates infection.

Treatment is the same as that for acute pyelonephritis and the correction of any predisposing causes, e.g. urethral stricture.

Heat to the suprapubic area may relieve pain. Large quantities of fluid should be given except when an antibiotic is used (the effect of the antibiotic would be diluted).

Incontinence of Urine
Urinary incontinence is involuntary loss of urine from the bladder.

Causes: It may be due to overactivity of the detrusor muscle or inadequate closure of the urethra by the urethral sphincter.

1 Neuropathy. An upper motor neuron lesion (Chapter 13) produces a hypertonic bladder which has a small capacity and contracts frequently without voluntary control; e.g. a stroke, multiple sclerosis, lesions of the spinal cord above the centre controlling the micturition reflex (at sacral 2, 3 and 4), e.g. myelitis. A lower motor neuron lesion destroys the spinal centre or the motor nerves to the bladder, e.g. a prolapsed intervertebral disc, abdominoperineal resection of the large bowel.

2   Loss of cerebral control over the bladder as in a major epileptic fit, cerebral arteriosclerosis, confusion due to sedatives and tranquillisers, and psychological (anxiety).

3   Damage to the sphincter of the bladder causes stress incontinence, e.g. multiparity, perineal tears, or occasionally following operation such as vaginal hysterectomy or prostatectomy.

4   Local obstruction to urinary excretion by an enlarged prostate, bladder calculus or tumour, or urethral stricture causes dilatation of the bladder and eventually dribbling overflow of urine and the bladder does not empty completely on micturition. The urine remaining in the bladder is called residual urine.

5   Other causes include a congenitally short urethra and a vesical (bladder) fistula.

Predisposing Causes include failure to reach the toilet in time (arthritis in the legs), cystitis, polyuria (diuretics, chronic nephritis, diabetes mellitus, diabetes insipidus).

Clinically: incontinence may occur at rest or on straining (stress incontinence). Urgency indicates increased bladder tone, as in cystitis. The stream is diminished and there is dribbling afterwards in urethral obstruction. Social effects are isolation, depression and anxiety.

Investigations: urine microscopy and 24-hour volume. Cystoscopy. Micturition cystogram shows ureteric reflux and leakage. Cystometrogram measures the pressure in the bladder as it is being filled with water and the volume at which the desire to micturate is felt and the final capacity is noted.

Treatment is of the cause. Weight reduction if obese, to reduce the intra-abdominal pressure.

Drugs: antispasmodic for detrusor overactivity e.g. emepronium (Cetiprin) 200 mg t.d.s., propantheline (Pro-Banthine) 15 mg t.d.s., or flavoxate (Urispas) 200 mg t.d.s. Side-effects: dry mouth, blurred vision, constipation.

Regular two- to four-hourly emptying plus parasympathomimetics (cholinergics) for detrusor hypotonicity e.g. bethanechol (Myotonine) 10–30 mg t.d.s., distigmine (Ubretid) 0·5 mg b.d., i.m. or 5 mg orally daily a.c. Side-effects: adbominal colic, bronchoconstriction (therefore they must not be used in asthmatics). Mechanical devices (penile clamps, indwelling catheter) or electrical devices.

Surgery for 3, 4 and 5 above.

Enuresis

Enuresis is incontinence of urine. The word is usually restricted to children who do not have organic bladder disease.

Causes:

1   A disorder of learning.

2   A small bladder capacity due to lack of training to hold the urine for increasingly longer periods. A small bladder may be due to disease, e.g. tuberculosis.

3   Psychological disturbance due to, e.g. social stress.

4 Urinary infection.
5 Neurological disease (Chapter 13), e.g. spina bifida.
6 Deep sleep was thought to be a cause but electroencephalography does not support this, and normal people remain dry when in deep sleep.

Treatment: guide the inadequate or fussy parents over toilet-training (they should not fuss or be scolding). Early 'potting' gives early bladder control. Restrict fluid intake in the evening and ensure an empty bladder before retiring. Conditioning with pad and bell, Anticholinergic antidepressant drugs, e.g. imipramine (Tofranil) 25–50 mg o.n.

11 THE REPRODUCTIVE SYSTEM

The Male Reproductive System

The male reproductive system consists of a pair of testes and epididymes in the scrotum, paired spermatic cords, seminal vesicles and ejaculatory ducts, the prostate gland and the penis (Fig. 11.1).

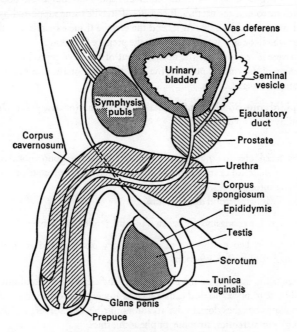

FIG. 11.1 The male reproductive system

The scrotum is a pouch of skin lined within by the dartos muscle and containing the testes (male gonads) and epididymes. The testes are surrounded by the tunica vaginalis, a double fold of serous membrane, and are suspended by the cremasteric muscle. Each testis consists of seminiferous tubules lined with germinal epithelial cells which, stimulated by the follicle-stimulating hormone (F.S.H.) from the pituitary gland, produce spermatozoa (the male egg cells). Between the tubules there are groups of interstitial cells which, under the influence of luteinising hormone from the pituitary, secrete testosterone (male sex hormone). The tubules join to become efferent ducts and these join each other to form the epididymis which continues as the vas deferens in the spermatic cord. The vas deferens passes upwards from the testis to the inguinal canal, along which it runs and turns towards the bladder where it joins the duct from the seminal vesicle to form the ejaculatory duct.

The seminal vesicles are two pouches lying behind the bladder, their lower parts continuing as a duct which joins the vas deferens. They are lined by columnar epithelium which secretes sticky fluid. This fluid and spermatozoa form the semen.

The ejaculatory ducts run through the prostate to join the urethra.

The prostate lies below the bladder and between the symphysis pubis and the rectum and surrounds the beginning of the urethra. It has an outer fibrous capsule and consists of follicles of columnar epithelium which line ducts opening into the urethra. Prostatic secretions are added to the semen.

The penis begins at its root in the perineum and continues as the body of the penis which surrounds the urethra. It consists of erectile tissue supported by fibrous tissue and surrounded by skin. At its end the erectile tissue expands into the glans penis over which the skin is folded to form the prepuce (foreskin).

Testosterone is required for the development of the male reproductive system, the deepening of the voice at puberty, the growth of hair on the face and trunk, and the formation of spermatozoa.

Acute Epididymo-orchitis. Inflammation of the testis (or ovary) is orchitis, and of the epididymis is epididymitis.

Causes:
1   Bacterial infection may spread from a urethritis (e.g. gonorrhoea) or cystitis (e.g. coliforms) or may complicate operations on the prostate or urethra.
2   Virus infection, e.g. mumps.
3   Sterile inflammation due to trauma.

Clinically: there is pyrexia and the organ is painful, tender and swollen.

Treatment: rest in bed or the use of a suspensory bandage and an analgesic to relieve pain. Antibiotic for infection.

Impotence is the inability of the male to erect sufficiently for sexual intercourse. It is usually due to psychological causes such as anxiety, but occasionally occurs in diabetes mellitus or tabes dorsalis due to autonomic nerve disorder; it may also be due to drugs, e.g. narcotics, atropine, or phenothiazines.

The Female Reproductive System
This consists of the vagina, the uterus, paired Fallopian tubes and ovaries (*Figs. 10.13 and 11.2*).

The vagina is a fibromuscular tube lined with stratified squamous epithelium. It lies behind the urethra and bladder and in front of the rectum.

The uterus is a hollow muscular organ between the bladder and the rectum. It is described in three parts; the fundus which is the rounded upper end, the body, and the cervix. Part of the cervix protrudes into the vagina. The uterus has three layers: the outer layer of peritoneum covering the fundus and body, the thick muscular layer (myometrium) and the inner lining of endometrium. The endometrium consists of columnar epithelium and tubular glands. The function of the uterus is to

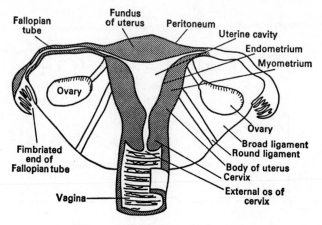

FIG. 11.2 The female reproductive system

nourish and protect the fertilised ovum and to expel the fully developed fetus. On each side near the fundus arise the Fallopian tubes which lie in the broad ligament, a double fold of peritoneum on each side of, and supporting, the uterus. Each tube is 10 cm (4 inches) in length and its free end (fimbriated end) opens into the peritoneal cavity. The tubes have three layers: peritoneal, muscular and an inner layer of ciliated epithelium. They convey ova from the ovary to the uterus.

The ovaries are the female gonads and are attached to the broad ligament. They consist of fibrous connective tissue containing numerous follicles and are covered with a layer of cubical epithelial cells, the germinal epithelium.

The function of the ovary is to produce ova, oestrogen and progesterone. During fertile adult life each month one follicle is stimulated by the follicle-stimulating hormone from the anterior pituitary and grows, producing oestrogen, while a mature ovum develops in it. This follicle ruptures and releases the ovum (ovulation) into the peritoneal cavity near the open end of the Fallopian tube. The remains of the follicle, under the influence of luteinising hormone from the anterior pituitary develops into a corpus luteum (yellow body) which secretes progesterone.

The menstrual cycle takes about 28 days. The first day of the cycle is calculated from the first day of menstruation. The cycle consists of the proliferative phase of 14 days followed by the secretory phase of 14 days. Menstruation is due to a fall in the level of progesterone in the blood and occurs during the first four days of the proliferative phase. It consists of the sloughing (shedding) of the endometrium except the deeper layer. The endometrium grows and thickens, under the influence of oestrogen from the ovarian follicle, from the fourth to the 14th day of the proliferative phase. On the 14th day ovulation takes place. After ovulation and under the influence of progesterone the endometrial glands coil and become secretory (*Fig. 11.3*) and the endometrium is ready to receive a fertilised ovum. If the ovum is not fertilised the production of luteinising hormone by the pituitary is inhibited, the corpus luteum degenerates into a white scar (corpus albicans) and ceases to produce progesterone, causing menstruation.

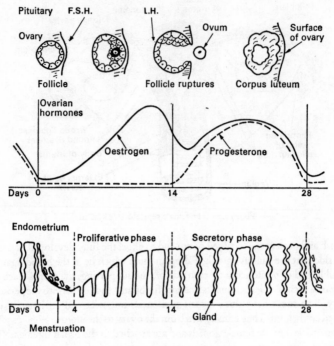

FIG. 11.3   The menstrual cycle

HYPOGONADISM

Hypogonadism is a deficient function of the testes or ovaries. In the male it may be due to pituitary deficiency, which causes a deficiency of gonadotrophic hormones (follicle-stimulating and luteinising hormones) with secondary failure of testicular function, disease of the testis such as syphilis, tuberculosis, mumps, orchitis, or bilaterally undescended testes (cryptorchidism), abnormality of the sex chromosomes as in Klinefelter's syndrome—the presence of an extra X chromosome (*see* Chapter 1), or to treatment with oestrogen for carcinoma of the prostate.

In the female hypogonadism may be due to pituitary failure to produce gonadotrophins causing secondary ovarian failure, the deficiency of an X chromosome (ovarian dysgenesis, Turner's syndrome), thus the patient has only one X chromosome (= XO) instead of two (XX), or to ovarian infection or irradiation.

INFERTILITY (STERILITY)

Infertility is failure to produce a fetus. Causes in the male include defective formation of spermatozoa, obstructed vasa deferentia (e.g. epididymitis), or hypogonadism. Infertility in the female is due to defective ovulation, hypogonadism, obstruction of the Fallopian tubes as in salpingitis, and sometimes to hyperthyroidism, diabetes mellitus, or antibodies to spermatozoa in the cervix. Pseudo-infertility is due to impotence or a faulty technique of sexual intercourse.

CONTRACEPTION

Contraception is the prevention of conception (prevention of pregnancy). The methods include the 'safe period' (avoidance of coitus from the ninth to the 19th day of the cycle), coitus interruptus (the male withdrawing before ejaculation), mechanical devices such as the vaginal diaphragm (dutch cap) used with a spermicide, penile sheath, or intra-uterine coil (e.g. copper wire), the 'pill', or sterilisation of the male or female. All have disadvantages or difficulties, e.g. intra-uterine devices may be expelled or be complicated by infection or bleeding, and the contraceptive pill may cause depression, headache, water retention, increase in blood pressure, liver damage (cholestasis), or thrombosis of arteries or veins.

12   THE ENDOCRINE SYSTEM

The endocrine system consists of the hypothalamus, pituitary, thyroid, parathyroids, thymus, islets of Langerhans in the pancreas, adrenals, and the ovaries or testes. These are ductless glands which secrete substances called hormones directly into the bloodstream. A hormone is a substance which is secreted by one organ and travels via the blood to act on another organ. *Note:* the pancreas also produces an exocrine secretion, i.e. the digestive juices, and the gonads produce germ cells, in addition to hormones.

The Hypothalamus
The hypothalamus is part of the brain and consists of groups of nerve cells below the thalamus and above the midbrain and pituitary gland. The non-endocrine part of the hypothalamus controls many functions of the body including hunger, thirst, body temperature and the autonomic nervous system. The endocrine part controls the posterior lobe of the pituitary by nerve fibres and the anterior lobe of the pituitary by factors (hormones, *Table 12.1*) secreted into a local portal system of blood vessels in which capillaries in the hypothalamus join to form larger vessels which run to the pituitary where they subdivide into a second set of capillaries.

The Pituitary Gland
The pituitary is the size of a small pea, lies in the pituitary fossa (sella turcica) in the sphenoid bone of the skull (*Fig. 7.1*) and is attached to the hypothalamus by a stalk consisting of nerve fibres and blood vessels. Above and in front is the optic chiasma.

The anterior lobe of the pituitary (adenohypophysis) consist of three types of secretory epithelial cells: acidophil (α), basophil (β) and chromophobe. The posterior lobe of the pituitary (neurohypophysis) consists of secretory cells derived from nerve cells. The anterior lobe secretes the thyroid stimulating hormone (thyrotrophin, T.S.H.), growth hormone (somatotrophin, S.T.H., G.H.), adrenocorticotrophic hormone (corticotrophin, A.C.T.H.), two gonadotrophic hormones: follicle-stimulating hormone (F.S.H.) and luteinising hormone (L.H.), (interstitial-cell stimulating hormone, I.C.S.H.), and lactogenic hormone (prolactin, luteotrophin, L.T.H.). The posterior lobe stores oxytocin and antidiuretic hormone (A.D.H., vasopressin) which are secreted by the hypothalamus and pass down the nerve fibres to the posterior pituitary. The actions of these hormones are shown in *Table 12.1* and are described under the appropriate gland.

The pituitary secretion of trophic hormones is regulated partly by the hypothalamus and partly by the 'feed–back' mechanism whereby the blood level of the hormone secreted by the target gland (e.g. thyroid, adrenal) controls the release of its trophic hormone by the pituitary; for example the hypothalamus secretes corticotrophin-releasing hormone (C.R.H.) which stimulates the secretion of

TABLE 12.1   *The hormones and their actions*

Hypothalamic hormone	Pituitary hormone	Gland and hormone	Action
Thyrotrophin releasing factor (T.R.H.)	Thyrotrophin (thyroid stimulating hormone, T.S.H.)	Thyroid, thyroxine and tri-iodothyronine	Increased tissue metabolism
Growth hormone releasing factor (G.H.R.H., S.R.H.)	Growth hormone (somatotrophin, G.H., S.T.H.)		Increased tissue growth
Somatostatin (G.H.-I.H.)			Inhibits G.H.
Corticotrophin releasing factor (C.R.H., C.R.F.)	Corticotrophin (A.C.T.H.)	Adrenal cortex, cortisol	Action on protein, carbohydrate, fat and electrolytes
	slight action on	aldosterone	Retention of sodium and water
Follicle-stimulating hormone releasing factor (F.S.H.-R.F.)	Follicle-stimulating hormone (F.S.H.)	Testis	Spermatogenesis
		Ovary (Graafian follicle), oestrogen	Female secondary sex characteristics, menstrual cycle
Luteinising hormone releasing factor (L.H.R.H.)	Luteinising hormone (L.H., I.C.S.H.)	Ovary (corpus luteum), progesterone	Prepares uterus for ovum
		Testis, testosterone	Male secondary sex characteristics Protein anabolism
Prolactin inhibiting factor (P.I.F.)	Lactogenic hormone (prolactin, L.T.H., luteotrophin)	Ovary	Maintains corpus luteum
		Breast	Induces milk secretion in primed breast
Antidiuretic hormone (A.D.H., vasopressin)	via posterior pituitary		Water reabsorption by distal tubular cells of kidney
Oxytocin	via posterior pituitary		Uterine contractions

Other glands	Hormone	Action
Thyroid	Calcitonin	Inhibits reabsorption of calcium from bone
Parathyroids	Parathormone (P.T.H.)	Increased urinary phosphate excretion and mobilisation of calcium and phosphate from bone
Pancreas, β-cells of islets	Insulin	lowers blood glucose, inhibits protein catabolism, increases fat and glycogen deposition
Pancreas, α-cells of islets	Glucagon	mobilizes liver glycogen, forming glucose
Adrenal medulla and sympathetic nerves	Adrenaline Noradrenaline	stimulates α and β-adrenergic receptors stimulates α-adrenergic receptors
Endometrium	Luteolysin	limits life of corpus luteum
Thymus	Thymosin	formation of T-lymphocytes

corticotrophin (A.C.T.H.) by the anterior lobe of the pituitary. A.C.T.H. circulates in the blood to the adrenals where it stimulates the production of cortisol (hydrocortisone). If there is more cortisol in the blood than is required it inhibits the hypothalamic secretion of C.R.H., the pituitary secretion of A.C.T.H. falls, reducing the adrenal cortical output of cortisol. On the other hand a low cortisol level in the blood stimulates the secretion of C.R.H. by the hypothalamus and A.C.T.H. by the pituitary and raises the adrenal cortisol secretion. A similar system applies to most of the endocrine secretions.

Antidiuretic Hormone (A.D.H.) acts on the cells of the distal renal tubules to cause the reabsorption of water. Changes in the osmotic pressure (O.P.) of the blood are detected by osmoreceptors in the hypothalamus which adjust A.D.H. secretion. A high osmotic pressure causes the osmoreceptors to stimulate the secretion of A.D.H. by the hypothalamic endocrine cells (*Fig. 12.1*), a low O.P.

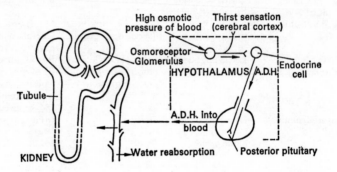

FIG. 12.1   The mechanism of water balance via antidiuretic hormone (A.D.H.)

inhibits the secretion of A.D.H. and increases urinary volume. Deficiency of A.D.H. causes diabetes insipidus.

Oxytocin causes the contraction of the pregnant uterus and of myoepithelial cells in the lactating breast squeezing milk into the ducts.

Prolactin causes the secretion of milk after childbirth.

Growth Hormone (Somatotrophin, G.H., S.T.H.) is secreted by the acidophil cells (α cells) of the anterior pituitary and stimulates the growth of epiphyseal cartilage and therefore of the long bones. Growth ceases when the cartilage ossifies (becomes bone) but the hormone continues to be secreted for tissue repair. Growth hormone stimulates the formation of protein and the conversion of glycogen to glucose. The secretion of growth hormone is controlled by somatotrophin-releasing factor (somatotrophin-releasing hormone, S.R.H.) secreted by the hypothalamus. Deficiency of growth hormone during growth causes pituitary dwarfism; an excess causes giantism during growth, or acromegaly in the adult.

DISORDERS OF THE PITUITARY–HYPOTHALAMIC SYSTEM

Underactivity of this system causes diabetes insipidus, dwarfism, or Simmond's disease (panhypopituitarism). Overactivity produces giantism, acromegaly, Cushing's syndrome, or water retention, depending on the situation and the type of disease.

Diabetes Insipidus

Diabetes (passing through) insipidus (tasteless) is rare and is polyuria due to failure of the distal convoluted and collecting tubules of the kidneys to reabsorb water owing to:

1 Deficiency of antidiuretic hormone caused by disease of the posterior pituitary or hypothalamus, or by surgical destruction of the pituitary.
2 Failure of the renal tubular cells to respond to antidiuretic hormone (nephrogenic diabetes insipidus).

Clinically: large volumes of urine are passed (polyuria), i.e. 5–20 l daily, of low specific gravity (1·003), i.e. 90 mosmol/kg. This results in a continued severe thirst, with rapid dehydration if water is withheld.

Treatment: sodium depletion reduces the polyuria, e.g. withhold salt from the diet or give a diuretic such as bendrofluazide 10 mg daily orally or frusemide 80 mg daily orally.

Desmopressin (Desamino arginine Vasopressin) 10–20 µg b.d. intranasally has superseded pituitary extract (Pitressin, Vasopressin). The hormone is absorbed from the nasal mucosa.

Fluid balance must be recorded.

Water Retention

Salt and water retention occurs in heart and kidney failure but must not be confused with retention only of water, which is due to an excessive intake of water when disease, e.g. a poor renal blood flow, prevents its excretion; or to an excess of antidiuretic hormone caused temporarily by head injury, the stress of an operation or pneumonia; or to carcinoma of the bronchus.

Dwarfism

Dwarfism is failure of growth during childhood. A short stature may be due to genetic causes (pygmies), abnormal chromosomes (Turner's syndrome), cretinism, severe malnutrition or malabsorption, or hypopituitarism. Pituitary dwarfism may be due to a pure deficiency of growth hormone (Lorain type) or to multiple defects (Frohlich's type).

Hypopituitary Dwarfism (Lorain type) is dwarfism due to a deficiency of growth hormone in childhood. The patient is minute, well-proportioned, and physically and mentally normal.

Treatment: human growth hormone 10 mg i.m. twice weekly until normal height is reached.

Frohlich's Syndrome (dystrophia adiposogenitalis) is dwarfism, hypogonadism, mental retardation and obesity due to deficiency of growth hormone, gonadotrophins and thyroid stimulating hormone. It is usually due to pressure on the pituitary and hypothalamus by a cyst or tumour, e.g. craniopharyngioma. The child is obese but fails to grow in height and the epiphyses do not unite. The secondary sex characteristics (changes of puberty) do not appear.

Treatment: human growth hormone, thyroxine, cortisone and testosterone (for boys) or oestrogens (for girls).

Giantism

Giantism is excessive growth in height, e.g. 2·4 m (7 ft 10 in), due to overgrowth of the long bones caused by an excessive secretion of growth hormone. Treatment is as for acromegaly.

Note: tall stature due to genetic or constitutional causes does not require treatment, except in unusually tall girls who have a psychological and social disadvantage. Their epiphyses can be fused with cyclical oestrogens started before the menarche.

Acromegaly

Acromegaly (acro = top or end, megaly = large) is due to excess of growth hormone in adults. Goliath had giantism with acromegaly and tunnel vision.

Clinically: further growth of the long bones cannot take place since the epiphyses have ossified, but the skull, jaw, hands and feet enlarge and larger sizes of shoes and gloves are needed. The skin becomes thick and coarse, the dentures do not fit, the voice is deep and husky due to enlargement of the larynx, the viscera enlarge and the spine becomes curved (kyphosis). If it is due to a pituitary tumour there are pressure symptoms such as severe headache due to stretching of the dura over the pituitary, visual defects from pressure on the optic chiasma, and deficiency of other hormones causing hypogonadism with impotence or amenorrhoea, or persistent lactation in male or female, due to excessive prolactin; and there may be diabetes insipidus. Death is from cardiovascular disease.

Complications (1) diabetes mellitus; (2) osteoarthrosis; (3) hypertension; (4) cardiac failure.

Investigations: a radiograph of the skull shows enlargement (ballooning) of the pituitary fossa and erosion of nearby bone. Radio-immunoassay shows high levels of growth hormone in the blood. A glucose tolerance test may show diabetes mellitus.

Treatment: radiotherapy to the pituitary, e.g. radioactive yttrium implanted into the pituitary or heavy particle irradiation, or hypophysectomy (excision of the pituitary), and replacement therapy for life with thyroxine, cortisone (or cortisol), and if there is sodium and water depletion despite cortisone, fluorohydrocortisone fludrocortisone). Analgesic for headache, vasopressin for diabetes insipidus, and anti-diabetic drugs (insulin or tablets) for diabetes mellitus. Bromocriptine suppresses growth hormone secretion, dose: 2·5 mg b.d. to 15 mg six-hourly.

Simmond's Disease (Panhypopituitarism)

Panhypopituitarism is deficiency of all the anterior pituitary hormones caused by infarction of the pituitary (Sheehan's syndrome) resulting from severe antepartum (before childbirth) or postpartum (after childbirth) haemorrhage, pressure from a tumour (craniopharyngioma, meningioma or secondary carcinoma), or by a granuloma (sarcoidosis, syphilis, tuberculosis).

Clinically: deficiency of thyrotrophin, corticotrophin, gonadotrophins and growth hormone lead to underactivity of the thyroid which causes anorexia, slight loss of weight, and a low temperature; underactivity of the adrenal cortex causing a low blood pressure, weakness and a low blood sugar; and hyposecretion by the gonads leading to loss of sexual desire and function, with amenorrhoea, atrophy of the genitals and breasts, and loss of axillary and pubic hair. Pallor of the skin is due to deficiency of corticotrophin. Coma is due to hypoglycaemia, hypothermia and hypotension and is followed by death if untreated.

Investigations: the serum cortisol and thyroxine and urinary steroids are low, and the glucose tolerance curve is flat.

Treatment is by substitution therapy for life, with cortisone 12·5–50 mg orally daily (or cortisol 20 mg mane + 10 mg o.n.), if necessary with fludrocortisone 0·1–0·2 mg orally daily. Thyroxine 0·5–3 mg orally daily (started after cortisone has been given, otherwise there is a danger of Addisonian crisis). Oestrogen for female, e.g. ethinyl oestradiol 50 µg orally daily. Androgen for male e.g. methyltestosterone 20–50 mg sublingually daily, or fluoxymesterone 1–5 mg orally daily, or testosterone implant of 600–800 mg in the abdominal subcutaneous tissues, which lasts for six months. Radiotherapy or excision of a tumour.

Pituitary Tumour

A tumour may be of the eosinophil, basophil, or chromophobe cells of the pituitary. Peter Pan was a hypogonadotrophic pituitary dwarf.

Tumours of, or near, the pituitary press on the optic chiasma and lead to visual defects and blindness. Enlargement causes increased intracranial pressure with headache and vomiting, and pressure on the third, fourth and sixth cranial nerves which lie nearby. It may also produce endocrine effects due to excessive production of one of the pituitary hormones (e.g. growth hormone causes acromegaly), or a non-secreting tumour may cause hypopituitarism by pressure on the normal part of the pituitary, causing atrophy of the secretory cells.

Pressure on the hypothalamus causes sleepiness (somnolence), obesity, polyuria and thirst (diabetes insipidus), hypothermia (low body temperature), hypotension, loss of body hair and libido (sexual desire) and atrophy of the breasts.

Treatment: radiotherapy or surgical excision.

THE THYROID GLAND

The thyroid gland consists of two lobes, one on each side of the trachea and over-lapping the thyroid cartilage, joined by a narrow portion, the isthmus, which lies in front of the second and third cartilaginous rings of the trachea. Behind it are the left and right recurrent laryngeal nerves supplying the larynx, four parathyroid glands and the fifth cervical to the first thoracic vertebrae (*Fig. 12.2*).

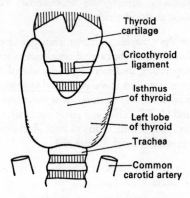

FIG. 12.2   The thyroid gland

The thyroid is composed of numerous follicles (acini, alveoli) each of which consists of a space containing colloid (thyroglobulin) surrounded by a layer of cubical epithelial cells (*Fig. 12.3*).

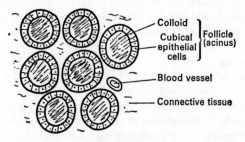

FIG. 12.3   The microscopic structure of the thyroid gland

Physiology. The thyroid takes up iodine from the blood to make the hormones thyroxine (T_4) and tri-iodothyronine (T_3) which are stored as thyroglobulin (T.G.). The thyroid secretes thyroxine and T_3 into the blood under the control of thyroid-stimulating hormone (T.S.H.) from the anterior pituitary. Fall in the thyroxine level of the blood stimulates the hypothalamus to release T.R.H. and the pituitary to secrete T.S.H. The T.S.H. stimulates the thyroid to secrete thyroxine and return the level in the blood to normal. Similarly a high blood level of thyroxine inhibits hypothalamic T.R.H. and pituitary T.S.H. secretion, thus decreasing the thyroid output and blood level of thyroxine (= feedback control, *Fig. 12.4*).

Thyroxine and tri-iodothyronine are required for the normal growth of the body and the brain, and for controlling the rate of metabolism in all the tissues of the body.

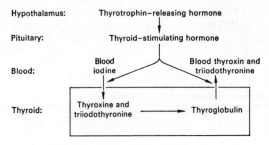

FIG. 12.4 Control of thyroid hormones

The thyroid also secretes a third hormone, calcitonin, from cells scattered between the follicles (parafollicular cells). Calcitonin lowers the calcium level in the blood by preventing the reabsorption of bone.

Goitre
Goitre is enlargement of the thyroid gland. Symptoms of hyperthyroidism may be present (toxic goitre) or absent (simple, non-toxic goitre). A large goitre may compress the trachea.

Causes:
1 Temporary enlargement of the thyroid may occur in girls at puberty and during lithium carbonate therapy for manic psychosis.
2 Iodine deficiency causes non-toxic goitre.
3 Tumour of the thyroid, adenoma or carcinoma.
4 Thyrotoxicosis.
5 Autoimmune thyroiditis.

Simple (Endemic, Colloid, Non-Toxic) Goitre
Simple goitre is due to iodine deficiency, the enlarged gland being able to take up a greater proportion of iodine from the blood and thus maintain thyroxine output. Iodine deficiency occurs in mountainous areas away from the sea, the rain having washed iodine from this soil, e.g. in the Alps, Himalayas and Derbyshire (hence the term 'Derbyshire neck'). Iodine is present in milk, eggs, sea fish, water and soil near the sea, and in vegetables grown in these soils.

Clinically: there is a goitre without signs of thyrotoxicosis, but if it is large it may produce pressure symptoms, e.g. dyspnoea due to pressure on the trachea.

Prevention: the Medical Research Council in 1944 recommended the addition of iodide to table salt.

Treatment: potassium iodide 100 mg orally daily prevents further enlargement.

Partial thyroidectomy if the enlarged thyroid is causing symptoms due to pressure on adjacent structures.

Tumours of the Thyroid

Thyroid tumours may be benign (adenoma) or malignant (carcinoma). An adenoma may produce thyroid hormones (toxic adenoma) and symptoms of hyperthyroidism (but not exophthalmos), or may be symptomless (non-toxic). Carcinoma is usually non-toxic.

Treatment is by surgical excision.

Hyperthyroidism (Thyrotoxicosis, Toxic Goitre)

Hyperthyroidism is due to excessive secretion of thyroxine or tri-iodothyronine due to a generalised overactivity of the thyroid (Graves' disease) or to a toxic adenoma.

Graves' Disease (Exophthalmic Goitre)

This is hyperthyroidism due to diffuse enlargement of the thyroid, often familial. The cause is unknown but it is not due to an excess of thyroid-stimulating hormone, nor is it due to fright or injury (although these may bring pre-existing thyrotoxicosis to notice). It may be due to autoimmune disease (antibodies produced by the body which act against the body's own tissues) since abnormal γ-globulin (antibodies) are present in the blood in many patients e.g. long-acting thyroid stimulator (L.A.T.S.) which it is thought release thyroxine from the thyroid.

Clinically: hyperthyroidism is eight times commoner in females than males and often appears between the ages of 15 and 30 years. A smooth goitre is present, with symptoms due to an increased metabolic rate, oligomenorrhoea (diminished menstruation), loose stools and eye signs. The increased metabolic rate is due to thyroxine or T_3 and causes weight loss despite an increased appetite; increased heat production which is lost by sweating and vasodilatation, hence the moist, warm, flushed skin and the patients' preference for cool weather and dislike of heat. The increased metabolism leads to an increased blood supply to the tissues by vasodilatation and by tachycardia which continues during sleep (unlike anxiety state). More oxygen is needed and more carbon dioxide is produced, increasing respiration.

Increased activity in the nervous system leads to restlessness, nervousness, brisk tendon reflexes, and a fine muscular tremor most easily seen in the outstretched fingers.

Eye signs are exophthalmos (protrusion of the eyeballs) giving a staring appearance, retraction of the eyelids, and lid lag which is exposure of the sclera, i.e. the white of the eye, between the lid and the iris on looking downwards.

Observations: record the weight, the pulse four-hourly at first, including the sleeping pulse, and both the radial and apex rates if fibrillating.

Complications: (1) atrial fibrillation; (2) cardiac failure; (3) thyrotoxic crisis; (4) 'malignant' exophthalmos.

Investigations: the serum thyroxine level is increased as is the serum protein-bound iodine (P.B.I., normal = 0·29–0·6 μmol/l = 3·5–8 μg%), which is mostly thyroxine. The radioiodine uptake by the thyroid is high. The P.B.I. gives false high results, and the radioactive uptake gives false low results, if the patient has recently taken iodine, as in certain cough medicines, fish, onions, Lugol's iodine, or after radiological contrast media containing iodine, as in a pyelogram. The basal metabolic rate (B.M.R.) is the rate of metabolism of the body at complete rest, and is measured by the rate at which oxygen is used by the patient from a special apparatus. The normal B.M.R. is within −10 to +15% of average. In hyperthyroidism it may be +50%. Results are unreliable unless the patient is relaxed. To allay apprehension the procedure is first explained and demonstrated to the patient, without fuss.

Treatment may be medical with antithyroid drugs or radioiodine, or surgical.

Medical Treatment: patients with severe disease must rest both physically and mentally. Visitors' stay should be brief. The bed should be in a quiet cool room away from radiators, and the bedclothes light. Bedbath daily for sweating.

Diet: high in calories, protein and vitamins. Adequate fluids but avoid coffee since it contains caffeine, which has many of the actions of thyroxine.

Antithyroid drugs for 12–24 months: carbimazole (Neomercazole) 5–10 mg eight-hourly. Side-effects are nausea, rash, fever and agranulocytosis. Patients should be warned to report a sore throat immediately, since it may be due to agranulocytosis, a low granulocyte (polymorph) count. Methyl or propyl thiouracil 100 mg eight-hourly orally has similar side-effects. Potassium perchlorate is seldom used since it may cause aplastic anaemia.

Other drugs: sedation with phenobarbitone 30 mg b.d. orally. Propranolol (Inderal) 10–40 mg t.d.s. orally inhibits sympathetic overactivity. Quinidine, digoxin, or direct current (D.C.) cardioversion for atrial fibrillation.

Radioactive Iodine: acts by irradiation destruction of the cells that concentrate it. It is given only to patients over the age of 40 years, since it may cause chromosomal changes, e.g. genetic damage to reproductive cells in the gonads. Its effect takes three to six months to reach a peak and antithyroid drugs may be needed meanwhile. It causes hypothyroidism in many patients.

Surgical: partial thyroidectomy for large goitres or nodules. An antithyroid drug may be given for several weeks before operation to help to prevent post-operative crisis, but is discontinued two weeks before operation since it makes the gland vascular and bleed excessively, and is replaced with Lugol's iodine 0·5 ml (= 65 mg iodine) t.d.s. given in milk. Iodine dampens thyroid activity but its action lasts only three weeks so it cannot be used for long-term treatment of thyrotoxicosis.

Thyrotoxic Crisis is rare but serious. It is a marked increase in all the signs of hyperthyroidism, with hyperpyrexia (41–42°C, 105–106°F), marked tachycardia, restlessness, delirium and finally coma and death unless treated urgently.

Treatment: the temperature is reduced by removing all clothing, sponging with cold water and the use of an electric fan, i.e. by hypothermia. Sedation with chlorpromazine. Propranolol to reduce β-sympathetic activity. Hydrocortisone 100 mg i.v. Dehydration is prevented by using an i.v. drip of glucose and saline.

Malignant Exophthalmos is protrusion of the eye which is sufficient to lead to ophthalmoplegia (paralysis of the muscles of the eyeball, causing diplopia) and inability to close the lids, which may cause corneal ulceration or conjunctivitis.

Treatment: the eyes should be shielded, or the lids may need to be stitched together.

Hypothyroidism

Hypothyroidism is underactivity of the thyroid. Material like mucus is deposited in the tissues and resembles oedema (myxoedema) but does not pit on pressure. True oedema shows pitting due to the displacement of fluid by the pressure.

Causes:

1 Auto-immunity. Antibodies slowly destroy the thyroid.
2 Deficiency of T.S.H. due to hypopituitarism (Simmond's disease).
3 Goitrogens, e.g. resorcinol used on varicose ulcers; certain hand creams.
4 Thyroiditis.
5 Following therapy for hyperthyroidism, especially radio-iodine, but may also follow partial thyroidectomy.
6 Severe iodine deficiency. Rare in the U.K.

Clinically: the onset is insidious. It is commonest in middle-aged women, often having menorrhagia. Deficiency of thyroxine reduces the metabolic rate of the tissues, thus weight is gained despite anorexia, less heat is produced and the patient has a pale dry yellow skin, prefers hot weather and dislikes the cold. There is also slowness of the pulse (bradycardia), muscles (slow in movement, and a feeling of 'stiffness'), speech, bowel (constipation), and brain (slow and forgetful), and thinning of the hair.

Deposition of myxoedema material in the larynx produces a croaky voice, in the ear causes deafness, and in the skin causes puffiness of the eyelids, broadening of the face and thick lips.

Complications:

1 Normochromic anaemia due to thyroxine deficiency, sometimes hypochromic or pernicious anaemia.
2 Congestive cardiac failure.
3 Atheroma, causing ischaemic heart disease, e.g. angina.
4 Psychosis with hallucinations and delusions ('myxoedema madness').
5 Carpal tunnel syndrome, i.e. compression of the median nerve at the wrist, causing paraesthesiae (tingling) in the thumb and fingers.
6 Hypothermia.

Investigations: the basal metabolic rate is low. The serum thyroxine level is low (below 55 nmol/l). The plasma cholesterol is raised to between 7·7 and 13 nmol/l (300 and 500 mg%); normal = 3·9–6·5 nmol/l (150–250 mg%). The serum T.S.H. is increased.

Treatment: L-thyroxine orally for life, begininng with 0·05 mg daily (0·025 mg if there is angina or cardiac failure) and increasing every two weeks by 0·05 mg until the patient is euthyroid, the maintenance dose is between 0·1 and 0·3 mg daily.

Hypothermia is a subnormal temperature. A special low-reading rectal thermo-meter must be used. In hypothyroidism it is due to a combination of low metabolic rate and neglecting to provide heat in the home. The patient becomes apathetic, confused and drowsy then unconscious and dies. While in coma the skin is icy cold and the patient may appear to be dead.

Treatment: gradual warming of the patient in a warm room but heat, e.g. hot water bottles, is NOT applied directly to the patient.

Triiodothyronine (liothyronine) 20 μg i.m., b.d. is given (it is more rapidly acting than thyroxine) and hydrocortisone 50 mg i.m., b.d. Antibiotic for broncho-pneumonia.

Cretinism (Infantile Hypothyroidism)
Cretinism is hypothyroidism in childhood.

Causes:
1 Mother with iodine deficiency goitre during pregnancy.
2 Antithyroid drugs given during pregnancy.
3 Severe iodine deficiency during childhood.
4 Congenital defects of the thyroid, e.g. recessively inherited enzyme deficiencies.

Clinically: the child is dwarfed and mentally retarded. It seldom cries (a 'good' baby) but is lethargic, sleeps excessively, feeds poorly yet is overweight, having a large abdomen with an umbilical hernia, coarse features, large tongue, constipation and anaemia. It is late in standing, walking and talking. The body is broad and the limbs are short. The dwarfism and mental retardation are permanent unless treated early.

Treatment must begin urgently; within the first six weeks after birth if possible. After this age the later the treatment is begun the greater is the degree of mental and physical retardation. Thyroxine for life, 12·5 μg orally daily at first for infants, 50 μg for children increasing weekly to between 50 and 300 μg daily.

THE PARATHYROID GLANDS

There are four parathyroid glands lying on the posterior surface of the thyroid (*Fig. 12.5*). Each is 5 mm (nearly 0·25 in.) in diameter and consists of columns of round cells which secrete parathyroid hormone (parathormone, P.T.H.).

Physiology. Parathormone controls calcium and phosphate metabolism. It increases the calcium level in the plasma by stimulating the release of calcium from bone, and decreases the plasma phosphate level by reducing the renal tubular reabsorption of phosphate, causing hyperphosphaturia. Calcium is needed for

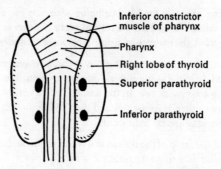

Fig. 12.5   The situation of the parathyroid glands

proper nervous conduction, muscular contraction, blood coagulation and for the skeleton. A low serum calcium stimulates the secretion of parathormone which raises the calcium level, and vice versa.

Hyperparathyroidism

Oversecretion of parathormone is rare. Primary hyperparathyroidism is often due to tumour(s) of the parathyroids, usually adenoma(s), sometimes to hyperplasia, and causes a high blood and urinary calcium (hypercalcaemia and hypercalciuria) and a low blood phosphate (hypophosphataemia). Secondary hyperparathyroidism is parathyroid hyperplasia due to a chronically low serum calcium caused by renal disease, or by rickets or osteomalacia due to malabsorption. 'Tertiary' hyperparathyroidism is the development of an adenoma following secondary hyperparathyroidism.

Primary (and Tertiary) Hyperparathyroidism.

Clinically: the excess of parathormone withdraws calcium from the bones and causes hypercalcaemia. The bones become soft, tender, cystic (osteitis fibrosa cystica, von Recklinghausen's disease of bone), bend, and fracture easily. Hypercalcaemia causes anorexia, nausea, vomiting, constipation, polyuria, thirst, calcification of soft tissues (cornea, arteries, kidneys), and hypercalciuria, producing renal calculi. There is muscular weakness due to hypotonia, and vague aches occur.

Complications: (1) peptic ulcer; (2) pancreatitis.

Investigations: the serum calcium (*Table 5.1*) is above normal, the serum phosphate is subnormal, and the alkaline phosphatase is raised. The urinary calcium is increased above 5 mmol (200 mg) in 24 hours (if the dietary intake of calcium is less than 12 mmol, 500 mg). Radiography of the kidneys shows calculi and nephrocalcinosis, and of the bones shows osteitis fibrosa cystica.

Treatment: surgical removal of tumour(s).

Secondary Hyperparathyroidism.
Symptoms are of the causative condition. The increased parathyroid activity is caused by hypocalcaemia and the serum

calcium may be low or become normal. The serum alkaline phosphatase is increased and the serum phosphate is low.

Treatment is with vitamin D.

Hypoparathyroidism
This is a deficiency of parathormone due to thyroidectomy with accidental removal of the parathyroids; or of unknown cause (idiopathic), possibly due to autoimmunity.

Clinically: hypocalcaemia causes lassitude, mental changes, cataracts, dry skin and hair, tetany and epileptiform convulsions. Tetany is muscular spasm due to hyper-excitability of nerves and muscles.

Treatment: 20 ml of 20% calcium gluconate i.v. immediately for tetany. For a prolonged action, calciferol (vitamin D) 1·25–5 mg orally daily or dihydrotachy-sterol (A.T. 10), which has a parathormone-like action, 4 mg daily at first, reducing to a dose which maintains a normal serum calcium level, e.g 1 mg twice weekly.

TETANY

Tetany is muscular spasm due to hyperexcitability of nerves and muscles because of a low concentration of calcium ions in the plasma. It must not be confused with the infection, tetanus.

Causes:
1   Hypoparathyroidism.
2   Vitamin D deficiency (i.e. rickets or osteomalacia).
3   Malabsorption (e.g. coeliac disease).
4   Chronic renal failure (diminished absorption of calcium).
5   Alkalosis (e.g. metabolic alkalosis due to severe vomiting or to an excessive intake of alkali), or respiratory alkalosis due to loss of carbonic acid by hyperventilation as in hysteria.

Clinically: altered conduction along nerves causes numbness and tingling in the fingers, toes and lips, and cramp in the limbs, larynx or gut. Carpopedal spasm is cramp in the hands and feet. Spasm of the muscle of the gut causes nausea, vomiting and abdominal pain, and of the larynx causes 'crowing' respirations. Convulsions (fits) may occur. In hypocalcaemia tetany is brought on in the hands (*Fig. 12.6*) by constricting the arm with a tourniquet (Trousseau's sign), and in the face by tapping the facial nerve in front of the ear (Chvostek's sign).

Investigations: the serum ionised calcium is low.

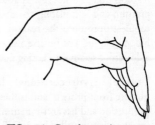

FIG. 12.6   Carpal spasm in tetany

Treatment is of the cause. A patient who is overbreathing is made to hold a bag over the nose and mouth for a few minutes so that carbon dioxide is rebreathed to replace that which has been lost. For hypocalcaemia give 20 ml of 10% calcium gluconate i.v. then calcium lactate 1–4 g six-hourly orally. Diet adequate in calcium and vitamin D (e.g. milk, cheese, egg yolk, liver).

THE ADRENAL (SUPRARENAL) GLANDS

The two adrenal glands are situated one on each side of the vertebral column on the posterior abdominal wall behind the peritoneum in contact with the upper poles of the kidneys and enclosed in the renal fascia (*Fig. 10.1*). Each consists of two parts: an outer part, the cortex, and an inner part, the medulla. The cortex is yellow and is composed of three layers of cells: the zona glomerulosa which produces aldosterone, the zona fasciculata which (when stimulated by A.C.T.H. from the pituitary) makes cortisol, and the zona reticularis which synthesises various steroids, including sex hormones, and is controlled by the pituitary.

The adrenal medulla consists of sympathetic ganglion cells which are stimulated by pre-ganglionic nerve fibres to produce the hormones adrenaline and noradrenaline.

Physiology. Steroids are substances with a similar basic structure to each other. Only certain steroids are hormones. Cholesterol is a non-hormonal steroid. The steroid hormones secreted by the adrenal cortex are corticosteroids; the most important are aldosterone and cortisol. Sex hormones, which are also steroids, are secreted by the adrenal cortex and the gonads.

Aldosterone controls electrolyte balance and is therefore a mineralocorticoid. Its secretion is controlled by the sodium level in the blood through the renin–angiotensin system. Fall in blood flow through the kidneys, for example due to a low blood volume (haemorrhage, burns, nephrotic syndrome, low salt diet), stimulates the kidneys to secrete renin into the blood. Renin converts the inactive angiotensinogen in the plasma into angiotensin which elevates the blood pressure and helps renal blood flow. Renin stimulates the adrenal cortex to secrete aldosterone. Aldosterone acts on the cells of the renal tubules to cause the reabsorption of sodium from the tubular lumen into the blood in exchange for potassium and hydrogen which are excreted in the urine. The reabsorption of sodium causes the reabsorption of water; partly automatically and partly by increasing plasma osmotic pressure and stimulating the secretion of A.D.H. which acts on the distal renal tubule to promote the reabsorption of water, thus increasing and restoring the blood volume. The reverse also occurs, thus a high salt intake depresses renin and aldosterone secretion, causing salt excretion (*Fig. 12.7*).

Cortisol (Hydrocortisone) has several actions including the formation of glucose from protein, and is therefore a glucocorticoid. It also decreases antibody production and has anti-inflammatory and mild sodium-retaining actions. Cortisol secretion is controlled by A.C.T.H. from the pituitary which in turn is controlled

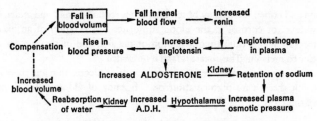

FIG. 12.7 The control of aldosterone secretion and its effects

by corticotrophin-releasing hormone (C.R.H.) from the hypothalamus. C.R.H. secretion is controlled partly by the level of cortisol in the blood (*Fig. 12.8*).

Deficient secretion of all the hormones of the adrenal cortex results in Addison's disease; deficiency of aldosterone alone results in hypoaldosteronism. Oversecretion of cortisol, with or without an excess of other hormones, leads to Cushing's syndrome; excess of aldosterone causes aldosteronism; and oversecretion of sex hormones in children causes precocious puberty, i.e. the development of the sexual organs and secondary sex characteristics at an unduly early age.

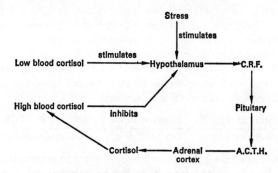

FIG. 12.8 The control of cortisol secretion

Addison's Disease (Hypoadrenocorticism)
Addison's disease is adrenal cortical insufficiency due to disease of both adrenals:

1 Adrenal atrophy, probably due to autoimmune disease.
2 Tuberculosis.
3 Metastatic (secondary deposits of) carcinoma.
4 Bilateral adrenalectomy for carcinoma of the breast.
5 Haemorrhage into the adrenals during septicaemia.
6 Amyloidosis.
7 Corticosteroid withdrawal, especially if sudden.

Clinically: deficiency of aldosterone and cortisol both lead to loss of sodium, chloride and water in the urine and retention of potassium and hydrogen; hence dehydration, hypotension (causing faintness), tachycardia, anorexia, nausea, vomiting, abdominal pain, loss of weight, weakness (asthenia) and fatigue. Cortisol deficiency also causes hypoglycaemia (a low blood sugar) which, if severe, leads to confusion and coma. Deficiency of sex hormones reduces bodily and axillary hair. The low level of cortisol in the blood stimulates the secretion of an excess of corticotrophin which causes pigmentation of the skin and of the mucosa of the mouth due to melanin. The disease is fatal if untreated.

Note: in hyopituitarism there is a deficiency of corticotrophin and therefore of cortisol, but there is no pigmentation or deficiency of aldosterone, electrolyte balance is therefore normal.

Complications: (1) uraemia due to dehydration; (2) Addisonian crisis, which is a sudden exacerbation of signs, precipitated by infection or drugs and the patient may die. Treatment is rest in bed, hydrocortisone 100 mg i.v. eight-hourly, glucose-saline i.v. and an antibiotic if there is infection. The pulse and blood pressure are recorded hourly and a fluid balance chart is kept.

Investigations: the serum cortisol and urinary hydroxysteroids and 17-ketosteroids (substances to which cortisol and other steroids are metabolised) and the blood glucose levels are low. The glucose tolerance curve is flat. The A.C.T.H. stimulation test does not cause an increase in the blood and urinary corticosteroids since the adrenals cannot respond. (Increased levels of steroids indicate functioning adrenals. An increase on previously low levels indicates pituitary or hypothalamic failure.) The blood urea increases due to dehydration. The serum potassium is increased and the sodium and chloride decreased in severe disease. Antibodies to the adrenal cortex are present in the serum.

The *Robinson–Power–Kepler Test* is based on the inability of patients with Addison's disease to excrete water quickly; the increased blood urea and the loss of chloride in the urine. The result, A, is calculated:

$$A = \frac{\text{urine urea mg\%}}{\text{plasma urea mg\%}} \times \frac{\text{plasma chloride}}{\text{urine chloride}} \times \frac{\text{largest volume of day urine}}{\text{volume of night urine}}$$

A result below 24 occurs in Addison's disease and above 30 in normal subjects. The patient fasts from 6 p.m. At 10.30 p.m. the bladder is emptied and urine discarded. All urine voided between 10.30 p.m. and 7.30 a.m. is collected and labelled 'night urine' and the patient drinks 20 ml of water or tea per kg body weight and empties the bladder at 8.30, 9.30, 10.30 and 11.30 a.m. The volume of the largest of the four specimens is measured. If the volume of one day specimen is greater than the night specimen the patient is unlikely to have Addison's disease. If the volume of the largest day specimen is less than the night specimen, the calculation, A, is made.

Treatment: cortisone 12·5–50 mg orally daily for life. The importance of continued treatment must be impressed upon the patient. A larger dose, e.g. 100 mg, is given during stress (injury, operation, infection). If the blood pressure remains low fluorohydrocortisone (fludrocortisone) 0·1–0·5 mg orally daily or salt 15 g daily is added.

Meals should be frequent and contain a high content of carbohydrate and protein.

A card should be carried by the patient showing his name and address, and the nature of the illness and treatment. The patient and his relatives must be warned about the serious consequences of stress and instructed to report infection or injury immediately so that the dose of cortisone can be increased. Exposure to sources of infection should be avoided.

Cushing's Syndrome

Cushing's syndrome is due to excessive secretion of cortisol, and sometimes of the other adrenal cortical steroids also.

Causes:
1. Hypothalamic oversecretion of corticotrophin-releasing hormone.
2. Pituitary oversecretion of corticotrophin (A.C.T.H.), sometimes due to a pituitary tumour (basophil adenoma).
3. Increased secretion of cortisol by the adrenals, due to adrenal tumour (adenoma or carcinoma) or hyperplasia caused by excess A.C.T.H., either from the pituitary or occasionally from a carcinoma of the bronchus or tumour of the ovary or thymus.
4. Corticosteroid therapy.

Clinically: excess of cortisol increases the breakdown of protein into glucose causing muscular wasting and weakness. Loss of protein from the skin leads to red cheeks and fragile blood vessels with bruising. The skin stretches easily and this produces purple striae over the thighs and abdomen. Lymphopenia (a low number of lymphocytes in the blood) leads to diminished antibody formation and predisposes to infection. Hyperglycaemia causes the deposition of fat, producing a round (moon) face and obesity of the trunk with a 'buffalo' hump over the lower part of the back of the neck, but the muscular wasting makes the limbs appear relatively thin. If insufficient insulin is secreted diabetes mellitus and glycosuria follow. The excess cortisol also leads to osteoporosis which causes kyphosis, and the bones fracture easily.

Increased cortisol or aldosterone causes hypertension due to sodium retention and potassium loss.

Amenorrhoea, hirsutes and acne in the female are due to an excess of sex hormones. Psychosis may occur.

Investigations: the serum cortisol and 24-hour urinary hydroxycorticosteroids are increased. The serum corticotrophin level is increased if there is a basophil adenoma.

Metyrapone Test: metyrapone (Metopirone) blocks the formation of cortisol by the adrenals, the low blood cortisol level stimulates the secretion of A.C.T.H. by the pituitary, which stimulates the formation of the precursors of cortisol, producing an increase in plasma and urinary 17-hydroxycorticosteroids. The absence of an increase indicates adrenal or pituitary disease.

Dexamethasone Test: dexamethasone, being a corticosteroid, inhibits the production of corticotrophin, reduces the output of steroids by the adrenals, and the serum cortisol level and 24-hour urinary steroid excretion fall. A fall does not take place if the Cushing's syndrome is due to an adrenal tumour, since tumours secrete independently of corticotrophin.

The urine may contain glucose and the glucose tolerance test may show diabetes mellitus.

Radiography of the skull shows enlargement of the pituitary fossa if there is a pituitary tumour. An intravenous pyelogram may show distortion of the kidney by an adrenal tumour.

Treatment: potassium chloride 6 g orally daily. Irradiation of a pituitary tumour. Removal of an adrenal containing a tumour, or bilateral adrenalectomy followed by lifelong cortisone therapy for adrenal hyperplasia.

CORTICOSTEROID THERAPY

Corticosteroids are used in the treatment of Addison's disease and hypopituitarism, and after adrenalectomy. In these conditions cortisone is the ideal replacement therapy since it is metabolised by the liver into cortisol (hydrocortisone), the natural hormone.

Corticosteroids, especially prednisolone, are also used in other conditions, e.g. to suppress inflammation, as in rheumatoid arthritis, ulcerative colitis, skin diseases (eczema) and allergies (asthma, drug sensitivity), and to inhibit lymphatic leukaemia, nephrotic syndrome, haemolytic anaemia, and the rejection of a graft such as a renal transplant. In these conditions artificial corticosteroids are used since they do not cause as much retention of salt and water as does cortisol.

When used as suppressives they produce the signs caused by cortisol in Cushing's syndrome. Their side-effects include the predisposition to infection, the masking of the signs of infection, hyperglycaemia, peptic ulcer which may bleed, osteoporosis and bone fracture, muscular weakness, gain in weight, salt and water retention, hypertension and psychosis. They suppress pituitary A.C.T.H. and adrenocortical secretion thus the adrenals may atrophy, and if corticosteroid therapy is suddenly discontinued the adrenals do not have time to recover and Addisonian crisis may be precipitated.

Anti-inflammatory drugs include corticotrophin 10–40 u i.m., b.d., and tetra-cosactrin (Synacthen) 0·25 mg i.m., b.d.

Corticosteroids and their daily dose (which should be divided into three or four doses) are: prednisolone or prednisone 5–60 mg, hydrocortisone 10–300 mg, betamethasone or dexamethasone 0·5–5 mg. Triamcinolone causes muscular wasting and is now seldom used. Other corticosteroids have no anti-inflammatory advantage over these, but fludrocortisone 0·1–1 mg daily orally is used for its action on electrolytes which is similar to that of aldosterone.

A patient receiving corticosteroids should be observed for oedema, gain in weight (weigh daily at first), 'moon face', and thrombosis of leg veins. The urinary output and blood pressure are recorded. The diet should be high in protein and low in fat and carbohydrate. Potassium chloride is given to prevent hypokalaemia.

ALDOSTERONISM

Excessive secretion of aldosterone by the adrenal cortex may be primary, e.g adrenal tumour, or secondary to cirrhosis of the liver, nephrosis, or renal artery stenosis.

In primary aldosteronism the kidneys excrete potassium and the blood and tissue levels of potassium fall, causing weakness, polyuria, and thirst. There is sometimes hypertension.

Treatment is of the cause.

Congenital Adrenal Hyperplasia (Adrenogenital Syndrome)
Congenital defects in the enzymes of the adrenal cortex may lead to an excessive secretion of androgens. This causes pseudohermaphroditism in the female child, the external genitals developing a partly male appearance (e.g. the clitoris is large). It causes virilisation in the female adult, and sexual precocity in boys, but the testes are small.

Treatment, often until puberty, is with oral cortisone 0·5 mg/kg body weight daily to suppress the excessive pituitary A.C.T.H. secretion.

Phaeochromocytoma
This is a rare tumour of the adrenal medulla which secretes an excess of catecholamines (adrenaline and noradrenaline), causing irregular hypertension, anxiety, tremor, weakness and sweating.

Treatment is by removal of the tumour.

THE PANCREAS

The pancreas has been described in Chapter 8. The islets of Langerhans in the pancreas contain three types of cells: delta, alpha and beta, which secrete gastrin, glucagon and insulin. Gastrin is secreted by the delta (δ) cells (as well as by certain cells in the stomach in response to fall in gastric acidity, e.g. by protein ingestion). The function of pancreatic gastrin is uncertain (gastric gastrin stimulates the secretion of hydrochloric acid in the stomach). Glucagon is secreted by the alpha(α) cells. It increases the blood glucose ('sugar') level by breaking down glycogen, and inhibits pancreatic enzyme secretion (it is given in pancreatitis for this purpose). Insulin is secreted by the beta (β) cells and lowers the blood glucose level by changing glucose into glycogen, which is deposited in the liver and muscles, and into fat, which is deposited in adipose tissues. A low blood glucose stimulates the secretion of glucagon. A high blood glucose stimulates insulin secretion. Thus glucagon and insulin control the blood glucose level (*Fig. 12.9*). Other hormones which increase the blood glucose level are adrenaline, cortisol and growth hormone.

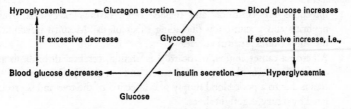

FIG. 12.9   The control of the blood glucose level

DIABETES MELLITUS

Diabetes mellitus ('flowing sweet') is a disturbance of carbohydrate, protein, fat, and electrolyte metabolism due to inadequate insulin.

Causes:

1 Insulin deficiency due to hereditary causes involving several genes. This causes the 'juvenile' type, the commonest type, of diabetes mellitus.
2 Insulin deficiency secondary to pancreatitis or haemochromatosis. Rare.
3 Relative insulin deficiency (insulin secretion may be higher than normal but is not sufficient to bring the blood sugar to normal) due to substances which antagonise the effects of insulin, such as growth hormone (acromegaly), cortisol (Cushing's syndrome), adrenaline (phaeochromocytoma) or glucagon (glucagon-secreting tumour of the pancreas). It also occurs in chronic liver disease, e.g. cirrhosis.
4 Obesity is associated with the 'adult' ('maturity onset') type of diabetes.

Symptomless diabetes may be unmasked by pregnancy or by thiazide diuretics. The blood sugar may be raised temporarily by subarachnoid haemorrhage or head injury.

Clinically: diabetes mellitus affects 1–2% of the population in the U.S.A. and U.K. The incidence increases with age. In the 'juvenile' type deficiency of effective insulin prevents the liver, muscle and adipose cells from taking glucose from the blood, resulting in hyperglycaemia (a high blood sugar), and for energy the muscles use fat and protein (brain cells are independent of insulin). Fat is mobilised from adipose tissue, causing a high level in the blood (hyperlipidaemia), and its breakdown causes ketosis and ketonuria (acetone and acetoacetic acid in the urine). (Ketosis also occurs in starvation and vomiting.) Severe ketosis causes vomiting, with loss of electrolytes and water; increased depth of respirations (hyperpnoea); and coma. The use of protein for energy causes muscular wasting, weakness, loss of weight and acidosis. A blood sugar above the normal renal threshold of 10 mmol/l (180 mg%) leads to glycosuria which causes an osmotic polyuria, hence thirst, dehydration and loss of electrolytes in the urine. Dehydration causes a dry tongue, constipation, tachycardia, fall in blood pressure and uraemia (*Fig. 12.10*).

In the obesity (adult, mature-onset) form the patient is over 40 years, without ketosis and the diabetes is often mild.

Complications:

1 Infections are common and include boils, carbuncles, cystitis, pyelonephritis and pneumonitis (including tuberculosis). Monilial infection of the vulva causes pruritus vulvae.
2 Atheroma causes angina, myocardial infarction, cerebral thrombosis and arterial disease in the legs (claudication and gangrene). Gangrene of the toes is due to a poor blood supply plus infection of the toes and is precipitated by injury, e.g. tight shoes.
3 Renal disease: (a) pyelonephritis; (b) 'diabetic' kidneys (Kimmelstiel–Wilson

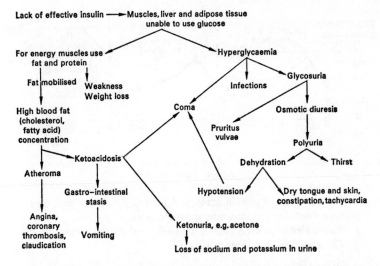

FIG. 12.10   The mechanism of symptoms in diabetes mellitus

syndrome), a chronic degeneration of the glomeruli which causes albuminuria and finally renal failure.

4   Eyes. Cataract (opacity of the lens); retinopathy, i.e. haemorrhages,
    exudates and micro-aneurysms in the retina; and optic atrophy. Any of
    these may lead to blindness.

5   Neuropathy. Peripheral neuropathy is damage to the peripheral nerves. It
    causes tingling in the fingers and toes, loss of tendon reflexes and painless
    ulcers of the skin. Autonomic neuropathy is malfunction of the autonomic
    nerves and causes impotence, diarrhoea and postural hypotension.

6   Untreated pregnant diabetics may have large babies, abortions or stillbirths.

7   Coma: (a) diabetic (hyperglycaemic, ketoacidotic) coma; (b) hypogly-
    caemic coma in a patient receiving insulin or hypoglycaemic drugs.

Investigations:

1   The fasting blood sugar is increased (normal = 4·4–6·7 mmol/l, 80–120
    mg%). Most of the blood sugar is glucose (normal = 3·4–5·6 mmol/l,
    60–100 mg%).

2   The glucose tolerance test is abnormal The patient should receive 250–300 g
    of carbohydrate daily for three days, then fasting blood and urine are
    tested for glucose, 50 g of glucose is given orally in 200 ml of water. Blood
    and urine are collected half-hourly for two and a half hours. The maximum
    normal blood sugar after carbohydrate is 10 mmol/l (180 mg%) (= 8·9
    mmol/l, 160 mg% of glucose) and glucose should be absent from the
    urine. *Figure 12.11* shows the normal and a diabetic curve.

3   Urine is increased in daily volume and is pale but has a high specific gravity
    (1·025–1·045), i.e. 780–1400 mosmol/kg, owing to the glucose which it

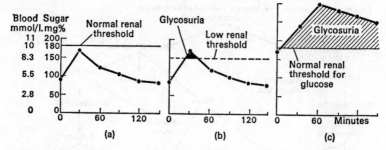

FIG. 12.11 Glucose tolerance tests: (a) normal curve; (b) normal curve with a low renal threshold; (c) diabetes mellitus

contains. It may contain ketones. Albumin, pus, blood and organisms should be tested for, since infection is common.

4 Plasma electrolytes and bicarbonate levels are abnormal in ketoacidosis.

5 Chest radiograph to show pneumonitis.

Treatment: the patient must be reassured and the condition explained to him so as to relieve his anxiety. Provided that he adheres to the diabetic regimen, which is essential, he can lead a normal life.

Therapy must:

1 Bring the body weight back to normal. Thus an obese patient receives a low calorie diet, e.g. 1000 kcal. (4·2 MJ) daily, until the weight is normal for the age, height and sex; then the calories are increased sufficiently to maintain that weight (Appendix 3). A young active diabetic may need e.g. 3000 kcal. (12·6 MJ) daily.

2 Provide enough carbohydrate to prevent ketosis.

3 If these two requirements increase the blood sugar, sufficient insulin or hypoglycaemic drug is given to return the blood sugar to normal.

Diet. Diet alone may be sufficient in the 'adult' (obesity) type of diabetes, but oral hypoglycaemic drugs or insulin may be needed. Insulin is always needed in the 'juvenile' type of diabetes. The daily number of calories is calculated from the patient's weight and occupation; more calories being needed in an active patient. The proportion of calories as carbohydrate, protein and fat are calculated; e.g. 40% as carbohydrate, 45% as fat and 15% as protein (a higher proportion of protein is taken if the patient can afford it). The amount of carbohydrate taken (between 100 and 250 g) should be the same each day so that the dose of insulin is constant, although an intelligent diabetic, once he has learned the subject, may vary food intake or insulin dosage according to circumstances. The diet, divided into three main meals and snacks if necessary, is based on the patient's daily routine, his activity, and his usual meal times. Its constituents must be weighed. The patient is given a diet sheet giving the caloric values of foods. Sugar is avoided since starch is more bulky and satisfying, and sweetening agents (e.g. saccharine) are used instead. Alcohol is permitted but counts as calories, e.g. 500 ml of beer = 300 kcal. (1·3 MJ). Non-starchy vegetables are unrestricted.

In the line ration scheme of Lawrence one black line is 10 g of carbohydrate and one red line is 7·5 g of protein and 9 g of fat, a total of 155 kcal., i.e. 0·7 MJ (*Table 12.2*).

TABLE 12.2 *Food portions for diabetics*

Carbohydrate Foods (containing sugars or starches) are **black** portions. Each of the following is equal to one black line (10 g carbohydrate = 42 kcal. = 178 kJ).

Raw fruit	g	oz	Cooked vegetables	g	oz
Dates	15	½	Potato, dried peas, kidney		
Currants (dried)	30	1	beans, lentils	60	2
Banana, grapes	60	2	Parsnip	90	3
Pineapple, cherries	90	3	Onion (fried), beetroot,		
			young peas	120	4
Peach, apple, peeled			Carrots, leeks, turnips,		
orange, plums	100	3½	artichokes	230	8
Gooseberries, pear,			*Cereal foods*		
grapefruit	120	4	Bread (all kinds, ½ large		
Strawberries,			slice)	20	⅔
raspberries	170	6	Breakfast cereals, plain		
Melon	200	7	biscuits	15	½
Stewed fruit			Rice, sago, tapioca, semolina	12	⅖
Apricots, prunes (29 g dry)	60	2	Ice cream	60	2
Plums, cherries	120	4	Barley sugar, sugar or glucose		
Pear, apple	140	5	(2 lumps or teaspoons)	10	⅓
Raspberries,			*Drinks*		
blackberries	170	6	Ovaltine, Horlicks	15	½
Fruit juices			Milk (also contains one red		
Orange juice	110 ml	4	line)	200 ml	7
Grapefruit juice	200 ml	7	Coca-cola, Pepsicola	86 ml	3

Protein and fat are **red** portions. 7·5 g protein plus 9 g fat equal one red line (113 kcal, 475 kJ) and are present in:

1 egg, 28·5 g (1 oz) sardines, lean ham, lean bacon, tongue, pork, duck;

or 7 g (¼ oz) fat plus 35 g (1¼ oz) beef, lamb, veal, liver, chicken, pigeon, crab, lobster, fish;

or 21 g (¾ oz) cheese or 7 oz milk (also contains one black portion);

or 21 g (¾ oz) fat plus 43 g (1½ oz) kidney, tripe, sweetbread;

or 7 g (¼ oz) fat plus 21 g pheasant, rabbit, hare.

Fats include meat fat, suet, dripping, lard, olive oil, butter, margarine.

NEGLIGIBLE carbohydrate and protein content in average helpings of asparagus, artichokes, French (string) beans, brussels sprouts, cabbage, cauliflower, celery, cress, cucumber, lettuce, marrow, mushrooms, radishes, spinach, rhubarb, seakale, coffee, tea, water.

No flour or breadcrumbs must be used in cooking and no sauces, thickened soups, custards or sweet chutneys taken.

Diabetic breads, jams, etc. *must not* be taken as extras. They must be weighed as ordinary bread and only an equivalent quantity taken.

No sugar must be used for sweetening drinks or for cooking, but tea, coffee and Bovril may be taken freely. No sweets, sweet biscuits, cakes or jam may be taken. Saccharine may be used for sweetening.

Diabetes may be stabilised by using a four-hourly scheme in which every four hours the urine is tested for glucose and the dose of soluble insulin given is related to the degree of glycosuria. Thus for a Clinitest showing blue no insulin is given;

green indicates 10 u, yellow 20 u, orange 30 u, and red 40 u. 40 g of carbohydrate is given four-hourly. Difficulties in using this scheme include a low renal threshold, when glucose would be present in the urine at lower blood sugar levels and too much insulin would be given; incontinence of urine preventing urine testing; and abnormal sensitivity to insulin.

Insulin. Insulin is made in different strengths and types and it is important that both the nurse and the patient know which strength and type is being used. It is given s.c. into the thighs, arms or abdomen. Its times of action are given in *Table 12.3.* Each division on the insulin syringe equals one unit of single-strength insulin (20 u/ml), two units of double strength insulin (40 u/ml), or four units of quadruple strength insulin (80 u/ml).

TABLE 12.3   *The onset and duration of action of the insulins*

	Action—hours	(depends on dose)	
Insulin	*Begins in*	*Maximum at*	*Ends at*
Soluble (S.I.)	$\frac{1}{2}$	2–4	6–10
Protamine zinc (P.Z.I.)	3–6	16–24	36
Isophane (N.P.H.)	3	8–12	24
Globin (G.I.)	2	6–8	18
Lente	1	8–12	24–30
Semilente (I.Z.S. amorphous)	1	6	8–16
Ultralente (I.Z.S. crystalline)	3–6	20	36

Soluble (Regular) Insulin (S.I.) should be used for stabilisation, and during infection, operation, ketosis or coma since it acts rapidly and is short-acting. It is given 30 minutes before meals, twice daily or more frequently if large doses are needed.

Nuso and Actrapid have a similar action to soluble insulin.

Protamine Zinc Insulin (P.Z.I.) is long-acting and is given once daily. It cannot be mixed with soluble insulin since it contains an excess of protamine which converts S.I. into P.Z.I. If used with S.I. the correct procedure for injection is to inject the S.I. first and leave the needle in the skin but reposition it (*Fig. 12.12*); draw the P.Z.I. into the syringe and re-attach it to the needle and inject. Thus the two insulins are injected close together but separately.

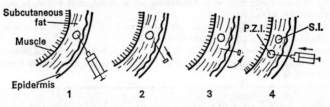

FIG. 12.12   Method of injection of soluble and protamine zinc insulins, pricking the skin only once: (1) soluble insulin injected; (2) needle partly withdrawn; (3) needle angled; (4) protamine zinc insulin injected after moving the needle slightly deeper

Isophane Insulin (N.P.H.) is protamine zinc insulin without an excess of protamine, and can therefore be mixed with soluble insulin and given as a single daily dose.

Globin Insulin is seldom used.

Insulin Zinc Suspension (I.Z.S.): semilente is the amorphous form acting like soluble insulin. Ultralente is slow-acting. Semilente and ultralente can be mixed in different proportions and a mixture of three parts of semilente with seven parts of ultralente is called lente and is given as a single daily dose of up to 50 units s.c. I.Z.S. should not be mixed with other insulins.

Oral Hypoglycaemic Drugs. These may be used in adult-type non-ketotic diabetes. They are effective only when some insulin is being secreted by the pancreas, since they release insulin from protein-binding both in the pancreas and in the plasma.

Sulphonylureas. Tolbutamide (Rastinon, Orinase) 0·5–1 g b.d. or t.d.s. Acts for six to 12 hours. Chlorpropamide (Diabinese) 100–500 mg single dose daily acts for 48 hours. Tolazamide (Tolanase) 100–500 mg daily. Glibenclamide (Euglucon, Daonil) 2·5–20 mg daily. Acetohexamide (Dymelor) 250–500 mg daily. Carbutamide may cause agranulocytosis and should not be used. They may all cause hypoglycaemia or skin rash. Chlorpropamide may also cause flushing of the face, jaundice and leucopenia. Hypoglycaemia due to chlorpropamide may be difficult to treat owing to its long action.

Glymidine 0·5–1·5 g daily. Similar action to the sulphonylureas. May cause leucopenia.

Biguanides (Diguanides). Phenformin (Dibotin) 25–100 mg b.d. with food. Side-effects: anorexia, nausea, vomiting, diarrhoea, lactic acidosis. Metformin 0·5–1·5 g b.d. with food. Biguanides may be given with sulphonylureas or with insulin.

Education of the Patient
The patient is taught his diet, how to give his injections and test the urine for sugar and keep a record in a notebook. It is more informative if the urine is tested before breakfast and after two meals on two days weekly rather than testing once daily. The patients should be made to experience a hypoglycaemic reaction so that they know the symptoms and that they should take sugar immediately. They should always carry sugar and a card stating their name, address and dose of insulin. An acute infection should be reported to the doctor immediately, since it needs treating in order to prevent ketosis and hyperglycaemia, and the dose of insulin may need to be increased. Booklets on diabetes may be obtained.

Diabetics should be seen regularly for life so as to detect the onset of complications and check the degree of control. The patient should never omit taking insulin, although a lower dose may be taken if there is anorexia, and some solid or fluid carbohydrate must be taken. If this is vomited he must report immediately to his doctor.

Advice on Social Aspects: diabetes has an hereditary predisposition, therefore if both parents are affected there is a risk of diabetes in their children. Diabetes increases the risk to the fetus and careful control of maternal diabetes is essential. The child is more likely to be born alive if birth is induced at 37 weeks than at term (40 weeks). Drivers must report diabetes to the driving licence department, since even transient confusion may be dangerous. They may drive unless hypoglycaemic attacks occur.

Treatment of Complications.

Good control of the diabetes may prevent complications.

Infection: antibiotic for pyogenic infection or tuberculosis.

Gangrene of the toes may be prevented by the avoidance of injury to the feet, however trivial, when cutting toenails or corns, and by avoiding tight shoes. Abrasions are painless if there is sensory neuropathy, and wounds heal poorly if there is arterial insufficiency. The feet should be washed in warm but not overhot water and dried carefully.

Cataract is treated surgically.

Diabetic (Hyperglycaemic, Ketoacidotic) Coma

Diabetic coma is often precipitated by infection and is usually due to ketosis (and therefore 'juvenile' diabetes). It is preceded by epigastric pain, nausea, vomiting, headache and anorexia. The blood pressure falls, the pulse is weak and rapid and the tongue is dry, due to dehydration caused by polyuria and vomiting. Ketoacidosis causes deep sighing respirations ('air-hunger'). The breath has a 'sweet' odour (new mown hay') due to acetone. Rarely coma occurs without ketosis but there is dehydration and hyperosmolarity of the blood and tissues. Untreated coma ends in death.

Treatment is urgent. The patient is laid on his side and the foot of the bed raised to combat shock and to help in preventing the inhalation of fluid from the stomach. The average comatose patient has lost six litres of water, up to 500 mmol (500 mEq) of sodium, up to 500 mmol (500 mEq) of potassium and 200 or more mmol (mEq) of bicarbonate. These need replacing, beginning with isotonic (0·9%) saline i.v., 1 l in 30 minutes, then 2 l of isotonic saline, each containing 1 g potassium chloride, in the next two hours. Isotonic (1·3%) sodium bicarbonate or sodium lactate (M/6) is given for ketoacidosis; then 5% glucose may be given.

Soluble insulin 20 units is given i.m., then 5–10 units hourly i.v. or i.m. according to the response. Other types of insulin are not used owing to their delayed action. The blood sugar is checked every 1–4 hours at first.

Gastric aspiration via a Ryle's tube prevents the inhalation of vomit.

So that urine can be tested hourly for sugar, an indwelling catheter is sometimes used; but catheterisation may cause cystitis and pyelonephritis, so is better avoided and blood sugar concentrations used as a guide to treatment until the patient recovers consciousness and is able to pass urine normally.

Record the pulse, blood pressure, temperature, respirations and fluid balance, and treat the dry mouth.

On recovery of consciousness oral fluids and carbohydrate are given and the diet and dose of insulin are stabilised. Sodium bicarbonate 2 g in a small amount of water orally two- to four-hourly helps to reduce acidosis and vomiting. The dose is repeated if lost by vomiting. Antibiotic for infection.

The differences between hyperglycaemic and hypoglycaemic comas are shown in *Table 12.4*.

TABLE 12.4   *Differences between hypoglycaemic and 'diabetic' coma*

	Hypoglycaemia	Ketoacidotic hyperglycaemic coma
History	Missing a meal, recent insulin overdose, unusual exercise	Missing insulin, infection Abdominal pain, vomiting
Onset	Sudden Well immediately before	Gradual
Tongue	Moist	Dry, furred
Skin	Moist, pale, cold	Dry, flushed
Pulse	Normal or rapid, good volume	Rapid, poor volume (dehydration)
Blood pressure	Normal	Low
Breathing	Normal or shallow	Deep ('air hunger'), acetone in breath
Urine	No ketones or glucose unless the bladder has not been recently emptied	Glycosuria
Blood sugar	Low (below 2·8 mmol/l, 50 mg%)	High (over 16·6 mmol/l, 300 mg%)
Plasma bicarbonate	Normal	Low

Hypoglycaemic Coma

This may occur in treated diabetics and is due to a low blood sugar caused by an overdose of insulin; by not taking adequate carbohydrate (e.g. missing or delaying a meal); or by excessive exercise. The onset is rapid. Hunger, weakness, faintness, mental confusion, diplopia, abnormal behaviour and headache may be followed by convulsions and coma, due to a deficient supply of glucose to the brain. Adrenaline is secreted to help to release glucose from liver glycogen, and causes sweating, tremor, palpitations and tachycardia. The blood pressure is normal or increased, and respiration shallow and rapid. The urine should be free from sugar but may contain sugar if the bladder has not been emptied since a previous episode of hyperglycaemia.

Treatment is urgent since hypoglycaemia may cause permanent brain damage. Carbohydrate is given orally if the patient is conscious. Glucose is the most rapidly acting, but cane sugar is also suitable. 25 g of glucose (50 ml of 50%) is given i.v. for coma, repeated if recovery is not immediate, then 30 g of sugar orally as soon as the patient can swallow. The dose of insulin should be reduced unless the hypoglycaemia was due to unaccustomed exercise or to not taking a meal at the correct time.

13 THE NERVOUS SYSTEM

The systems of the body for convenience are described separately, but they are completely dependent on each other and their functions are integrated, not only by hormones and the bloodstream, but also by the nervous system.

The nervous system comprises the cerebrum, cerebellum, brain stem, spinal cord, peripheral nerves and autonomic nerves. These parts consist of nerve cells (neurons) and their processes in a special type of connective tissue called neuroglia. The brain and spinal cord are surrounded by three membranes, the meninges, between two of which flows cerebrospinal fluid.

The Meninges

These consist of an outer tough layer of fibrous tissue, the dura mater; a middle delicate layer, the arachnoid mater; and an inner vascular membrane, the pia mater (*Fig. 13.1*). The dura mater is partly fused with the periosteum, the membrane lining the skull (which is sometimes wrongly called the outer layer of dura mater). Where the dura does not fuse with the periosteum there are spaces which form the venous sinuses into which the blood drains from the brain. The arachnoid mater is

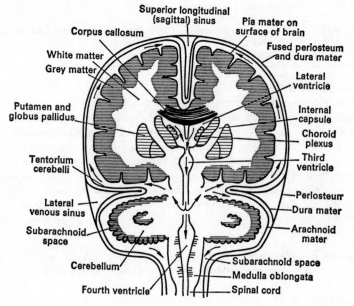

FIG. 13.1 The meninges, the ventricles and the flow of cerebrospinal fluid; anterior view

a serous membrane in contact with the dura. The potential space between the two is the subdural space. Attached to the brain is the pia mater, a fine vascular membrane. The pial and arachnoid membranes follow the convolutions of the brain and between them is a space, the subarachnoid space, through which cerebrospinal fluid flows.

The Cerebrospinal Fluid (C.S.F.)
In each half of the cerebrum there is a cavity, the lateral ventricle, containing a highly vascular body, the choroid plexus, which runs into the third ventricle. The cerebrospinal fluid is made by the choroid plexuses, flows from the lateral ventricles through the interventricular foramina (openings) into the third ventricle, then along the aqueduct of the midbrain into the fourth ventricle (*Fig. 13.2*). From the

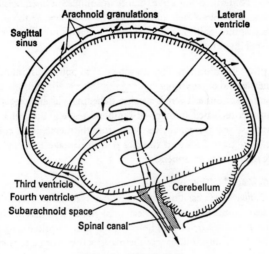

FIG. 13.2   The ventricles

fourth ventricle it flows downwards through the central canal of the spinal cord and also through openings (foramina) in the roof of the fourth ventricle into the subarachnoid space, hence flowing around the brain and spinal cord. The cerebrospinal fluid is reabsorbed into blood capillaries in the arachnoid mater.

Functions. The cerebrospinal fluid supports and protects the brain and spinal cord, acting as a shock-absorber for them, keeps them moist and allows the interchange of substances between the fluid and the nerve cells; but there is a barrier between the blood and the C.S.F., the blood–brain barrier, which protects the brain against toxic substances in the blood. The barrier is lost during inflammation of the meninges owing to vasodilatation, and this is the reason why antibiotics enter the C.S.F. in meningitis but not when the membranes are normal.

Normal C.S.F. is clear and colourless and contains protein 0·2–0·4 g/l, glucose 2·8–5 mmol/l (50–90 mg%); chloride 120–130 mmol/l; less than five lymphocytes per mm³, (5 × 10⁶/l) and does not precipitate colloidal gold. The normal pressure of C.S.F., with the patient relaxed and lying on his side is 0·5–1·5 kPa (50–150 mm of C.S.F.).   Queckenstedt's test is compression of both sides of the patient's neck with the flat of the hands. This occludes the venous return from the brain, increases the intracranial pressure and causes a brisk rise in the pressure of C.S.F., which falls to normal on releasing the compression. If there is pressure on the spinal cord by a lesion blocking the spinal canal the C.S.F. pressure does not rise.

DISORDERS OF THE MENINGES AND CEREBROSPINAL FLUID

Meningitis

Meningitis is inflammation of the meninges, which become inflamed, red and swollen. It may be sterile or infective. Sterile inflammation (meningism) is due to meningeal irritation by blood in a subarachnoid haemorrhage or to carcinomatous deposits. Infective meningitis is due to viruses, pyogenic organisms, tuberculosis, and rarely to syphilis or fungi.

Virus ('Aseptic') Meningitis. This may be due to poliovirus, mumps, ECHO, Coxsackie, measles and other viruses.

Symptoms are of the cause. There is also headache, pyrexia and photophobia. The C.S.F. contains an increased number of lymphocytes, e.g. 200 per mm^3 (200× 10^6/l), and its pressure is increased. Recovery from the meningitis is complete, but poliomyelitis may leave paralysed muscles due to damage to peripheral motor nerves. There is no specific treatment.

Pyogenic Meningitis. The commonest causes are the meningococcus, pneumo-coccus and *H. influenzae* (a bacillus which should not be confused with the influenza virus), but it may be caused by streptococci, staphylococci, or *E. coli*. The organism spreads to the meninges from middle-ear infection, mastoiditis, nasal sinusitis, compound fracture of the skull, or septicaemia associated with infection elsewhere in the body.

Clinically: the rapid onset of headache, pyrexia, rigors, vomiting, malaise, photo-phobia, irritability, restlessness, and pain in the back and limbs, is followed by confusion, drowsiness, coma, and slowing of the pulse rate due to increased intra-cranial pressure caused by inflammatory exudation into the C.S.F. The patient resents interference and lies curled up. Muscle spasm produces neck stiffness and prevents the neck from being flexed, and may be severe enough to bend the head backwards (head retraction). In infants the whole back may be arched and stiff (opisthotonos). With the thigh flexed to 90° to the abdomen the knee cannot be straightened (Kernig's sign) owing to reflex spasm of the hamstring muscles caused by stretching of the inflamed sciatic nerve roots. Epileptiform convulsions may occur.

Meningococcal meningitis is spread by droplets and may be sporadic or epidemic. The incubation period is one to four days. From the nasopharynx the meningococcus enters the blood to reach the meninges. Septicaemia may cause a petechial rash (hence the name 'spotted fever'), conjunctivitis, arthritis, and death from haemorrhage into the adrenals (Waterhouse–Friderichsen syndrome).

Infection by other organisms is due to spread from infection elsewhere in the body (e.g. pneumococcal pneumonia).

Complications: bronchopneumonia, hydrocephalus, damage to nerves causing deafness, blindness and various paralyses such as squint.

Prognosis: meningitis is serious, but most patients recover if treated urgently.

Investigations: C.S.F., obtained by lumbar puncture, is under increased pressure. It is turbid due to polymorph leucocytes; the protein level is high; the glucose concentration is low; and the causative organism is present. The blood shows a polymorph leucocytosis.

Treatment: rest in bed in a quiet, darkened room, using padded bedsides to prevent injury in the restless patient.

Strict isolation is needed for 48 hours in meningococcal meningitis but not in the other types.

Diet is fluid at first but should contain protein, e.g. milk, given via an intragastric Ryle's tube if swallowing is difficult, as in stupor. At least three litres of fluid is given daily. Fluid intake and output are recorded. As soon as C.S.F. has been taken antibiotic is given and is continued until four days after the patient has become apyrexial and the C.S.F. normal.

Drugs: For meningococcal meningitis sulphadiazine 6 g is given initially for an adult or 2 g for an infant, then 1 g four-hourly (adult) orally, or i.v. if vomiting, plus benzylpenicillin 6 mg (10,000 u) intrathecally mixed with 10 ml of C.S.F. Benzylpenicillin 300–600 mg i.m. four-hourly may be given in place of, or in addition to, the sulphonamide, and is suitable for pneumococcal meningitis.

This therapy is also given in other types of pyogenic meningitis until the type and sensitivity of the organism is known; then the antibiotic may need to be changed, e.g. to ampicillin or chloramphenicol for *H. influenzae.*

An analgesic is given for headache and a sedative for restlessness.

Septic foci are also treated, e.g. by incision and drainage. Acute retention of urine may occur and requires catheterisation. The pressure areas are treated. The mouth may ulcerate and should be cleaned and kept moist. The eyelids become sticky and require bathing with saline or boracic lotion.

Tuberculous Meningitis. This is due to spread from a focus of tuberculosis elsewhere in the body.

Clinically: the onset is insidious. The patient, commonly a child, shows lassitude, anorexia and constipation, with gradually increasing headache, pyrexia, neck stiffness, positive Kernig's sign, papilloedema, drowsiness and coma. It is fatal in a few weeks if untreated and 30% die even with treatment.

Complications: cranial nerve palsies, blindness, deafness, hemiplegia, hydrocephalus, mental defect, epilepsy.

Investigations: the C.S.F. is under increased pressure. It is clear but a fine fibrin clot may form in it; the protein is slightly increased; the glucose level is low; the lymphocyte count is increased up to 400 per mm^3 (400×10^6/l), and tubercle bacilli are present. Chest X-ray may show pulmonary tuberculosis.

Treatment is as for tuberculosis elsewhere (*see* Chapter 4). Streptomycin is also given intrathecally, 50 mg daily for 10 days. Prednisolone 10 mg q.i.d. orally or i.m., and hydrocortisone 10 mg intrathecally may be given since theoretically glucocortico-steroids may prevent spinal block (obstruction of the subarachnoid space) by adhesions. Nutrition and hydration must be improved. Complications of anti-tuberculous drugs must be watched for, especially giddiness and deafness due to streptomycin.

Meningovascular Syphilis. This occurs in the third (tertiary) stage of syphilis. Inflammation of arteries obstructs them (endarteritis obliterans) producing syphilitic ischaemic areas of necrosis (gummas). Inflammation of the meninges damages the cranial nerves. Peripheral motor and sensory nerves are also affected. The blood and C.S.F. Wassermann reaction is positive.

Treatment: penicillin 300 mg q.i.d. i.m. for 14 days.

Fungal Meningitis, e.g. *Cryptococcus neoformans*, is predisposed by Hodgkin's disease, sarcoidosis and corticosteroids.

Treatment is with amphotericin B 1 mg/kg daily i.v.

Hydrocephalus

Hydrocephalus ('water brain') is an increased amount of cerebrospinal fluid in the skull. It is due to obstruction to the outflow of C.S.F. from the ventricles, e.g. by congenital malformations or tumour, which causes dilatation of the ventricles (internal hydrocephalus); or to inadequate absorption of C.S.F. through the meninges into the venous sinuses owing to meningeal thickening following meningitis; or to thrombosis of the venous sinuses, which increase the amount of C.S.F in the ventricles and in the subarachnoid space (communicating hydro-cephalus).

Intracranial pressure is increased, the brain becomes compressed and thinner, the sutures are widened, the fontanelles bulge in infants and the skull enlarges in infants and children (*Fig. 13.3*). Fetal hydrocephalus may obstruct vaginal delivery. Infants fail to thrive. Death occurs within a few months or years in severe cases.

Complications: mental defect, blindness, spastic paralysis, epilepsy, pressure sores on the head.

Treatment is used for rapidly increasing hydrocephalus and consists of the insertion of a Spitz–Holter valve. One end of a tube is in the lateral ventricle, through the skull, the other end drains C.S.F. into the jugular vein. Treatment is often un-satisfactory since the valve may become infected and the tube blocked. When lifting a child the head must be supported before moving the trunk.

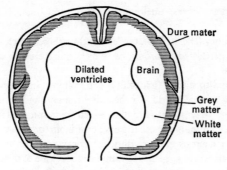

FIG. 13.3   Internal hydrocephalus

THE BRAIN, SPINAL CORD AND PERIPHERAL NERVES

The nervous system is artificially divided into the central and the peripheral nervous systems. The central nervous system consists of the brain and spinal cord and contains more than 10,000 million neurons and nerve fibres embedded in a special type of connective tissue called neuroglia. The peripheral nerves consist of bundles of nerve fibres which are distributed throughout the body and contain motor fibres (e.g. the fibres to the muscles of the eye), and sensory fibres (e.g. those carrying impulses from stretch receptors in tendons).

A Neuron consists of a nerve cell and its processes: an axon and dendrites (*Fig. 13.4*). The nerve cells form the grey matter of the nervous system and lie in the

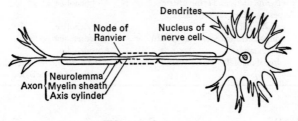

FIG. 13.4   A neuron

periphery of the brain, at the centre of the spinal cord, in ganglia outside the brain and spinal cord, and in the walls of the organs. The axons and dendrites form the white matter of the nervous system, which is deep in the brain but at the periphery of the spinal cord. The axons form the peripheral nerves and nerve fibres which carry impulses away from nerve cells and are usually longer than dendrites, e.g. the axons to the toes are 100 cm (40 inches) long.

An axon consists of the central axis cylinder surrounded by a fatty sheath, the medullary or myelin sheath, which speeds up nerve impulses, acts as an insulator and may supply nutrition to the axis cylinder. A delicate membrane, the neurolemma, surrounds the myelin sheath of the peripheral nerves.

Dendrites are nerve fibres, usually short, which carry impulses towards the cell body.

Nerves are sensory (afferent), motor (efferent) or those which link sensory and motor nerves (intercalated neurons) or which link cerebral cortical neurons (association fibres).

Neurons respond to stimuli (irritability) and conduct impulses (conductivity). Stimuli from the outside world, e.g. heat, light, sound and contact (touch), are changed by the special senses into impulses which are transmitted to the brain. The brain may then send impulses to other parts of the brain for the storage of information, or to motor neurons to cause muscular contraction for movement or the maintenance of balance, or to glands to stimulate the release of their secretions.

A nerve impulse is transmitted from its origin to its effector organ through more than one neuron. The site at which the axon of one neuron branches close to the dendrites of the next neuron is called a synapse. The impulse crosses the space at the synapse by the release, from the endings of the axon, of chemical transmitters such as noradrenaline (norepinephrine), serotonin and acetylcholine. These are rapidly inactivated by enzymes so that their action is brief. The sites of action of the different transmitters is shown in *Table 13.1*.

TABLE 13.1   *The sites of action of the chemical transmitters released at nerve endings*

Nerve ending	Chemical transmitter
In brain	Serotonin, dopamine
	γ-amino butyric acid
Motor nerve ending in voluntary muscle	Acetylcholine
Autonomic nervous system	
(1) In ganglia (preganglionic nerve endings),	
parasympathetic and sympathetic	Acetylcholine
(2) At postganglionic nerve endings:	
parasympathetic	Acetylcholine
sympathetic (except sweat glands)	Noradrenaline
sweat glands	Acetylcholine
adrenal medulla	Adrenaline and noradrenaline
	released into the blood

THE BRAIN

The brain lies in the cranial cavity and consists of the cerebrum (forebrain), the brain stem, and the cerebellum (hind brain). The brain stem consists of the midbrain, the pons varioli and the medulla oblongata (*Figs 13.5 and 13.6*).

The Cerebrum

The cerebrum is divided into left and right cerebral hemispheres by the longitudinal cerebral fissure. The two hemispheres are joined by the corpus callosum, a large bundle of association nerve fibres which connect similar areas in the two hemispheres. The outer layer of the cerebrum is the cerebral cortex. It consists of nerve cells (grey matter) and is infolded to form convolutions (gyri) which are separated by fissures (sulci). The infoldings increase the surface area of the cerebrum, are most numerous in the intelligent mammals such as man, whale and dolphin, and are absent in the lower animals. Each hemisphere is divided into lobes named frontal, parietal, occipital and temporal (*Figs 13.5 and 13.6*). The sulcus between the frontal

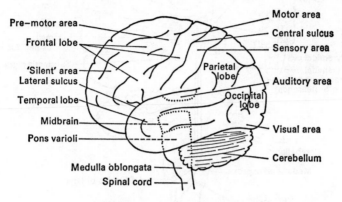

FIG. 13.5   Lateral view of the brain

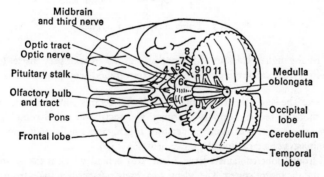

FIG. 13.6   The brain from below (4 to 11 are cranial nerves)

and parietal lobes is the central sulcus (fissure of Rolando) and that separating the temporal from the frontal and parietal lobes is the lateral sulcus (fissure of Sylvius). From the neurons in the cerebral cortex run nerve fibres which form groups (tracts) and make up the white matter of the brain.

The fibres which link different parts of the cerebral cortex are association fibres, those linking the two hemispheres are commissural association fibres, those connecting parts of the brain with each other and continuing into the spinal cord are projection fibres. Most projection fibres converge into one area in each hemisphere, called the internal capsule (*Figs 13.1 and 13.7*), which lies between the thalamus and the basal ganglia, and contains fibres carrying impulses descending from, and ascending to, the cerebral cortex in that hemisphere.

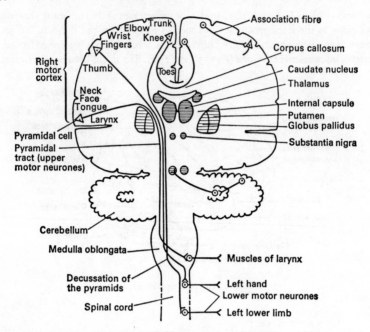

FIG. 13.7   Transverse section of the brain

The basal ganglia, thalamus and hypothalamus are areas of grey matter (nerve cells) which are synaptic relay stations deep in the cerebral hemispheres.

Function. The cerebral cortex contains the higher centres which provide intelligence, thought, reason, memory, learning, and social and moral conscience. It perceives the sensations of pain, temperature, touch, taste, smell, hearing and sight and it initiates voluntary muscular movement (*Fig. 13.8*).

Each frontal lobe contains a large 'silent' area behind which is the pre-motor cortex and the motor cortex. The 'silent' area receives association fibres from other parts of the brain and probably controls thinking, initiative, complex learning, character and behaviour. The premotor area of the cortex lies immediately in front of the motor area which it controls and co-ordinates to ensure that movements are carried out in their correct order and to provide manual dexterity. The motor area lies in front of the central sulcus. Its nerve cells (upper motor neurons) are large and are called pyramidal cells. They initiate voluntary muscular movements.

The Motor Pathway: the axon from each pyramidal cell passes downwards through the internal capsule to the medulla, where it crosses to the opposite side, then descends in the spinal cord where, at a suitable level, it synapses with a second neuron (lower motor neuron) which transmits impulses to the muscle. Thus the motor area of the left hemisphere controls voluntary muscles on the right side of the body and vice versa. Damage to either the upper or the lower motor neuron

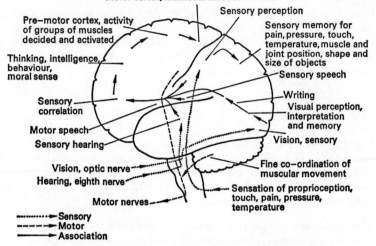

Motor cortex, individual muscles activated

Sensory perception

Pre—motor cortex, activity
of groups of muscles
decided and activated

Sensory memory for
pain, pressure, touch,
temperature, muscle and
joint position, shape and
size of objects

Thinking, intelligence,
behaviour,
moral sense

Sensory speech

Sensory
correlation

Writing
Visual perception,
interpretation
and memory

Motor speech

Sensory hearing

Vision, sensory

Vision, optic nerve

Hearing, eighth nerve

Fine co—ordination of
muscular movement

Motor nerves

Sensation of proprioception,
touch, pain, pressure,
temperature

Sensory
Motor
Association

FIG. 13.8   Simplified diagram of the functional organisation of the brain

causes paralysis. The cells in the upper part of the motor cortex control the feet and
the cells in the lower. deeper part control the fingers, head and neck.

The Sensory Pathway: from the different types of sensory nerve endings, e.g. pain
receptors in the skin, sensory stimuli pass along the axons of the sensory nerves to
the posterior horns of the spinal cord where, after giving off branches, the nerve
fibres ascend in the sensory tracts of the spinal cord and brain stem to the thalamus.
Here they relay to the cerebral cortex where the sensation is interpreted and stored.
Sensation from the rods and cones in the retina is relayed through the lateral
geniculate bodies of the brain before reaching the cerebral cortex.

In the parietal lobe behind the central sulcus is the sensory area where the sensations of pain, temperature, touch, taste, pressure, positions of the joints and muscular
movements from the opposite side of the body are received and interpreted. Behind
this area is the interpretation and memory of objects. In the lower part of the
parietal lobe and extending into the temporal lobe lies the sensory speech area
where the spoken word is interpreted. In a right-handed person the dominant
area is in the left hemisphere. and vice versa.

In the temporal lobe lies the auditory (hearing) sensory area which receives and
interprets impulses transmitted from the inner ear by the auditory nerve. Deep in
the temporal lobe is the sense of smell.

The occipital lobe is the site of vision.

The basal ganglia are deep in the brain and consist of several groups of nerve cells
including the caudate nucleus, the lenticular nucleus (putamen and globus pallidus),
and the substantia nigra. They control skeletal muscular tone. Disorder of their
function causes Parkinsonism.

The thalamus lies below the corpus callosum and receives the sensations of pain,
temperature, touch and pressure in a crude form; finer discrimination being inter-

preted in the sensory area of the cerebral cortex. The *hypothalamus* is below and in front of the thalamus and above the pituitary gland. It is linked by nerve fibres to the posterior lobe of the pituitary, and by blood vessels (the hypophyseal portal tract) to the anterior lobe of the pituitary. Through these it controls the secretion of hormones by the pituitary. The hypothalamus also controls hunger, thirst, body temperature, and defence (fear, rage).

THE BRAIN STEM

The brain stem joins the cerebrum to the spinal cord and consists of the midbrain, that part of the brain below the cerebrum, the pons varolii below the midbrain and in front of the cerebellum, and the medulla oblongata below the pons and continuous with the spinal cord. The third to the twelfth cranial nerves arise from the brain stem (the first and second are attached to the cerebrum).

The Midbrain consists of two cerebral peduncles which are composed of nerve fibres passing through it, upwards to the cerebrum or downwards to the cerebellum, pons, medulla oblongata and spinal cord. It also contains groups of nerve cells which act as relay stations including the lateral and medial geniculate bodies which relay impulses from the optic nerves and the vestibular portion of the auditory nerves to the cerebellum. These impulses help to maintain the balance of the body.

The Pons Varolii consists of nerve fibres passing through it from one half of the cerebellum to the other and ascending and descending fibres passing between the cerebrum and the spinal cord. Groups of nerve cells (grey matter) within the pons act as relay stations; other groups are the nuclei of the cranial nerves.

The Medulla Oblongata consists of ascending and descending nerve fibres running between the brain and the spinal cord, and nerve cells. Most of the nerves from the motor area of the cerebral cortex to the spinal cord cross (the decussation of the pyramids) from right to left or left to right in the medulla; hence the cerebral hemispheres control the muscles of the opposite side of the body. Some sensory nerves ascending to the cerebrum also cross here (the sensory decussation). The nerve cells within the medulla include relay stations for sensory nerves ascending to the cerebrum, the nuclei of cranial nerves, and the vital centres (i.e. cardiac, vasomotor, respiratory), and reflex centres for vomiting, swallowing, sneezing and coughing.

The cardiac centre controls the rate of cardiac contraction via sympathetic nerve fibres, which increase the rate and force of the heart, and via parasympathetic nerve fibres which decrease the heart-rate.

The respiratory centre controls the rate and depth of respiration by sending impulses along the phrenic and intercostal nerves to the diaphragm and intercostal muscles.

The vasomotor centre receives impulses from baroreceptors (pressure-sensitive receptors) in the walls of the carotid arteries and controls the tone of the smooth muscle, and therefore the diameter of blood vessels, via sympathetic nerves.

Stimulation of the vasomotor centre constricts blood vessels (except the coronary arteries) and increases the blood pressure.

The Cerebellum (*Figs 13.5 and 13.6*)
This consists of two hemispheres connected by a narrow strip, the vermis. Grey matter forms the outer layer of the cerebellum; white matter lies within. The cerebellum is situated behind the pons varolii, below the posterior part of the cerebrum, and in the posterior cranial fossa. Cerebellar action is unconscious and automatic. It controls voluntary muscular co-ordination which ensures smooth and accurate movement, and maintains body balance assisted by sensory information received from the muscles and joints (proprioception—proprioceptive sensation indicates the positions of muscles and joints), the eyes, and the semicircular canals in the temporal bone which sense the position of the head in space. Damage to the cerebellum results in inco-ordination which produces clumsiness, staggering gait (ataxia) and loss of muscular tone (flaccidity).

THE SPINAL CORD

The spinal cord (*Figs 13.9 and 13.10*) is a long cylinder of nervous tissue situated in the neural canal of the vertebral column and surrounded by the dura, arachnoid and pia maters. C.S.F. circulates in the subarachnoid space and along the central canal of the spinal cord which is continuous with the fourth ventricle of the brain. The spinal cord extends from the upper border of the atlas to the lower border of the first lumbar vertebra and is 45 cm (18 inches) in length. It is continuous above

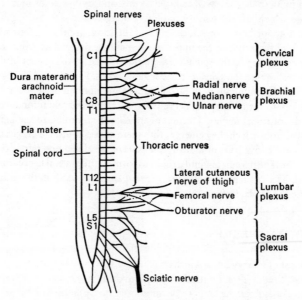

FIG. 13.9   The spinal nerves, plexuses and peripheral nerves

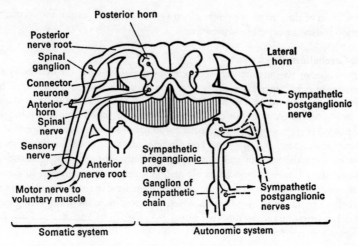

FIG. 13.10   Transverse section of the spinal cord

with the medulla oblongata and below with the cauda equina ('horse's tail') and filum terminale. The right and left halves of the spinal cord are separated in front by the median fissure. The spinal cord consists of central grey matter (nerve cells) and peripheral white matter (nerve fibres). The grey matter projects like horns behind (posterior horns) and in front (anterior horns) and is therefore H-shaped. The posterior horns receive sensory impulses from the body and transmit them to the brain in ascending axons in the spinal cord, and to connector neurons in the spinal cord which link the sensory and lower motor neurons to form spinal reflex arcs. The anterior horns contain the cells of the lower motor neurons which are stimulated by the axons of the upper motor neurons descending from the brain. Impulses descending in the spinal cord are transmitted to the organs of the body along nerves leaving the spinal cord at suitable levels. From each half-segment of the spinal cord, continuous with each horn, the anterior and posterior nerve roots arise and join to form the spinal nerve lying in the intervertebral foramen. There are 31 pairs of spinal nerves. The nerves are named according to the part of the neural canal from which they emerge; thus there are eight pairs of cervical, twelve pairs of thoracic, five pairs of lumbar, five pairs of sacral and one pair of coccygeal spinal nerves. The nerves join into groups to form the peripheral nerves running to the tissues. The last ten pairs of spinal nerves pass downwards in the neural canal to become the cauda equina.

PERIPHERAL NERVES

These consist of sensory fibres which convey impulses from sensory organs (in, e.g. the ear, eye, tongue, skin, muscles and joints) to the brain, and motor nerves which convey impulses from the brain to the motor organ, e.g. muscle. Each nerve fibre is surrounded by the endoneurium, bundles of fibres are surrounded by the perineurium, and many bundles are surrounded by the epineurium. The peripheral nerves include 12 pairs of cranial nerves arising from the brain and the nerves continuing from the spinal nerves or their plexuses. A nerve plexus is a network of nerves formed by the union of certain spinal nerves and their subdivisions. Branches of the plexus join to become the peripheral nerves; e.g. the first to the fourth cervical nerve roots join to form the cervical plexus, the fourth cervical to the first thoracic form the brachial plexus, and the fourth lumbar to the third sacral roots form the sacral plexus (*Fig. 13.9*).

The cervical plexus supplies nerves to the head and neck and forms the phrenic nerve which supplies the diaphragm. The brachial plexus gives off the nerves to the upper limb of the same side, including the circumflex, musculocutaneous, radial, median and ulnar nerves. The thoracic nerves do not form a plexus and are called intercostal nerves since they pass between the ribs to supply the chest wall. The lumbar plexus supplies the femoral nerve to the front of the thigh and supplies the leg. The sacral plexus gives rise to the sciatic and other nerves to the lower limb.

Cranial Nerves (*Table 13.2*)

TABLE 13.2   *The cranial nerves and their function*

Nerve	Function	Origin and ending
1 Olfactory	Smell	Mucosa of nose via olfactory bulb to temporal lobe
2 Optic	Sight, balance	Retina of eye via optic chiasma to occipital lobe and cerebellum
3 Oculomotor	Eye movement, pupillary size and focussing	Midbrain to external muscles of eye and ciliary muscle
4 Trochlear	Eye movement	Midbrain to superior oblique muscle of eye
5 Trigeminal	Sensation from face Chewing Lacrimation	Skin, teeth, gums and muscles to pons Pons to muscles of mastication and lacrimal gland
6 Abducens	Eye movement	Pons to lateral rectus muscle of eye
7 Facial	Facial expression Taste	Pons to facial muscles Anterior two thirds of tongue to pons and cerebral cortex
8 Auditory 　Cochlear	Hearing	Cochlea (inner ear) to auditory area of temporal lobe
Vestibular	Balance	Semicircular canals (inner ear) to cerebellum
9 Glossopharyngeal	Sensory Motor	Posterior third of tongue and pharynx to cerebrum Medulla oblongata to parotid gland and muscles of pharynx
10 Vagus	Motor	Medulla oblongata to pharynx, larynx, heart, lungs, stomach, intestine, gall bladder
11 Accessory	Motor	Medulla oblongata to muscles of pharynx, larynx, sternomastoid, trapezius
12 Hypoglossal	Motor	Medulla oblongata to muscles of tongue

The 12 pairs of cranial nerves arise from the brain. Some are sensory; some are motor; and some, like the peripheral spinal nerves, are mixed, i.e. contain motor and sensory fibres.

Reflex Action is an automatic motor response to a sensory stimulus without conscious control, e.g. coughing due to irritation of the trachea or larynx, blinking when the eye is threatened or touched, withdrawal of a limb on contact with heat, maintenance of balance, variation in heart-rate, respiratory rate and vascular tone. A reflex action requires the presence of a **reflex arc.**

A Simple Reflex Arc consists of a sensory neuron, a connector neuron and a motor neuron (*Fig. 13.11*). When stimulated, sensory endings in the organ pass

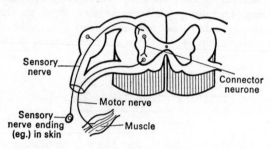

FIG. 13.11   A reflex arc

impulses along the sensory (afferent) nerve fibre to the posterior horn of the spinal cord where the connector (junctional) neuron passes on the impulse to the anterior horn (motor) cell. This transmits the impulses along its axon to the motor end-plate in the muscle and causes muscular contraction. Many reflex arcs are usually involved in an action. Impulses also reach the brain which becomes aware of what is happening. The knee jerk is a stretch reflex; tapping the tendon at the knee stretches it and causes reflex contraction of its attached muscles. Micturition and defaecation are reflexes which, with training, come partly under voluntary control, i.e. impulses reach the brain and the reflex is controlled. Reflexes which cannot be controlled include the secretions of glands and the alimentary, cardiac, and vaso-motor reflexes. Damage to the spinal cord prevents spinal sensation from reaching the brain, thus the bladder and rectum empty reflexly without control (reflex incontinence).

THE AUTONOMIC NERVOUS SYSTEM

The autonomic (involuntary) part of the nervous system (*Fig. 13.12*) controls those functions of the body which do not normally reach consciousness, e.g. the heart-rate, alimentary movements and secretions.

Efferent (motor) impulses arise from neurons in the brain. The axons leave the brain stem and spinal cord, usually with the peripheral nerves, to innervate the

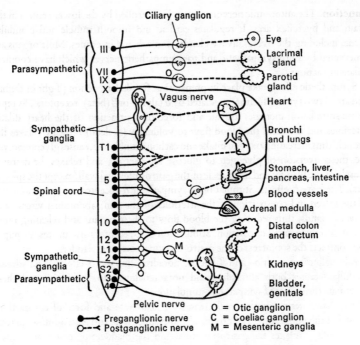

FIG. 13.12   The efferent autonomic nervous system

heart, blood vessels, bronchioles, gut, bladder and glands. The autonomic nervous system is divided into sympathetic and parasympathetic parts.

The Sympathetic Nervous System conveys impulses from the hypothalamus and medulla oblongata to the organs and tissues via cells in the lateral horns of grey matter of the spinal cord (*Fig. 13.10*) between the levels of the first thoracic and the fifth lumbar vertebrae. The axons (preganglionic fibres) of the lateral horn cells leave the cord by the anterior root and end in a ganglion outside the spinal cord. The ganglia contain relay neurons, the axons (postganglionic fibres) of which convey impulses to the organs. The ganglia form a chain, the sympathetic chain, lying outside the neural canal on the lateral surfaces of the bodies of the vertebrae. Other sympathetic ganglia lie in the abdomen, forming the coeliac and the superior and inferior mesenteric ganglia and the adrenal medulla.

The Parasympathetic Nervous System (craniosacral outflow) conveys impulses from:
1   The midbrain, pons varioli and medulla oblongata via preganglionic fibres in certain cranial nerves, e.g. the vagus nerve, to ganglia in the walls of the organs from which postganglionic fibres pass to innervate the smooth muscle or glandular cells.
2   The second to fourth sacral segments of the spinal cord via the pelvic nerves to postganglionic neurons in the walls of organs in the bony pelvis.

Function. The autonomic nervous system is controlled by the lower centres in the brain and by reflex arcs. It regulates cardiac and smooth muscle and glandular tissue, including the liver, salivary glands, stomach and intestines. Most organs are innervated by both sympathetic and parasympathetic nerves which have counter-balancing actions.

Sympathetic effects take place in preparation for skeletal action ('fight or flight') and are of two types which are mediated by α (alpha) or β (beta) 'receptors'. Sympathetic stimulation increases the rate and force of contraction of the heart, dilates arterioles and increases the blood flow to voluntary (skeletal) muscles, relaxes the bronchi thus increasing oxygen intake and carbon dioxide loss, causes glycogenolysis (i.e. the conversion of glycogen to glucose for energy), and relaxes the detrusor muscle of the bladder and the muscle of the gastro-intestinal wall (except the sphincters). These are β-effects. Stimulation of sympathetic α-receptors causes contraction of the spleen and constriction of the arterioles of the skin, abdominal viscera and salivary glands, thus reducing the blood flow to these organs and releasing more blood into the general circulation. Stimulation of α-receptors also dilates the pupils and contracts the sphincters of the gastro-intestinal tract and bladder.

Adrenaline has both α- and β-effects; noradrenaline has α-effects. The adrenal medulla secretes both adrenaline and noradrenaline into the blood and these potentiate the effects of sympathetic stimulation.

Parasympathetic stimulation decreases the heart rate and force of contraction, constricts the pupils, increases bronchial and bladder tone and gastro-intestinal tone and motility; relaxes the gastro-intestinal and the bladder sphincters and causes glandular (salivary, lacrimal, pancreatic, gastro-intestinal) secretion and thus favours the digestion and absorption of food.

Afferent (Sensory) Fibres run with the autonomic nerves and send visceral sensation to the brain via the posterior root ganglia of the spinal nerves.

Damage to the sympathetic supply to the skin produces atrophic changes; the skin becomes shiny, dry and red, ulcerates easily, but heals slowly.

The Blood Supply

The blood supply to the brain is provided through the right and left internal carotid arteries and the right and left vertebral arteries. The right common carotid artery arises from the innominate artery, a branch of the aorta. The left common carotid artery arises directly from the aorta. The common carotid arteries ascend on either side of the neck to branch into the external and the internal carotid arteries. The internal carotid artery passes into the skull through the carotid foramen of the temporal bone, gives off the ophthalmic artery supplying the eye, then branches into three arteries which supply the brain: the anterior cerebral, the middle cerebral and the posterior communicating arteries. Each subclavian artery gives off a branch, the vertebral artery, which ascends in the foramina in the traverse processes of the cervical vertebrae (*Fig. 13.13*), and enters the skull through the foramen magnum. The right and left vertebral arteries join to form the basilar artery which divides into two posterior cerebral arteries. The latter are joined by the posterior communicating arteries to form a circle of arteries, the circle of Willis, at the base

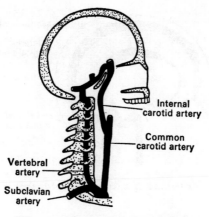

FIG. 13.13   The arterial supply to the brain

of the brain in front of the brainstem (*Fig. 13.14*). The circle of Willis consists of an anterior communicating artery, two anterior cerebral arteries, two posterior communicating arteries, and two posterior cerebral arteries.

Venous blood from the brain enters the venous sinuses (*Fig. 13.15*) which consist of dura mater lined with endothelium. The inferior sagittal sinus continues as the straight sinus which joins the superior sagittal sinus. This junction then divides into the right and left transverse sinuses which continue as the right and left internal jugular veins in the neck. The blood from the jugular veins passes via the brachio-cephalic (innominate) veins into the superior vena cava.

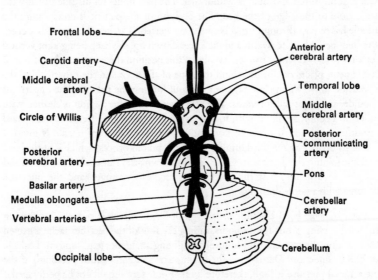

FIG. 13.14   The blood supply to the brain, showing the circle of Willis

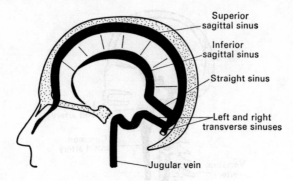

FIG. 13.15   The venous sinuses of the skull

INVESTIGATIONS IN DISEASES OF THE NERVOUS SYSTEM

Clinical Examination. The size and equality of the pupils, their reaction to light and accommodation, ophthalmoscopic examination of the retina and optic disc, the cranial nerves, the reflexes (tendon, abdominal and plantar), muscular tone and bulk, sensation of pain, temperature, touch and vibration, and coordination.

Cerebrospinal Fluid is obtained by lumbar or cisternal puncture.

Lumbar Puncture: a lumbar puncture needle is introduced between the spines of the third and fourth lumbar vertebrae into the subarachnoid space, the pressure of the C.S.F. is measured and fluid is withdrawn. The patient lies on his side (usually the left), close to the edge of the bed. The position of the patient is crucial since the needle has to pass through a gap between the vertebral arches. The spine is arched, the chest being bent forwards and the knees drawn up, the back being kept vertical (otherwise the vertebrae rotate). To obtain this position the nurse stands in front of the patient, places one hand behind the nape of the neck and the other behind the knees and draws them close together without hurting the patient. The uppermost shoulder must not fall forwards. The skin over the lumbar region is cleaned with ether or alcohol, sterilised with iodine and surrounded with sterile towels. Local anaesthetic is injected into the skin and the lumbar puncture needle is inserted immediately below the third lumbar vertebral spinous process which is at the level of a line joining the iliac crests. C.S.F. is withdrawn after removal of the stylet, and allowed to drip into a sterile bottle. The needle is removed and the puncture covered with a sterile dressing.

Complications: headache, due to leakage of C.S.F. which is reduced by keeping the patient lying prone for six hours, raising the foot of the bed (headache is caused by lowering the intracranial pressure) and giving analgesics (e.g. aspirin). Leakage of C.S.F. Infection. Damage to the brain stem and cerebellum ('coning') if the intracranial pressure is high, therefore lumbar puncture should not be performed if there is raised intracranial pressure.

Uses: (1) In the diagnosis of nervous disease; (2) for the injection of drugs, e.g. penicillin or streptomycin in meningitis; (3) to produce spinal anaesthesia by injecting spinal anaesthetic into the epidural space (the space surrounding the dura); (4) for the injection of radio-opaque solution ('dye') prior to X-ray to detect space-occupying lesions pressing on the spinal cord.

Cisternal Puncture: a needle is introduced into the subarachnoid space at the base of the brain between the occiput and the spine of the axis vertebra.

Plain Radiographs of skull, spine and chest. The skull may show bony erosion or displaced contents due to a tumour. The spine shows tuberculosis, fracture, Paget's disease, or bony erosion by a tumour. The chest may show a carcinoma of the bronchus producing secondary deposits in the brain.

Myelography is the injection of radio-opaque solution into the spinal subarachnoid space via lumbar or cisternal puncture. It demonstrates the presence and site of any filling defect, e.g. tumour pressing on the spinal cord.

Pneumoencephalography. Air is injected into the subarachnoid space (after removing 25 ml of C.S.F.) and radiographs are taken. The size and any displacement of the cerebral cortical gyri and ventricles can be seen. In **Ventriculography** air is injected directly into the ventricles through a burr-hole made in the skull. The ventricles are dilated in hydrocephalus and are displaced by tumours.

Echoencephalography. Ultrasonic waves are aimed at the brain and their reflections are recorded. These show space-occupying lesions.

Electroencephalography (E.E.G.) is a record of the electrical activity of the brain. It is abnormal in epilepsy, brain injury and if there is increased intracranial pressure.

'Brain-scanning' in **Radio-isotope Encephalography** a trace of radioactive isotope such as technetium is given i.v. Its concentration is measured in the different parts of the brain and is greater in tumours than in normal tissue. In **EMI scanning** (computerised tomography) a beam of x-rays, passed through the body, is interpreted by computer to provide image reconstruction.

Cerebral Arteriography. Radio-opaque material ('dye') is injected into the carotid or vertebral artery to make the cerebral vessels visible on X-ray. It demonstrates aneurysms or displacement of vessels by cerebral tumour.

DRUGS ACTING ON THE NERVOUS SYSTEM

Drugs used for specific diseases (epilepsy, Parkinsonism) are described under the disease concerned. Antiemetics are listed in Chapter 8.

Hypnotics, Sedatives and Tranquillisers

Hypnotics are drugs which aid sleep by sedation. Sedatives and tranquillisers relieve anxiety and restlessness. The same drugs are hypnotics with large doses, sedatives with medium doses, and tranquillisers with small doses, although theoretically tranquillisers allay anxiety without altering alertness and should not cause sleepiness.

Barbiturates. Amylobarbitone (Amytal), butobarbitone (Soneryl), pentobarbitone (Nembutal), quinalbarbitone (Seconal), phenobarbitone. Hypnotic dose: 100–200 mg orally o.n.; tranquillising dose 30–60 mg orally t.d.s. (phenobarbitone) or 50 mg t.d.s. (amylobarbitone). Side-effects: tolerance (a higher dose being required for the drug to be effective), habituation, stimulation of liver enzymes so that the barbiturates and other drugs are metabolised more rapidly, 'hangover', depression.

Chloral Hydrate 1 g in 50 ml water orally o.n. Side-effects: unpleasant taste, gastric irritation. Dichloralphenazone (Welldorm) (0·6 to 2 g) and triclofos (1 to 1·5 g) are similar.

Paraldehyde 5–10 ml i.m. is rarely used as an hypnotic but is useful in status epilepticus, delirium or mania. Side-effects: offensive odour, irritant. Inflammable.

Benzodiazepines. Nitrazepam (Mogadon), hypnotic dose 2·5–10 mg orally o.n., does not cause a 'hangover'. Side-effects: nausea, rash, respiratory depression. Benzodiazepines used as tranquillisers include: Chlordiazepoxide (Librium, Tropium) 5 mg b.d. to 25 mg q.i.d. orally, diazepam (Valium) 2–10 mg t.d.s. orally (or 2–10 mg i.m. as hypnotic), medazepam (Nobrium), oxazepam (Serenid-D). Side-effects: rash, dizziness.

Phenothiazines. Chlorpromazine (Largactil) 25–100 mg orally. Up to 800 mg daily is used in psychiatric states. Promazine (Sparine) 50–800 mg daily; perphenazine (Fentazin) 2–8 mg single dose as antiemetic, or t.d.s. in psychiatric states, prochlorperazine (Stemetil), trifluoperazine (Stelazine). Side-effects: drowsiness, hypotension, hypothermia, Parkinsonism (including oculogyric crises), jaundice, rash. They should not be given with tricyclic antidepressants since they have opposing actions.

Others. Glutethimide (Doriden) 250–500 mg orally o.n., meprobamate (Miltown) 400 mg orally o.n.

Antidepressives
Tricyclic Drugs take two to three weeks to become effective, and three to 12 months' treatment before spontaneous remission occurs. Side-effects: sedation, hypotension (causing dizziness), anticholinergic action (dry mouth, urinary retention, glaucoma, constipation). They neutralise the antihypertensive action of guanethidine, bethanidine and clonidine. Imipramine (Tofranil), amitriptyline (Tryptizol, Limbitrol), and nortriptyline (Allegron, Aventyl). Dose: 25 mg t.d.s. orally increasing by 25 mg each week to 75 mg t.d.s. (10–30 mg t.d.s. in the elderly). If there is anxiety or agitation a benzothiadiazine (but not a barbiturate) hypnotic or tranquilliser may be added. Protriptyline (Concordin) 5–20 mg t.d.s. orally. Doxepin (Sinequan) also has a tranquillising action. Dose: 10–25 mg b.d. or t.d.s. plus 20–50 mg o.n. as an hypnotic. Maprotiline (Ludiomil) 25–150 mg daily.

Monoamine Oxidase Inhibitors (M.A.O.I.) inhibit the enzyme monoamine oxidase (which destroys monoamines such as noradrenaline) and allows the concentration of monoamines, which are cerebral stimulants, to build up, taking two to three weeks to become effective.

Phenelzine (Nardil) 15 mg t.d.s. orally, iproniazid (Marsilid), nialamide (Niamid), tranylcypromine (Parnate), isocarboxazid (Marplan). Side-effects: interaction with many foods which contain amines (cheese, Marmite, wines and beers), with drugs (amphetamines, ephedrine, fenfluramine), causing hypertension, headache, and sometimes cerebral haemorrhage, and with tricyclic antidepressants and pethidine. The action persists for 10 days after stopping the M.A.O.I.

Cholinergics

These increase the action of acetylcholine, usually by inhibiting cholinesterase, the enzyme which destroys acetylcholine. They therefore increase sweating, salivary and gastric secretions, urinary and gastro-intestinal tract motility; slow the heart-rate and constrict the pupils. These effects are antagonised by atropine. Neostigmine methylsulphate (Prostigmin) 0·5–2 mg s.c., or i.m., or neostigmine bromide 15 mg orally. Pyridostigmine (Mestinon) 60–240 mg orally is less powerful but longer-acting. Carbachol 250–500 μg s.c.

Analgesics

These are drugs which relieve pain:

Opium Derivatives (these are controlled drugs, *see* Chapter 19).

Morphine 10–20 mg s.c., i.m., or i.v. is analgesic and sedative. Side-effects: vomiting, respiratory depression (therefore it is not used in emphysema or asthma), spasm of smooth muscle (therefore not used in colic), addiction. It is used in coronary thrombosis, terminal illness, and after operation or injury.

Heroin (diamorphine) 5–10 mg s.c. or i.m. Similar action to morphine but causes less nausea, vomiting and constipation.

Pethidine (Demerol) 25–100 mg s.c. or i.m., 25–50 mg i.v., 50–100 mg orally. Side-effects: vomiting, respiratory depression, fall in blood pressure causing dizziness and sweating.

Methadone (Physeptone) 5–10 mg s.c. or orally. Side-effects: dry mouth, dizziness, sweating.

Papaveretum (Omnopon) is a mixture of morphine alkaloids. Dose: 10–20 mg oral or s.c.

Pentazocine (Fortral) 30–60 mg i.m. or i.v., 25–100 mg orally four-hourly. Side-effects: nausea, hallucinations, dependency, respiratory depression.

Dihydrocodeine (DF 118, Paracodin) 30–60 mg orally. Side-effects: constipation.

Codeine Phosphate, 10–60 mg orally, is the weakest opium derivative. It is an analgesic and is also used to suppress cough and diarrhoea. Side-effects: constipation.

Codeine Compound is a mixture of codeine phosphate, aspirin and phenacetin.

Other Analgesics

Aspirin 0·3–1 g up to four times daily orally is analgesic, antipyretic and anti-inflammatory. Side-effects: peptic ulceration, haematemesis (therefore it should not be used with anticoagulants). It is unsatisfactory in cardiac, urinary tract, or gastro-intestinal pain.

Soluble Aspirin: as for aspirin, but is less likely to cause haematemesis.

Sodium Salicylate Mixture (0·5 g in 10 ml) or strong mixture (1 g in 10 ml). Dose: 5 to 10 ml orally, up to four times daily. Actions similar to aspirin.

Paracetamol (Panadol) 0·5–1 g orally up to four times daily. Side-effects: overdose is toxic to the liver.

Phenylbutazone (Butazolidine) 100 mg b.d. to q.i.d. orally. Side-effects: rash, peptic ulceration, nausea, oedema, agranulocytosis, thrombocytopenia.

Phenacetin is toxic to the kidney.

NOTE: Sometimes non-analgesic drugs are more suitable than analgesics for pain; thus trinitrin relieves angina pectoris, antispasmodics relieve ureteric or biliary colic.

SYMPTOMS, SIGNS AND DISEASES OF THE NERVOUS SYSTEM

Headache
The extracranial tissues and intracranial blood vessels and dura are sensitive to pain but the brain is not.

Causes:
1   Anxiety. Headache is due to tension in the muscles of the scalp and neck.
2   Dilatation of intracranial or extracranial blood vessels. This may be due to general infection (typhoid, influenza), pyelonephritis, anaemia, high altitude, migraine, severe hypertension, vasodilator toxins and drugs such as trinitrin, nitrate in food e.g. 'hot-dog' headache, tyramine in chocolate and cheese, glutamate ('Chinese-restaurant' syndrome), and lead-poisoning. Headache follows an epileptic attack. Vascular headache is throbbing, and worse on moving the head or stooping.
3   Inflammation of the meninges, e.g. by infection (meningitis), blood (subarachnoid haemorrhage), or air (pneumoencephalography).
4   Cranial arteritis (inflammation of cranial arteries). The temporal artery is inflamed and tender.
5   Traction on intracranial structures such as vessels and dura, e.g. by increased intracranial pressure from cerebral oedema (head injury), abscess or tumour. Worse on change of position, non-throbbing.
6   Referred pain from diseases of the nose (sinusitis), teeth (caries), eye

(glaucoma, iritis, ciliary spasm caused by a refractive error), ear (otitis media), temporo-mandibular joint (arthritis) or cervical spine (spondylosis).

7 Psychogenic. Hysteria.

Treatment:

1 Of the cause, e.g. prednisolone for cranial arteritis.

2 Analgesic such as aspirin 600 mg or paracetamol 500 mg. Morphia and pethidine should be avoided owing to the possibility of addiction.

3 Tranquilliser for muscle tension headache, e.g. chlordiazepoxide (Librium) 10–30 mg t.d.s. or phenobarbitone 30 mg t.d.s.

Migraine. This is periodic unilateral headache associated with visual disturbance and vomiting.

Cause: the predisposition to migraine is inherited, probably as a defect in catecholamine metabolism, thus there is often a family history of headaches or 'biliousness'. Attacks are due to changes in the walls of cranial arteries and are precipitated by emotional stress and by pressor amines such as tyramine (in cheese and chocolate).

Clinically: the patient is typically conscientious, obsessional and tense. Attacks begin in young adulthood and become less common after middle age. An attack often begins with a visual aura such as wavy lines or defects in the visual fields (scotomata) lasting a few minutes and are due to cerebral or retinal ischaemia. This is followed by a throbbing headache lasting several hours, photophobia, sweating and vomiting. Fluid retention is common during an attack, ending in a diuresis.

Treatment: avoid precipitating factors. Rest in a quiet dark room. Cold compresses to the head. Analgesic such as aspirin 0·6–1 g orally. Prophylactic or therapeutic sedation with phenobarbitone 30 mg t.d.s. or prochlorperazine (Stemetil) 5–15 mg t.d.s orally. Ergotamine tartrate (a vasoconstrictor) 0·5 mg s.c. or i.m. or as an aerosol used early in an attack, repeated in one hour if necessary. Side-effects: gangrene of fingers or toes, abortion. Avoid in pregnancy and arteriosclerosis. Methysergide (Deseril) a serotonin antagonist, 2 mg t.d.s. orally. Side-effects: retroperitoneal and pleuropulmonary fibrosis, and peripheral vascular constriction. These are prevented by giving the drug for three months then omitting it for one month.

Vertigo

Vertigo is a feeling of rotation or swaying, with loss of balance, and is not simple light-headedness. It is caused by motion sickness, glaucoma, disorders of the middle and inner ears, Menière's disease, toxins such as salicylates, alcohol, nicotine and streptomycin, cerebral tumours and head injury.

Menière's Disease. This is progressive unilateral deafness with recurrent sudden attacks, lasting minutes or hours, of vertigo, tinnitus, nausea and vomiting, and the patient may fall.

Treatment: sedation, e.g phenobarbitone 200 mg i.m., antiemetic, diuretic. The patient should lie still. Surgical or ultrasonic destruction of the labyrinth or division of the vestibular branch of the eighth nerve for severe disease.

Cerebral Compression

This is compression of the brain due to increased pressure within the rigid skull caused by cerebral oedema, as in head injury, and by cerebral haemorrhage, tumour or abscess. It causes headache followed by vomiting, a slow pulse, rising blood pressure, coma and stertorous breathing.

Insomnia (Sleeplessness)

Adequate sleep is necessary for health. Insomnia is due to psychological upset such as depression, anxiety or excitement, to physical disorder such as pain or discomfort due to injury, inflammation, dyspnoea, pruritus (itching), frequency of micturition, gastro-intestinal or cardiac disorders, or excessive external stimulation such as noise or light. Insomnia causes irritability and impaired concentration.

Treatment: the bedroom must be quiet, dark, warm and well ventilated, the bedclothes warm but light and the patient comfortable. A hot bath, warm milky drink or a little carbohydrate food helps. Tea and coffee contain caffeine, a stimulant, and should be avoided. Alcohol is not advisable. The cause should be treated, e.g. linctus codeine for a cough, antacid for peptic ulcer pain, analgesics for other types of pain. Hypnotics aid sleep but may lead to habituation or addiction and are not analgesic.

Delirium

Delirium is temporary acute mental disturbance with confusion, tremor, restlessness, insomnia, disorientation, impaired memory, hallucinations and a feeling of fear. The patient may be dirty, abusive and violent.

Causes: infections (typhoid, smallpox, pneumonia, encephalitis), drugs (alcohol, cannabis), injury to the brain, cerebral hypoxia (cardiac failure, pneumonia), mania, or toxins from hepatic or renal failure.

Treatment is of the cause, e.g. tepid sponging for pyrexia, oxygen for cyanosis; prevention of injury to the patient and others using mechanical restraint until sedatives have become effective. Vitamin B i.m. for delirium tremens.

Involuntary Movements

Tremor. Causes include Parkinsonism, multiple sclerosis, thyrotoxicosis, chronic alcoholism, and familial tremor.

Choreiform Movements are jerky and without purpose although they give the impression of interrupted purpose.

Athetosis is a slow writhing.

Agnosia (no knowledge)

Agnosia is inability to recognise the meaning of sensory perceptions, e.g. inability to recognise a known object despite normal sensation.

Apraxia (inaction)
Apraxia is loss of the ability to perform a movement although the patient understands its purpose and has normal sensation and musculature.

Aphasia (no speech) and **Dysphasia** (hard speech).

Motor Dysphasia: the patient knows what he wishes to say and forms the correct sentences in thought, but cannot speak them although the muscles of speech are normal. It is due to abnormality of the lower frontal convolution.

Sensory Dysphasia is impaired understanding of spoken language.

Dysarthria is faulty articulation of speech due to inco-ordination of the lips, tongue and palate, a cleft palate, or upper or lower motor neuron lesions.

Dyslexia is loss of the ability to read.

Dysphonia
Dysphonia is a reduced volume of speech due to weak respiratory movements caused by lesions of the brain (e.g. Parkinsonism), peripheral nerves, or respiratory muscles.

Tinnitus
Tinnitus (noises in the ear) may be due to drugs (quinine, salicylates), diseases of the ear (otitis media), or tumour (neuroma) of the eighth nerve.

Ataxia
Ataxia is inco-ordination of muscular movement. For accurate movement muscles must be co-ordinated with each other. From sensory endings in the muscles and joints sensory impulses (proprioception) inform the brain of the position and tension of each muscle. The brain decides what movements are required and sends impulses down the pyramidal and extrapyramidal nerves to the muscles. The cerebellum provides fine co-ordination of these movements. Ataxia may be due to faulty proprioception (sensory ataxia) or to cerebellar disease (motor ataxia). It occurs in alcoholic intoxication.

Tabes Dorsalis (locomotor ataxia) is a chronic degeneration of sensory nerve roots and posterior columns of the spinal cord due to syphilis.

Friedreich's Ataxia is an hereditary degeneration of the nervous system with ataxia, fits, optic atrophy, sphincter disturbances, club foot and kyphoscoliosis.

Spasm
A spasm is an involuntary contraction of a muscle. Tonic spasm is a continuous spasm due to, e.g. tetanus, strychnine or the onset of an epileptic fit. Clonic spasms are repeated contractions and relaxations of muscles, as seen in epilepsy after the tonic phase. Habit spasm (tic) is psychological in origin and is a repeated peculiar movement, e.g. grimacing.

Muscular Weakness

Weakness may be due to paralysis caused by a disorder of nerves, either upper or lower motor neuron; abnormality at the neuromuscular junction as in myasthenia gravis; disorders of the muscle, e.g. muscular dystrophy; or to general causes such as hypokalaemia or hypoglycaemia.

Paralysis

Paralysis is loss of movement; paresis is partial paralysis. Paralysis may affect one limb (monoplegia), one side of the body (hemiplegia), both legs (paraplegia), a single cranial nerve as in facial palsy, several cranial nerves as in bulbar palsy, or may take various other forms.

Paralysis may be spastic or flaccid. Spastic paralysis is due to damage to upper motor neurons in the brain or pyramidal tracts. The muscles are rigid due to increased tone, the tendon reflexes are increased (brisk), the abdominal reflexes are absent, the plantar response is extensor (the great toe turns upwards and the toes fan out on stroking the sole of the foot), and clonus (a repeated jerking movement) is present on passive dorsiflexion of the foot, due to the brisk tendon reflexes (*Fig. 13.16a*).

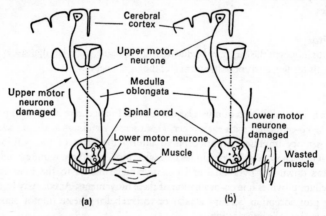

FIG. 13.16   (a) Upper motor neuron lesion: spastic paralysis, no muscular wasting; (b) lower motor neuron lesion: flaccid paralysis, muscular wasting

Flaccid paralysis is due to damage to lower motor neurons, either in the anterior horns of the spinal cord, as in poliomyelitis, or in the peripheral nerves, as in peripheral neuritis. The tendon reflexes are diminished or absent; the plantar response is flexor (normal, i.e. the great toe turns downwards on stroking the sole of the foot) or absent; and the muscles have a poor tone and are soft and limp (*Fig. 13.16b*).

Hemiplegia

Hemiplegia is paralysis of one side of the body. It may be caused by:

1   A stroke (cerebrovascular accident).

2 An intracranial space-occupying lesion such as tumour, abscess or subdural haematoma.
3 Head injury damaging one side of the brain.
4 Multiple sclerosis.
5 Temporary (Todd's) paralysis following an epileptic attack.

A Stroke is an abrupt loss of function of part of the nervous system due to a vascular lesion. Brain cells die if their blood supply is lost for four minutes or longer. The dead (infarcted) area of brain may become scar tissue or a cyst. A stroke is caused by cerebral thrombosis, embolism or haemorrhage and is predisposed by anaemia or hypotension (dehydration, shock).

Thrombosis is obstruction of a blood vessel by clotting, usually on a plaque of atheroma, in a cerebral, carotid or vertebrobasilar artery. Polycythaemia and the contraceptive pill predispose to thrombosis. Loss of the blood supply through one artery can be partly compensated by a supply from the other arteries joining the circle of Willis.

Clinically: symptoms depend upon the size of the clot and the portion of brain affected, and vary from a transient weakness of a limb to coma with hemiplegia. The onset is over hours or days. Paralysis affects the opposite side of the body and is flaccid (limp) at first but soon becomes spastic with hypertonic muscles, brisk tendon reflexes, clonus, extensor plantar response and loss of abdominal reflexes. The paralysed cheek blows out on expiration. There is dysphasia or aphasia if the dominant hemisphere is affected (the left in a right-handed person), sensory loss (hemianaesthesia) on the paralysed side and there may be blindness (hemianopia) on the same side as the thrombosis.

The carotid artery supplies blood to the frontal lobe and parts of the parietal and temporal lobes, its obstruction therefore causes forgetfulness, defective judgement, confusion, blindness (hemianopia) on the same side, dysphasia, and paralysis of the opposite side. The patient may lose intellect and become selfish, paranoid and emotionally labile.

The vertebrobasilar arteries supply the medulla oblongata, pons, midbrain, cerebellum and occipital lobes. Their obstruction causes giddiness, dysarthria, ataxia (cerebellar), and hemiparesis (pyramidal tracts damaged) and occasionally blindness.

Drop attacks: the patient drops to the ground, without loss of consciousness, for a few minutes. Attacks are due to kinking of the vertebral arteries and sudden loss of posture sense. The patient should not wear tight collars and should avoid excessive movement of the head.

Investigations: a blood count detects anaemia or polycythaemia. Lumbar puncture may show bloodstained C.S.F. in cerebral haemorrhage. Carotid or vertebral arteriography shows the site of narrowing or obstruction. Thermography shows a cold area on the forehead on the same side as an internal carotid arterial obstruction. Echoencephalography within 24 hours shows displacement of midline structures in haemorrhage (or infarct oedema after 24 hours).

Cerebral Embolism is obstruction of a cerebral artery with a fragment of blood clot which has detached from thrombus on the inner wall of the heart (as in atrial fibrillation, atrial myxoma, mitral stenosis or myocardial infarction), from a detached vegetation in bacterial endocarditis, from clot on a patch of atheroma in the aorta or carotid artery (*Fig. 6.39*), or obstruction by a septic embolism from pulmonary suppuration. The onset is sudden, otherwise symptoms are as for thrombosis. **Cerebral Haemorrhage** (apoplexy) is haemorrhage into the brain from a ruptured cerebral artery or a bleeding tumour. A lenticulostriate artery ruptures into the internal capsule. Haemorrhage is predisposed by hypertension (commonly), or by a blood-clotting defect caused by leukaemia, thrombocytopenia or anticoagulants. The rupture of an aneurysm, which usually causes subarachnoid haemorrhage, sometimes occurs into the brain and causes intracerebral haemorrhage.

Clinically: there is a rapid onset of headache, vomiting and loss of consciousness. The pulse is slow, breathing is stertorous (snoring) or Cheyne–Stokes, and the face is congested. At first the face and eyes deviate to the side of the lesion; later they deviate to the opposite, paralysed, side. Paralysis is flaccid at first, with low muscular tone and absent reflexes, but the plantar response is extensor. Spasticity appears after cerebral shock wears off. The pupils may be unequal. Neck stiffness occurs if blood breaches the subarachnoid space and irritates the meninges. In pontine haemorrhage the pupils are pinpoint and pyrexia is common, e.g. 40°C, owing to damage to the temperature-regulating centre.

Treatment of a Stroke is in three phases: preservation of life and prevention of complications, rehabilitation as soon as recovery begins, and teaching the patient and his relatives how to manage at home.

Care of the Comatose Patient

Preservation of life and prevention of complications: rest in bed, preferably in the room where the stroke occurred, until shock wears off. Side-rails if confused. The greater the depth of coma the greater are the losses of protective reflexes such as coughing and swallowing; in order to keep the airway clear the patient should lie prone, or on the side and slightly prone, with the face clear of pillows so that gravity prevents the tongue from falling backwards and prevents the inhalation of vomit, and not supine (on the back facing upwards). A pharyngeal airway may be used. Saliva and mucus are cleared from the cheek and pharynx by suction. Oxygen is given for cyanosis. Raising the foot of the bed aids the drainage of secretions but tends to increase the venous pressure in the head. Sandbags or frames are used for correct limb position.

Tepid sponging for hyperpyrexia; otherwise the patient should be kept warm with blankets, since heat is rapidly lost from the unconscious patient owing to impairment of the vasomotor and shivering reflexes; however, the application of heat, e.g. hot-water bottles, is avoided because it may cause serious burns. The temperature, pulse rate, respirations, blood pressure, pupillary size and equality, the colour of the patient, and the grade of consciousness are recorded at intervals varying from 15 minutes to 4 hours. The fluid intake and output are also recorded.

Dehydration is prevented by giving 2·5 l of fluid daily via a nasogastric tube (eggs, milk, sugar, soya-bean oil and minerals) or 5% glucose 2 l plus saline 0·5–1 l every 24 hours i.v. if in coma, or feed by mouth using a spoon feeder or drinking straw when conscious—the first drink being given with great caution if difficulty in swallowing is suspected. The conscious patient with motor aphasia should be spoken to normally, not loudly or in babytalk, since he can usually understand although he cannot speak, and should be offered a urinal and bedpan regularly in order to avoid 'incontinence'.

Care of the Skin, Bladder and Bowels: paralysed patients are very liable to develop bedsores since they are unable to move away from damaging stimuli. To prevent pressure sores a 'ripple'-mattress is used, the distribution of pressure of different sections being varied by alternate inflation and deflation by an automatic pump. The undersheet should be free from wrinkles, crumbs or other objects which cause local pressure on the skin and lead to ischaemic necrosis. The patient's position is changed every two hours, and at the same time the pressure points are washed with soap and water or treated with spirit, massaged, and fine talc or silicone cream or spray applied. Sheepskin elbow- and heel-pads may be used. The bladder is watched for distension, and catheterised if necessary. The catheter should not be trapped beneath the leg where it predisposes to pressure sores and leakage. Constipation is treated with enemata (or aperients when conscious), or digital removal of scybala if necessary. If incontinence is present scrupulous cleanliness is essential in preventing ulceration of the skin; the buttocks and thighs being washed each time incontinence occurs. An indwelling catheter may be used.

Drugs should be used with caution and hypnotics avoided if possible since they may cause confusion and predispose to incontinence (during deep sleep) and pneumonitis.

Antibiotic for infection, but not prophylactically. Respiratory infection should be watched for, and treated according to the sensitivity of the organisms isolated from bronchial aspirate. Antibiotic cannot be mixed with intralipid.

Anticoagulants are given for six months in embolism to prevent further clotting and embolism, but are contra-indicated both in haemorrhage, which would be made worse, and in cerebral thrombosis, owing to the possibility of causing haemorrhage into the infarcted brain.

Diazepam 10 mg o.n. for muscle spasm. Phenytoin for muscle twitching ('latent epilepsy').

Rehabilitation: all joints should be put through their full range of movement three or more times daily; passively in paralysed limbs, actively in unparalysed limbs. The aim is to maintain full function of all joints and power in all muscles, especially those of locomotion, and to prevent muscular contractures (shortening). A Balkan beam or Guthrie–Smith frame may be used to suspend and extend affected limbs, or a bed-cradle used to take the weight of the bedclothes off paralysed feet.

The patient is propped up within 48 hours of regaining consciousness; is taught how to turn in bed and how to sit up; and gets out of bed as soon as he can support himself in a chair. A patient kept in bed becomes apathetic, curls up and develops muscular wasting and contractures. Exercises are performed in rising from sitting to standing, walking with nursing help, then with mechanical aids (tripod, sticks, toe-spring or below-knee caliper). Correctly fitting shoes should be worn, not slippers.

Skilled movements are redeveloped by occupational therapy. If the dominant hemisphere is involved the patient should learn to write with the other hand and should have speech therapy.

Frustration and depression are common and need sympathetic reassurance.

Teaching and advice to the patient and his relatives on how to manage at home begins in hospital and is continued by the relatives, district nurse, health visitor and social worker. The patient may need a non-slip mat in the bath, handrails to the bath or lavatory, a pulley over the bed, a special chair, walking aids, or incontinence bags or pads. Rubber mats to stop plates from slipping. If there is intellectual loss, activities requiring good judgement are prohibited.

Other Treatment: endarterectomy (removal of clot and atheroma) or anticoagulants for carotid thrombosis of slow onset.

Prevention: treatment of hypertension and sources of emboli, avoidance of excessive physical strain in hypertension.

Prognosis: atheroma is slowly progressive. Embolism is rarely fatal and some improvement is likely. Haemorrhage is commonly fatal within a few hours, but if the patient survives some function returns over days or weeks. Recovery begins in the face, then the leg and finally the arm. Fine movements of the hand return last or not at all.

Vascular and Ischaemic Diseases of the Brain

Causes:

1 A stroke is due to atheroma, thrombosis, embolism or haemorrhage and has been described above.
2 Severe anaemia.
3 Hypotension, e.g. shock due to myocardial infarction or haemorrhage.
4 Venous sinus thrombosis.
5 Intracranial haemorrhage: (*a*) meningeal—extradural, subdural, subarachnoid; (*b*) intracerebral.

Venous Sinus Thrombosis is the clotting of blood in the venous sinuses within the skull.

Causes:

1 Malnutrition and dehydration; cachectic children, adults with cancer.
2 Septic embolism via the vertebral veins from pelvic venous sepsis after childbirth.
3 Infection spreading from otitis media, nasal sinusitis, osteomyelitis of the skull, infections of the scalp and face.

Clinically: there is swinging pyrexia, tachycardia, sweating, headache, vomiting, rigors, confusion, coma and death. In addition, fits, hemiplegia and epistaxis in superior longitudinal sinus thrombosis; exophthalmos (protrusion of the eyes), swelling of the eyelids, pain behind the eyes, papilloedema and retinal haemorrhages in cavernous sinus thrombosis; pain, tenderness and swelling in the mastoid region and thrombosis extending into the internal jugular vein in sigmoid sinus thrombosis.

Complications: cerebral abscess; hydrocephalus.

Treatment: antibiotic; anticoagulant or surgical removal of the thrombus.

Extradural Haematoma (*Fig. 13.17*) is bleeding between the skull and the dura mater due to rupture of the middle meningeal artery caused by a fracture of the skull. The pupil on the same side dilates. The patient rapidly loses consciousness and dies if untreated. Treatment is surgical.

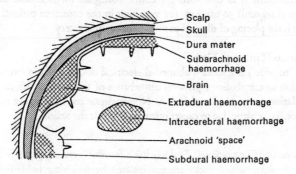

Scalp
Skull
Dura mater
Subarachnoid haemorrhage
Brain
Extradural haemorrhage
Intracerebral haemorrhage
Arachnoid 'space'
Subdural haemorrhage

FIG. 13.17   Sites of intracranial haemorrhage

Subdural Haematoma (*Fig. 13.17*) is a blood clot, beneath the dura, caused by bleeding from veins and capillaries following a blow on the head. The patient may appear to recover from the blow as bleeding ceases (lucid interval) but over several days the intracranial pressure increases, because the haematoma absorbs fluid by osmosis, and causes headache, vomiting, drowsiness, coma, fits and paralysis of the opposite side of the body.

Investigations: carotid angiography. Ventriculography.

Treatment: surgical removal of the haematoma.

Subarachnoid Haemorrhage is bleeding into the subarachnoid space. It is commonly due to a ruptured berry aneurysm on the circle of Willis or on a cerebral artery, but may be due to a ruptured arteriovenous abnormality, 'mycotic' aneurysm or atheroma. An aneurysm is a swelling of an artery. A berry aneurysm is a small berry-like projection from an artery due to a congenital weakness in the wall. A 'mycotic' aneurysm is due to an infected embolus from, e.g. infective endocarditis.

Clinically: there may be previous signs of pressure on cranial nerves due to an aneurysm, e.g. diplopia, squint. Rupture of the aneurysm causes increased intra-cranial pressure with sudden severe headache, confusion, restlessness, irritability, vomiting, photophobia (dislike of light), papilloedema, slow pulse, bilateral extensor plantar responses and Cheyne–Stokes breathing. Meningeal irritation by blood causes neck stiffness and Kernig's sign (spasm of the hamstring muscles on extending the leg at the knee with the thigh flexed to a right angle). 33% of patients die within three days. Those recovering are liable to bleed again within a few weeks.

Investigations: lumbar puncture reveals evenly bloodstained C.S.F., and xanthochromia (yellow colouration due to altered blood) appears after six hours. Carotid angiography shows the abnormality.

Treatment: the patient is nursed in a quiet, darkened room; in bed for four to six weeks. Treatment is as described for coma. Analgesic for headache and chlorpromazine (Largactil) 50 mg i.m. for vomiting in the conscious patient. Surgical treatment is the placing of silver clips on the aneurysmal artery.

Convulsions (Epilepsy, Fits)

Epilepsy ('to seize') is a sudden abnormal electrical discharge from over-excitable neurons due to metabolic or physical disturbance of the brain. It affects 0·5% of the population in the U.K. and U.S.A. Non-epileptic convulsions are attacks due to a neuronal discharge due to causes primarily outside the brain.

Causes:

    A *Idiopathic (Constitutional) Epilepsy* has a familial (genetic) predisposition but the cause is unknown. Attacks are precipitated by flickering lights (television), emotion, alcohol and relaxation. The first fit usually occurs before the age of 30 years.

    B *Symptomatic (Secondary) Epilepsy* is caused by:

      1 Head injury, birth trauma (head injury, hypoxia, haemorrhage).

      2 Space-occupying lesion (brain tumour, abscess, haematoma, angioma, cyst).

      3 Inflammation (meningitis, cysticercosis, encephalitis, syphilis, i.e. general paralysis of the insane).

      4 Acute cerebral oedema due to acute glomerulonephritis, Henoch–Schönlein syndrome.

      5 Malignant hypertension.

    C *Non-epileptic Convulsions:*

      1 Cerebral hypoxia or ischaemia, e.g. atheroma, hypotension, Stokes-Adams syndrome (in heart block or ventricular asystole).

      2 Metabolic disorders such as hypoglycaemia, uraemia, alkalosis (e.g. hyperventilation), hypocalcaemia (as in newborn infants fed on cows' milk, the excessive phosphate intake lowering the serum calcium).

      3 Inborn errors of metabolism such as porphyria, phenylketonuria and lipidosis.

      4 Poisons, e.g. alcohol, lead, cocaine, i.v. lignocaine, i.v. penicillin, aminophylline.

      5 Eclampsia (toxaemia of pregnancy).

      6 Withdrawal of sedatives, e.g barbiturates in patients used to large doses.

      7 Fever in children under the age of three years.

Types depend on the site of origin of the abnormal discharge.

   A   *Generalised:* (1) grand mal; (2) myoclonic epilepsy; (3) petit mal.

   B   *Local (focal):* (1) Jacksonian; (2) psychomotor; (3) others, e.g. uncinate, cerebellar, myoclonic.

Observations in Epilepsy: note the patient's behaviour, whether disordered; the mode of onset of the attack, whether local or bilateral, gradual or sudden, the presence of fainting, the mode of spread, the presence of external injury, bitten tongue, or incontinence. History from a witness.

Grand Mal (major epilepsy) may begin with a brief **aura** (e.g. tingling, noises) followed by the **tonic** stage in which the patient loses consciousness and falls, and there is tonic spasm of all the muscles which forces air through the glottis producing a 'cry'. The jaws are closed, the pupils are dilated and breathing is arrested, causing cyanosis. The tonic stage lasts 20–30 seconds and is followed by the **clonic** phase which lasts half a minute. The face, body and limbs jerk, the jaw opens and closes and the tongue may be bitten. There is sweating due to the muscular exertion, saliva forms foam in the mouth, and urinary or faecal incontinence may occur. The patient relaxes, unconscious, for a few minutes, then passes into normal sleep. Prior to sleeping the patient may be confused and perform actions which he cannot later remember (post-epileptic automatism).

Investigations: chest and skull X-ray, electroencephalogram, cerebrospinal fluid, blood Wassermann reaction, carotid angiogram, brain-scanning.

Treatment: protect from injury: if possible, catch the patient before he falls, lay him on the ground, remove spectacles and dentures, place a padded wedge between the teeth (without force) to prevent the tongue being bitten. Do not use restraint (except to prevent injury). Clear the airway: loosen the collar and tie, clear the mouth of saliva or vomitus. Change clothing and turn the patient on his side after an attack. Treat the cause; give glucose for hypoglycaemia, oxygen for persistent cyanosis; avoid alcohol; surgical excision of cerebral scars, drainage of abscesses, removal of tumours.

   Drugs are given to reduce the number of fits but may not prevent them all, and are not given for an isolated fit. They should be continued for three years after the last attack and then reduced gradually (if they are suddenly stopped, fits may recur). Phenobarbitone (Luminal) 30–120 mg orally t.d.s. Side-effects: sedation, rash. Primidone (Mysoline) 250 mg b.d. to 500 mg orally q.i.d. Side-effects: sedation, rash, confusion, nausea, ataxia. Carbamazepine (Tegretol) 100–300 mg t.d.s.

   Hydantoins: phenytoin (Epanutin, Dilantin) 50–200 mg orally t.d.s.; side-effects: gum hypertrophy, rash, reversible cerebellar inco-ordination (ataxia, dysarthria), headache, folate-deficient megaloblastic anaemia, lymphadenopathy; methoin (Mesantoin) 100 mg orally t.d.s.; ethotoin (weak action). Sulthiame (Ospolot) 100–600 mg orally daily.

   Social Aspects: explain the cause; i.e. 'an electrical upset', and that controlled epilepsy does not cause mental deficiency. Driving a vehicle and unaccompanied swimming, sailing, horse-riding or cycling in traffic are prohibited. Open fires must be heavily guarded. Bathe under observation. Education at an ordinary school unless attacks are frequent, when a special school is preferable. Employment out of danger to themselves and others, away from fire, water, heights, machinery and traffic. The patient should tell the employer of his epilepsy and both decide if any risk is to be taken. Suitable occupations include printing, book-binding, packing, store-keeping, clerical work or light assembly work. Marriage and parenthood; if both parents are epileptics there is an increased risk to the child. Parental epilepsy is not a legal indication for abortion.

Status Epilepticus is a succession of grand mal fits without recovery of consciousness between them. It causes anoxic cerebral damage. The patient should be under continuous observation to prevent injury or obstruction of the airway. The temperature is recorded hourly since the excessive muscular activity may cause fever.

Treatment: induce light anaesthesia with paraldehyde 10 ml i.m. then 5 ml every 30 minutes until fits stop, 50 ml paraldehyde in 500 ml isotonic saline by i.v. drip, sod. phenobarbitone 200 mg i.m. two-hourly, sod. amylobarbitone 500 mg i.v., or diazepam 10 mg i.v., repeat 20 mg in a few minutes if fits continue, then 5 mg hourly i.v. in a saline drip. Maintain a clear airway. Tepid sponging for hyperpyrexia, abundant fluids orally on recovery.

Myoclonic Epilepsy. Myoclonic jerks occur without loss of consciousness or with the brief loss of consciousness associated with petit mal. Treatment is with diazepam (Valium) 2–10 mg orally t.d.s. or nitrazepam (Mogadon) 5–15 mg orally daily.

Petit Mal ('Absences'). There is fleeting unconsciousness lasting five to 20 seconds, arrest of movement and loss of attention ('dazed') with amnesia. Seldom fall. It begins in childhood and often ends during adolescence. The E.E.G. shows three spikes and waves a second.

Treatment: troxidone (Tridione) 150–300 mg orally t.d.s. Side-effects: rash, photophobia, agranulocytosis, nephrotic syndrome. Give with phenytoin to prevent grand mal. Ethosuximide (Zarontin) 250–500 mg orally t.d.s. Side-effects: sedation, dizziness, rash, vomiting, photophobia. Phensuximide (Milontin) 250–1000 mg t.d.s. Methsuximide (Celontin) causes pancytopenia, and phenacemide (Phenurone) is hepatotoxic. Sodium valproate (Epilim) 200–600 mg t.d.s.

Akinetic Epilepsy (drop attacks). The patient falls unconscious but recovers immediately. Treat as for petit mal.

Jacksonian Epilepsy may be motor and/or sensory. Attacks begin at one point and spread slowly; e.g. twitching begins in the thumb and spreads to the fingers, hand and arm. Consciousness is not lost unless most of the brain becomes involved. Treatment is as for grand mal.

Psychomotor (Temporal Lobe) Epilepsy. Hallucinations occur and are commonly of smell, but may be visual, auditory (of hearing) or gustatory (of taste). Memory disturbance includes 'déjà vu' (the feeling of reliving an experience), dream states, and feelings of unreality. Treatment is as for grand mal, or with diazepam (Valium) 2–10 mg orally t.d.s., pheneturide (Benuride) 200 mg orally t.d.s., or carbamazepine (Tegretol) 100–300 mg orally t.d.s.

Narcolepsy
Narcolepsy consists of sudden short attacks of sleep from which the patient can be awakened as from normal sleep. Attacks may be prevented with amphetamine sulphate 10–50 mg orally b.d.

Cataplexy
Cataplexy is sudden muscular weakness, the patient falling to the ground fully conscious but unable to move or speak for several seconds. It is often due to sudden emotion.

Multiple (Disseminated) Sclerosis
Multiple sclerosis is a patchy demyelination in the nervous system, followed by gliosis (fibrosis). The cause is unknown but there is a genetic predisposition, probably to a specific virus infection.

Clinically: it begins in young adults. There are exacerbations lasting days or weeks and remissions of months or years. 60% of patients have no residual disability at five years; others recover partially and a few become severely paralysed, incontinent, and chair-borne and die of pneumonia or urinary infection. Symptoms depend on the situation of the plaques of demyelination and include depression, anxiety, euphoria (optimism) and transient diplopia. Acute retrobulbar neuritis is due to a plaque in the optic tract which causes blurred vision, pain, tenderness and a central scotoma in one eye. It recovers within six weeks. Involvement of corticospinal (motor) tracts causes spastic paralysis of one or more limbs, with weakness, stiffness, brisk tendon reflexes and extensor plantar response. It may cause paraplegia, in extension (lower limbs extended) at first, in flexion later. Painful flexor spasms may occur.

Sensory lesions include paraesthesiae (abnormal sense of touch, e.g. tingling), diminished proprioception and vibration sense, and numbness. Damage to the autonomic tracts in the spinal cord causes urinary retention, precipitancy or incontinence, and constipation or faecal incontinence. Cerebellar lesions produce nystagmus (a jerking movement of the eyes on lateral fixation), intention tremor (tremor absent at rest but appearing on voluntary movement), inco-ordination, ataxia and dysarthria (slurred syllables and staccato or scanning speech, i.e. slow deliberate speech with equal emphasis on each syllable). Dysarthria may be of the cortical spastic type.

Investigations: the C.S.F. may show a slightly increased protein (up to 100 mg%), an increased lymphocyte count (up to $50 \times 10^6/l$) and an abnormal gold curve due to increased globulin. X-ray the spine to exclude other causes for symptoms, e.g. paraplegia.

Treatment: rest in bed during an acute relapse. The patient should stay at work between attacks but avoid undue fatigue. Good nutrition, vitamins.

Psychotherapy; i.e. encourage morale with sympathy and a willingness to help the patient with his problems.

The patient should not be told the suspected diagnosis in the first attack since needless anxiety may be created even when recovery is complete; but the truth should be told if permanent disability develops.

General nursing care as for the paralysed patient (see 'Stroke'), with physiotherapy (massage, passive or active movements and re-educational exercises). Catheterisation for urinary retention, laxative for constipation. Skin care; change position two-hourly; bed-cradle. For pressure sores, remove dead tissue, clean with saline, antibiotic by mouth if infected, and relieve the area from pressure.

Drugs: symptomatic, to improve bladder and bowel function; e.g. ephedrine 15 mg or propantheline 15 mg t.d.s. orally for frequency or incontinence of urine, carbachol 250–500 µg s.c. for retention of urine. Antibiotic for urinary, skin or pulmonary infection. Corticotrophin may provide mild benefit; dose: 40 u i.m., b.d. for one week, then gradually reduce to zero over three weeks. For spasticity baclofen (Lioresal) 5 mg orally t.d.s. increasing by 5 mg daily until effective, but not more than 100 mg daily. Side-effects: sedation, nausea, hypotension, increased number of fits in epileptics.

Surgical for severe spasticity in flexion and painful reflex spasms; the lumbosacral motor nerve roots are blocked with intrathecal phenol or sectioned.

Parkinsonism

Parkinsonism is a syndrome comprising hypokinesia (impaired movement), rigidity and tremor due to deficiency of dopamine in the basal ganglia. Normally there is a balance between dopamine (inhibitory) and acetylcholine (stimulatory). Deficiency of dopamine leaves a relative excess of acetylcholine, hence spasticity.

Causes:

1 Paralysis agitans, the commonest type, is due to idiopathic degeneration of the substantia nigra which normally produces dopamine.
2 Damage to the brain by anoxia, as in cerebrovascular atheroma, carbon monoxide poisoning, and cardiac arrest.
3 Encephalitis lethargica, which follows encephalitis due to certain viruses which especially damage the basal ganglia.
4 Poisons such as mercury, manganese, and copper (Wilson's disease).
5 Drugs such as phenothiazines, e.g. chlorpromazine, benzodiazepines, reserpine, methyldopa.
6 Others: trauma (the 'punch-drunk' professional boxer), rarely cerebral tumour, syphilis.

Clinically: paralysis agitans affects patients over 50 years of age. Hypokinesia is shown by the immobile face, unblinking eyes, monotonous speech, shuffling small steps, difficulty in chewing and slow movements. The knees and elbows are flexed and the posture is stooping. There is no weakness but the muscles show 'cogwheel' and 'lead-pipe' rigidity; i.e. rigidity throughout the full range of movement, associated with tremor. Tremor is present at rest and disappears on voluntary movement. The fingers and thumb show a 'pill-rolling' movement. Depression is common but mental ability is retained in paralysis agitans and the unwary should not be misled by the mask-like face and slow movement. Intellectual loss is common in the other types of Parkinsonism. The patient may become bed-ridden and die of infection.

Treatment: treat the cause if possible, e.g. penicillamine 300 mg t.d.s. orally to excrete copper in Wilson's disease, discontinue phenothiazines.

Physiotherapy, regular exercise but avoid fatigue, speech therapy, maintenance of good nutrition and social interests.

Drugs: Levodopa is converted into dopamine in the brain. Dose: 250 mg orally daily initially, increasing by 250 mg every third day until effective (1–8 g daily). Side-effects: nausea, vomiting, insomnia, agitation, confusion, dizziness due to postural hypotension, involuntary movements. Smaller doses may be given with a dopa decarboxylase inhibitor, e.g. Carbidopa 200 mg daily.

Anticholinergic drugs: benzhexol (Artane, Pipanol) 2–10 mg t.d.s., benztropine (Cogentin) 0·5–2 mg t.d.s., orphenadrine (Disipal) 50–100 mg q.i.d. Side-effects: dry mouth, constipation, drowsiness, blurred vision.

Diphenhydramine (Benadryl, Histex), 25 mg b.d. to 50 mg q.i.d. orally.

Surgical: stereotactic destruction of the 'overactive' part of the basal ganglia.

Chorea

Chorea is involuntary movement due to extrapyramidal disorder.

Sydenham's Chorea (St. Vitus' Dance) is related to rheumatic fever. It affects highly-strung children aged five to 15 years. The child is nervous, fidgety, clumsy; drops things and grimaces. Irregular violent movements may occur. Movements are absent during sleep. Sensation is normal. Most recover in two to three months.

Treatment is as for rheumatic fever (Chapter 4) with rest in bed in quiet surroundings and in warm clothing since blankets will not remain in position. To prevent injury the bed is padded, and padded sides are used. Bony points such as wrists, elbows, and ankles are padded. Unbreakable feeding utensils are necessary. If swallowing is affected tube feeding is used. Soluble aspirin and a sedative, e.g. phenobarbitone, are given. During and after convalescence skilled muscular exercises are performed.

Huntington's Chorea is a degeneration of the basal ganglia and the cerebral cortex of Mendelian dominant inheritance. It begins after the age of 35 years with choreiform movements and dementia, slowly progressing until the patient becomes chairborne or dies of pneumonia within 20 years. There is no specific treatment but tetrabenazine or thiopropazate (Dartalan) may reduce the chorea. The irregular movements chafe the skin and cause bedsores, therefore skin care is important.

Kernicterus

Kernicterus is damage to the basal ganglia caused by neonatal jaundice as in prematurity and 'rhesus' babies. The liver of the premature baby is immature and cannot conjugate haemobilirubin to cholebilirubin for excretion in the bile, the blood bilirubin level rises and at 34 μmol/l (20 mg%) the basal ganglia, which stain yellow, are damaged. In the 'rhesus' baby (one cause of haemolytic disease of the newborn) maternal antibodies destroy the fetal rhesus-positive red cells, causing haemolytic jaundice.

Clinically: jaundice is followed by convulsions and coma or athetosis, deafness, spastic paralysis and mental deficiency.

Treatment is by early detection of haemolytic jaundice of the newborn and by exchange transfusion.

Prevention: anti-D globulin is given i.m. to Rh-negative women within 72 hours of the birth of a Rh-positive child.

Motor Neuron Disease

This is a degeneration of motor neurons, both upper and lower (*Fig. 13.16*), of unknown cause. Sensation is normal.

Clinically: symptoms begin at age 40–60. There are three main types according to the site of greatest damage. In **progressive muscular atrophy** lower motor neuron damage in the spinal cord predominates and the small muscles of the hands and feet are first affected, producing 'claw hand' and 'club foot'. In **amyotrophic lateral sclerosis** both lower and upper motor neurons are affected, causing a mixture of progressive muscular atrophy and spasticity. In **progressive bulbar palsy** the damage mostly affects the motor nuclei of the pons and medulla causing dysarthria and dysphagia and the danger of aspiration pneumonia. (In pseudobulbar palsy upper motor neurons to the cranial nerves are damaged; usually by cerebrovascular disease.)

The muscles are weak and waste. The patient dies within a few years.

Treatment is symptomatic, with sympathetic support and mechanical aids. There is no specific treatment.

Intracranial Neoplasm ('Tumour')

Types: primary neoplasms arise from brain tissue and include gliomas e.g. astrocytoma, medulloblastoma (malignant); pituitary tumours; ependymoma from the lining of the ventricles, and neurofibroma (benign) from the sheaths of cranial nerves. A meningioma (benign) arises from the meninges, is hard and erodes the skull.

Secondary metastases are from elsewhere in the body, e.g. lung, breast, stomach.

Clinically: increased intracranial pressure produces headache, which is worse on coughing and is due to stretching of vessels and the dura, vomiting, drowsiness, diplopia, mental changes such as apathy and loss of memory and intellect, and papilloedema (swelling of the optic disc) due to increased pressure in the veins draining the eye. A rapid rise in pressure increases the blood pressure and reduces the pulse rate.

Focal signs depend on the site and size of the tumour, e.g. ataxia if it is in the cerebellum, paralysis if affecting the motor tracts, or deafness from an acoustic (eighth nerve) neuroma.

Fits, often focal(Jacksonian) in type.

Similar signs are produced by cerebral abscess, encephalitis, and accelerated ('malignant') hypertension.

Investigations: radiograph of the skull to detect bony erosion or brain displacement. Electroencephalogram. Carotid or vertebral arteriogram. Air encephalogram. Ventriculogram. Brain-scanning using i.v. radioactive material which is taken up by tumours and detected from outside the skull. Ultrasonic scan. Lumbar puncture may be dangerous if there is increased intracranial pressure since sudden release of C.S.F. jams the medulla into the foramen magnum ('coning').

Treatment: surgical excision of a meningioma, neurofibroma or pituitary tumour. Radiotherapy for tumours deep in the brain. Decompression, i.e. remove a plate of bone from over the tumour. Dehydration to relieve pressure, e.g. 150 ml hypertonic (50%) magnesium sulphate p.r., up to 500 ml 50% sucrose i.v., or 40 g urea in 130 ml 10% dextrose i.v. Diuretic for cerebral oedema. Analgesic such as codeine phosphate (NOT morphine since it depresses the central nervous system). Antiemetic.

Cerebral Abscess

An abscess in the brain is commonly due to staphylococci, streptococci or pneumococci and is caused by spread from infection in the middle ear, frontal sinuses, scalp, jaw (dental sepsis) or a compound fracture of the skull.

Clinically: there are symptoms of the original lesion, of suppuration (malaise, fever, rigors, anorexia), of increased intracranial pressure (headache, vomiting, drowsiness, confusion, coma, slow pulse rate, papilloedema) and localising signs depending on the site of the abscess. In chronic cerebral abscess the temperature is normal.

Treatment: antibiotic, e.g. benzylpenicillin 1·2 g i.m. then 600 mg i.m. four-hourly. Surgical aspiration of pus through a burr hole made in the skull and the instillation of antibiotic.

Neurosyphilis

Syphilis of the nervous system may be any one, or any combination of: pupillary abnormalities, meningovascular syphilis (*see* 'Meninges'), general paralysis of the insane, and tabes dorsalis.

Pupillary Abnormalities. Argyll Robertson pupils are small, irregular and unequal pupils which do not react to light but react to convergence.

General Paralysis of the Insane (G.P.I., dementia paralytica) is a chronic syphilitic infection of the brain (encephalitis) which causes degeneration of neurons, cerebral atrophy and thickening of the meninges.

Clinically: symptoms appear five to 15 years after the primary infection and begin with dementia (deterioration of memory, reasoning and intellect), irresponsibility, and neglect of personal appearance. Delusions of grandeur (power or wealth, causing extravagance and euphoria), poverty or disease may develop. Spastic paralysis, with weakness and brisk reflexes, is due to bilateral upper motor neuron degeneration. Speech becomes slurred, lips and head tremble and fits may occur. If untreated the patient becomes bedridden and dies of status epilepticus or respiratory infection.

Investigations: blood W.R. is positive in most patients. C.S.F. contains an increase in cells and protein, the W.R. is positive and the gold curve paretic, i.e. 5554321100.

Treatment: benzylpenicillin 1·2 g im. daily for 20 days. This may produce a Herxheimer reaction (fever, headache, tachycardia and vasodilatation) within two hours, due to the release of Treponemal material into the circulation. The patient should be warned of this and kept in bed. C.S.F. is examined every six months for two years and repeat courses of penicillin given if necessary.

Tabes Dorsalis (Locomotor Ataxia) is a chronic progressive degeneration, first of the lumbosacral sensory (posterior) nerve roots, later of the posterior columns (sensory tracts) of the spinal cord.

Clinically: symptoms begin five to 30 years after the primary infection. The first symptoms are attacks of sharp shooting pains ('lightning pains') in the legs, around the body ('girdle pains') or in the viscera ('visceral crises'), usually the stomach, rectum (with tenesmus) and bladder, often with vomiting, thus resembling an abdominal emergency. Laryngeal crises cause stridor. Loss of sensation in the bladder produces retention of urine with dribbling overflow incontinence. Because of sensory loss the limbs feel heavy and numb. The patient cannot feel the position of the limbs (proprioceptive loss) and lifts his feet too high, slams them down, and walks with an ataxic gait with his feet widely apart. He has to rely on vision for knowledge of the position of his body and finds it difficult to get about at night. Trophic changes lead to ulcers of the big toe or the foot which may perforate to the bone. Sensory loss leads to arthritis of large joints which enlarge but are painless (Charcot's joints). Tendon reflexes are lost and the muscles are hypotonic. Bilateral ptosis (drooping of the eyelids) is typical.

Investigations: the blood W.R. is positive in 50%. C.S.F. contains an increase in cells and protein, the W.R. is positive and the gold curve 0123454321.

Treatment: penicillin 1·2 g i.m. daily for 20 days, repeated if necessary, using the C.S.F. as a guide. Analgesic for pain. Walking exercises for ataxia. Urinary antibiotic for cystitis.

Cerebral Palsy
Cerebral palsy is paralysis due to damage to the growing brain, either before, during or after birth.

Causes:
1   Genetic abnormalities affecting the brain.
2   Intra-uterine infection, e.g. German measles, hypoglycaemia, kernicterus, radiation.
3   Cerebral injury or hypoxia during birth.
4   Encephalitis or meningitis.

Clinically: newborn infants are pale, cyanosed or jaundiced, according to the cause, and may have difficulty in sucking or breathing. Spastic paralysis may affect one limb (monoplegia), both arms or both legs (cerebral diplegia), three limbs (triplegia) or all limbs (quadriplegia). Involuntary movements may be athetoid (slow, writhing), or choreic (jerky). Mental retardation and epilepsy are common.

Treatment: physiotherapy, speech therapy and education in a special school. Drugs to control epilepsy.

Injuries of the Brain

Injury of the brain varies from mild concussion to severe laceration and haemorrhage.

Concussion is sudden brief physiological paralysis of the function of the brain. On regaining consciousness the patient has a headache and is drowsy and confused, but recovers completely in minutes or hours.

Treatment: Rest. Analgesic for headache.

Amnesia is loss of memory. It may be retrograde, i.e. amnesia for events before the injury, or post-traumatic, i.e. for events between the injury and recovery of consciousness.

Post-concussional Syndrome occurs in neurotics and in malingerers when compensation for injury is pending and consists of headache, anxiety, difficulty in concentration and giddiness. The patient may have periods of hysterical or psychopathic amnesia and wander from home.

Contusion of the brain is bruising or oedema which damages some neurons. Unconsciousness is more prolonged than in concussion and focal damage is present.

Laceration of the brain causes confusion or coma and is usually fatal.

Compression of the brain is due to increased intracranial pressure caused by oedema of the brain, acute hydrocephalus due to obstruction to the flow of C.S.F. by blood clot, or to intracranial haemorrhage.

Post-traumatic Epilepsy occurs in 4% of brain injuries; usually within two years.

Post-traumatic Dementia occurs especially in the elderly and in boxers ('punch-drunk').

Congenital Malformations of the Nervous System

Anencephaly is absence of most of the brain. The infant dies at birth.

Microcephaly is an abnormally small brain. The child has a small cranium and mental deficiency.

Platybasia is a congenital flattening of the base of the skull.

Arnold-Chiari Malformation is the projection of the medulla and part of the cerebellum through the foramen magnum, often causing hydrocephalus and associated with meningocele.

Tuberous Sclerosis (Epiloia) is of dominant inheritance and consists of epilepsy, mental deficiency and tumours (fibromas) of the skin.

Spina Bifida is failure of closure of the vertebral arches in the fetus. The defect varies from mild to severe. In spina bifida occulta a bony defect is seen on X-ray of the spine, but no external defect is visible, except sometimes a small dimple in the skin over the defect. In severe spina bifida a meningocele or a meningomyelocele is present (*Fig. 13.18*). A meningocele is a dural sac containing C.S.F. The sac

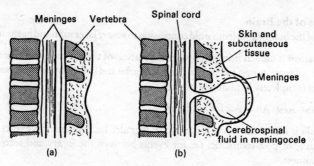

FIG. 13.18   (*a*) Spina bifida occulta; (*b*) meningocele

protrudes between the vertebrae and forms a soft bulge in the cervical or lumbar region. A meningomyelocele is a sac containing spinal cord which is liable to injury, thus there is deformity of the limbs, e.g. clubfoot, and often paraplegia and incontinence. The skin over the sac is likely to ulcerate and allow infection to enter and produce meningitis.

Treatment is surgical closure of the gap and the correction of deformities.

Coma
Loss of consciousness may be partial (drowsiness, stupor) or complete (coma).

Causes:

1 Damaged brain, e.g. head injury, intracranial haemorrhage.
2 Inflammation, e.g. brain abscess, meningitis, encephalitis (viral, malarial).
3 Reduced blood supply to the brain (ischaemia), e.g. fainting, Stokes–Adams attacks, cerebral thrombosis or embolism.
4 Intracranial tumour.
5 Epilepsy.
6 Electric shock.
7 Hypoxia, e.g. asphyxia.
8 Hypercapnia.
9 Poisoning, e.g. alcohol, carbon monoxide, anaesthetics, drugs (morphine, barbiturates).
10 Metabolic, e.g. diabetic acidosis, hypoglycaemia, uraemia (renal failure), liver failure.
11 Hypothermia.

Symptoms, Signs and Treatment are of the cause. The general treatment of coma is described under 'Stroke'.

Fainting (Syncope)

Fainting is sudden brief loss of consciousness due to inadequate cerebral blood flow due to a fall in the blood pressure. It is often not considered to be 'coma' since recovery rapidly occurs on falling (lying) down.

Causes:

1 A vasovagal attack (simple faint) is due to overactivity of the vagus nerve which slows the heart and allows blood to collect (pool) in the abdominal organs, leading to a fall in the blood pressure.

2 Postural hypotension is a fall in the blood pressure due to suddenly rising from the lying or sitting position, sympathectomy (when postural vascular reflexes are abolished), prolonged standing (when blood collects in the lower limbs), antihypertensive drugs, or pressure on the carotid sinus in the neck.

3 Pathological, due to haemorrhage, heart disease (myocardial infarction, arrhythmia), or disease of the autonomic nervous system.

Clinically: there is pallor, sweating, lightheadedness and brief loss of consciousness.

Treatment: rest lying down for a few minutes.

Syringomyelia

Syringomyelia is a cystic degeneration in the spinal cord which produces a dilated central canal. Syringobulbia is extension of the disease to the medulla oblongata.

Clinically: it begins before the age of 30 years and causes degeneration of adjacent anterior horn cells, resulting in wasting of the small muscles of the hand, and degeneration of tracts in the spinal cord, producing spastic paralysis of the legs. There is dissociated sensory loss, i.e. loss of pain and temperature sensation with retention of touch, vibration and position. Loss of protective pain sensation leads to burns and ulcers of the hands and to damaged painless (Charcot's) joints. The disease is slowly progressive.

Treatment: prevent injury.

Vitamin B$_{12}$ Deficiency Neuropathy (Subacute Combined Degeneration of the Spinal Cord)

This is a degeneration of the posterior and lateral columns of the spinal cord and peripheral neuropathy due to cobalamin (vitamin B$_{12}$) deficiency usually caused by a deficiency of the 'intrinsic factor' and is often associated with pernicious anaemia.

Clinically: bilateral numbness and paraesthesiae (tingling and burning sensations) in the feet and fingers, and loss of vibration sensation in the legs are followed by ataxia and spastic or flaccid weakness in the legs. Symptoms of anaemia are present if there is also pernicious anaemia.

Investigations: blood count to detect megaloblastic anaemia. Serum vitamin B_{12} is low. Gastric juice to detect achlorhydria.

Treatment: hydroxo-cobalamin (Neocytamen) 1 mg i.m. on alternate days in the first week then 1 mg i.m. weekly until recovery is occurring, then 250 µg i.m. monthly for life. Peripheral neuropathy recovers completely but myelopathy improves only slightly.

Encephalitis
Encephalitis is inflammation of the brain.

Causes include virus infection (measles, chickenpox, rabies, influenza) and measles vaccination.

Clinically: there is headache, pyrexia, restlessness and drowsiness, and fits may occur. The prognosis varies from complete recovery to permanent disability or death.

Treatment: analgesic for headache. Sedation for fits.

Hepatolenticular Degeneration (Wilson's Disease)
This is a rare hereditary disorder in which an excess of copper is absorbed and deposited in the tissues. Damage to the basal ganglia in the brain causes choreo-athetosis or Parkinsonism. The liver becomes cirrhotic, the renal tubules are damaged and a ring of copper (Kayser-Fleischer ring) is deposited in the eye. Treatment is with D-penicillamine 300 mg t.d.s. orally or dimercaprol (B.A.L.) which attach to copper and cause its excretion.

Neurofibromatosis (von Recklinghausen's Disease)
This is an hereditary disease in which tumours (neurofibromas) grow in the skin and elsewhere. Treatment is unnecessary except for removal of tumours compressing the brain or spinal cord.

Paraplegia
Paraplegia is paralysis of both legs and often of the sphincters of the bladder and rectum, causing incontinence.

Quadriplegia is paralysis of all four limbs due to a lesion of the cervical part of the spinal cord.

Causes: A Pressure on the spinal cord.
1. Injury, e.g. fractured vertebra.
2. Prolapsed intervertebral disc.
3. Spina bifida.
4. Cervical spondylosis.
5. Inflammation e.g. tuberculosis of the spine (Pott's disease) and extradural abscess.
6. Paget's disease of bone.
7. Tumours—myeloma, angioma, osteoma, meningioma, glioma, Hodgkin's disease, secondary deposits of carcinoma.

B *Disease of the spinal cord.*
1 Inflammation, e.g. myelitis, poliomyelitis, syphilis.
2 Degenerations such as multiple sclerosis, motor neuron disease, vitamin B_{12} deficiency neuropathy (subacute combined degeneration of the spinal cord), syringomyelia.
3 Thrombosis of the anterior spinal artery.

Clinically: symptoms are of either acute injury to the cord or of slow compression.

Acute Injury causes spinal shock lasting for three weeks. There is complete flaccid paralysis with loss of reflexes and sensation below the level of injury. Paralysis of the bladder and rectum leads to retention of faeces and urine since the internal sphincters are not involved. Trophic changes develop in the affected parts producing a blue, cold skin and a liability to bedsores and urinary infection. After the spinal shock wears off the flaccid muscles become spastic, the tendon reflexes are increased and the plantar responses become extensor. Reflex micturition develops. Sensory loss remains.

Slow Compression. Pressure on dorsal nerve roots produces root or girdle pain, worse on coughing and sneezing. Pressure on the spinal cord results in upper motor neuron (spastic) paralysis below the lesion, and bladder disturbance, i.e. precipitancy and incontinence at first, later retention with dribbling overflow, and ulceration of the moist skin.

Lesions Below the Second Lumbar Vertebra damage the cauda equina and cause lower motor neuron paralysis, anaesthesia and bladder dysfunction.

Investigations: urine to detect infection. X-ray of the spine to show bony lesions. Myelogram. Lumbar puncture: complete block of the subarachnoid space produces Froin's syndrome (the C.S.F. is yellow and contains an excess of protein), and Queckenstedt's test does not increase the pressure of the C.S.F.

Treatment is as for any paralysed patient (*see* 'Stroke') and of the cause, e.g. surgery for abscess, prolapsed intervertebral disc and meningioma. Prevent bedsores by changing the patient's position two-hourly, skin care, use of an air, water or ripple-mattress and lying face-down for six out of every 24 hours. In acute paraplegia the flaccid limbs must be kept in a good position, especially the feet, which should be dorsiflexed. Physiotherapy, encouragement to use and strengthen the arms, occupational therapy. Attention to the bladder and bowels. For retention of urine the bladder is catheterised eight-hourly if attempts fail to induce automatic reflex emptying of the bladder by suprapubic pressure and carbachol $250–500\,\mu g$ s.c.

Poliomyelitis ('Infantile Paralysis')
Acute anterior poliomyelitis is due to polioviruses types 1, 2 or 3 which are spread by droplets, flies, and infected food and water. It occurs sporadically or in epidemics.
    The virus invades the nasopharyngeal or intestinal mucous membrane to reach the blood. The patient may overcome the infection at this stage but excretes the virus in the faeces as a symptomless carrier. Poor immunity allows the virus to

enter the nervous system and destroy the motor neurons of the anterior horns of the spinal cord and the brain stem.

Clinically: children and young adults are affected. The incubation period is five to 14 days. Viraemia causes the pre-paralytic stage with fever, malaise, aching in the muscles, headache and sore throat. Meningeal irritation produces vomiting, neck stiffness and a positive Kernig's sign. The paralytic stage, if it occurs, begins after one to seven days. Paralysis varies from slight weakness of a muscle to complete paralysis of one or more limbs. Paralysis is maximum within 24 hours and is of lower motor neuron type (*Fig. 13.16b*), with flaccidity, loss of tendon reflexes and wasting of affected muscles. Paralysis of the respiratory muscles, if untreated, results in asphyxia and death. Urinary retention is common. Involvement of the brain stem (bulbar poliomyelitis) leads to difficulty in swallowing and coughing and to nasal speech due to paralysis of the muscles of the pharynx and palate, and secretions collect in the throat. Paralysis of the larynx causes difficulty in speaking, of the eye muscles causes squint, and of the facial muscles produces a flaccid immobile face. The patient remains conscious.

Recovery is gradual, begins in one week, and with physiotherapy, may continue for months. It is often incomplete since partly damaged neurons recover but those destroyed completely do not. In children paralysed limbs do not grow normally and are short. Deformity may be produced by the pull of unaffected muscles. One attack provides lifelong immunity.

Investigations: C.S.F. contains an increase in lymphocytes and protein.

Treatment: isolation for six weeks. Complete rest in bed. Vaccination of contacts. Virus is present in faeces for two to six weeks, and in the upper respiratory tract for five days. To prevent spread of infection to others, faeces and urine are disinfected before disposal, paper handkerchiefs are burnt and barrier nursing is used (Chapter 4). Nutrition and fluid intake are maintained. An analgesic is given for pain and a sedative for restlessness.

A paralysed muscle is stretched by the pull of its antagonists, leading to deformity. Stretching is prevented by supporting the limbs so as to relax paralysed muscles. Sandbags and splints are used to prevent foot and wrist drop, the foot being dorsiflexed; the arm is slightly abducted if the deltoid muscle is paralysed. A pad is placed in the palm of the hand to keep the thumb abducted and the fingers slightly flexed.

Physiotherapy is begun when the patient is apyrexial, beginning with putting the limbs through their full range of movement, passively if paralysed, actively if not, and later providing re-educational exercises, e.g. occupational therapy.

Appliances may be needed, e.g. surgical boots, walking calipers; or operation, e.g. tendon transplant or arthrodesis, to correct deformity or instability.

For bulbar paralysis the foot of the bed is raised to allow postural drainage of secretions, pharyngeal suction is used, and feeding is by nasogastric tube.

For respiratory paralysis tracheostomy (Chapter 7) and positive pressure ventilation are used.

Prevention: poliomyelitis is notifiable to the area community medical officer. γ-globulin gives temporary passive immunity for a few weeks. Vaccination with a drop of oral Sabin vaccine (live attenuated virus) on a lump of sugar every three weeks for three doses, then every three years, or by i.m. injection with Salk vaccine killed virus).

In an epidemic, public swimming pools are closed, mass vaccination is performed, and nose and throat operations are avoided since they predispose to bulbar poliomyelitis.

Peripheral Neuropathy

Mononeuropathy is disorder of a single nerve. It is commonly due to compression, e.g. compression of the median nerve in the carpal tunnel at the wrist (carpal tunnel syndrome) which occurs in middle-aged women or may complicate hypothyroidism, rheumatoid arthritis, pregnancy or acromegaly.

Multiple mononeuropathy may be due to systemic lupus erythematosus, rheumatoid arthritis, or amyloidosis.

Polyneuropathy ('Polyneuritis') is a bilateral dysfunction of both motor and sensory nerves beginning peripherally.

Causes:
1. Hereditary: peroneal muscular atrophy.
2. Metabolic: diabetes mellitus, uraemia.
3. Infections: leprosy, diphtheria, certain viruses (acute infective polyneuritis).
4. Toxins: mercury, lead, arsenic,
5. Deficiency of vitamin B_{12} or of thiamine (beriberi, alcoholism).
6. Others: carcinoma of the bronchus.

Clinically: there is sensory and lower motor neuron disturbance. Paraesthesiae (tingling, pins and needles) and numbness begin in the toes and fingers and spread proximally. The patient cannot perform fine movements such as fastening buttons, and is ataxic. Muscular weakness begins in the hands and feet, producing wrist and foot drop, and spreads proximally. Tendon reflexes are absent. The muscles are tender to pressure.

Treatment is of the cause, prevention of pressure sores, splints for foot-drop.

Acute Infective Polyneuritis (Guillain-Barré syndrome, Landry's paralysis) is rare. It follows certain virus infections. There is generalised muscular weakness and the respiratory muscles may be affected. C.S.F. protein is increased. Recovery is usually complete. There is no specific treatment. Corticosteroids are ineffective. Artificial respiration may be needed.

Peroneal Muscular Atrophy (Charcot-Marie-Tooth disease) is an inherited disease beginning in childhood. The posterior columns and the lower motor neurons degenerate and the distal muscles become paralysed and wasted, and deep sensation is impaired.

Disorders of the Cranial Nerves
The cranial nerves are listed in *Table 13.2.*

Olfactory Nerves. The sense of smell is temporarily lost when the mucosa of the nose is swollen by a cold, and may be permanently lost if the nerves are torn by a fracture of the base of the skull. Taste sense may seem to be partially lost since many flavours are really odours.

Optic Nerves. Nerve fibres receiving impulses in the retina converge to form the optic disc, which is the blind spot since it does not contain nerve cells. From the optic disc the optic nerve passes backwards through the sphenoid bone to meet the nerve from the opposite side to form the optic chiasma in front of the pituitary gland. The optic tracts continue backwards to reach the visual centres in the occipital lobes. The optic disc and the retina can be seen by using an ophthalmoscope.

Papilloedema is swelling of the optic disc and is seen in severe hypertension and when the intracranial pressure is increased, as in cerebral tumour, meningitis or cerebral injury.

Optic Neuritis causes visual loss and is due to multiple sclerosis, syphilis, methanol, quinine, ethambutol, vitamin B_{12} deficiency or smoking strong pipe-tobacco.
Optic Atrophy results in loss of sight and is due to optic neuritis, glaucoma, trauma, diabetes mellitus and pressure on the optic nerve by tumours or aneurysms.

The Oculomotor, Trochlear and Abducens Nerves supply the muscles that move the eyes. Injury to one nerve results in paralytic squint (ophthalmoplegic strabismus) and diplopia (double vision). The third nerve contains the autonomic fibres that control the pupil. The pupil dilates if the third nerve is damaged.

The Trigeminal Nerve has three main divisions, which receive sensation from the face. The ophthalmic branch supplies the forehead, the eye (including the cornea), and the front of the nose. The maxillary branch supplies the cheek, the upper lip and the side of the nose. The mandibular branch supplies the side of the head. This also has a motor branch to the muscles of mastication.

Trigeminal Neuralgia mainly affects the elderly. Attacks of severe unilateral stabbing pain affect the face and last seconds or minutes. Pain is triggered by a stimulus to the face, e.g. shaving, eating, washing, or a cold wind. Paroxysms may last for days and are followed by temporary remissions.

Treatment: carbamezepine (Tegretol) 200 mg t.d.s. Phenytoin 100–200 mg t.d.s. For persistent pain, alcohol or phenol is injected into the nerve or the Gasserian ganglion, but leaves an unpleasant numbness.

Herpes Zoster virus (shingles) may attack any sensory nerve, but ophthalmic herpes is the most serious since it involves the cornea and may lead to corneal scarring and blindness.

The Facial Nerve leaves a canal in the skull to run through the parotid gland before branching to the muscles of the face, except those of mastication. Paralysis of the face may be upper motor neuron (as in hemiplegia) or lower motor neuron (due to trauma, Bell's palsy, mastoid infection, operation on a parotid tumour) in type. Lesions of the facial nerve cause paralysis of the same side of the face and fore-head.

Bell's palsy is the commonest cause of facial paralysis. The cause is unknown but paralysis is due to compression of the nerve by inflammation in the facial canal and comes on suddenly. One side of the face is paralysed, the eye cannot be closed, tears run down the face, and food collects in the cheek. The paralysis usually clears completely over a few months.

Treatment: the patient should be reassured about recovery. An eyeshade is used if the eye cannot be closed, and a wire splint applied to support the corner of the mouth and prevent stretching of the muscles. Electrical stimulation maintains muscle tone but does not hasten recovery. Facial exercises should be performed in front of the mirror once recovery begins. Corticotrophin 40 u b.d., s.c. or i.m. or prednisolone 20 mg q.i.d. for five days, reducing to zero over the next five days, may reduce the inflammation.

The Auditory (Acoustic) Nerve receives the impulses of hearing and balance (position of the head). Damage to the cochlear nerve causes tinnitus (ringing in the ears) or deafness. Damage to the vestibular nerve causes vertigo (giddiness) and loss of balance, and may be caused by Ménière's disease, neuroma, meningitis, strepto-mycin or kanamycin.

14 MENTAL ILLNESS

Mental illness is abnormality of the mind. Psychiatry is the study of mental illness. Psychology is the study of normal mental behaviour.

Mental and physical illnesses are not separate entities. Many 'mental' illnesses have a physical cause; e.g. dementia due to degeneration or faulty metabolism of cells in the cerebral cortex, caused by, e.g. atherosclerosis, trauma, or severe hypothyroidism.

Mental illness may be classified as:

1 Neuroses (psychoneuroses): anxiety state, hysteria, obsessional-compulsive state.
2 Psychosomatic.
3 Psychopathic.
4 Psychoses: schizophrenia, dementia, affective disorders, and mental illnesses due to alcoholism, brain infection or injury.

Drugs used in mental illness are listed in Chapter 13.

Anxiety State

A certain amount of anxiety is a normal response to danger and stress and keeps us alert and ready for fight (resistance) or flight (running away); but in anxiety state the anxiety is excessive or prolonged. Anxiety is often associated with overactivity of the autonomic nervous system. Normally adrenaline is released during danger and redirects blood from the skin (by vasoconstriction) to the muscles (vasodilatation) where it is needed. Adrenaline also increases the heart-rate so as to supply increased amounts of oxygen and nutrients to the muscles which are more tense and ready for action.

Cause: anxiety state has a genetic predisposition, and is precipitated by environmental stress with which the patient is unable to cope.

Clinically: a family history of anxiety may be present. There is apprehension (fear), tension, irritability, inability to concentrate, insomnia, headache, dizziness, fatigue and frequency of micturition. Release of adrenaline causes tremor, sweating, dry mouth, dilated pupils and tachycardia (which are absent during sleep).

A patient may become conditioned to a particular stimulus, e.g. having been involved in a car accident he develops acute anxiety whenever in traffic.

Treatment: attempt to find the cause by sympathetic listening and by taking a history. Psychotherapy: reassurance, suggestion, psychoanalysis. Sedation with a tranquilliser, e.g. phenobarbitone 30–60 mg t.d.s., chlordiazepoxide (Librium, Tropium) 5–20 mg t.d.s., diazepam (Valium) 2–10 mg t.d.s., or chlorpromazine (Largactil) 25–100 mg t.d.s.

Hysteria

Hysteria is suppressed stress or frustration converted into a physical symptom.

Cause: failure of satisfaction of the patient's wish causes stress. This causes the hysteric to unconsciously suppress the wish, i.e. to dissociate it from the conscious mind (dissociation), and to release the stress as a conversion symptom. Owing to dissociation the hysteric is unaware of the motive causing the symptom, unlike the malingerer who knowingly pretends he has a symptom. Both have the motive of personal gain. Dissociative reactions occur in hysterics, schizophrenics and psychopaths.

Clinically: the hysterical personality is easily influenced by people or ideas that appeal to him, i.e. he is easily suggestible, immature in thought, emotionally unstable, shallow, self-centred and goes to any ends to gain attention. Conversion symptoms include 'paralysis' of a limb, 'aphonia' ('loss' of voice), 'anaesthesia', 'blindness', vomiting, stupor, amnesia (loss of memory for people and events so as to avoid unpleasant situations), and hysterical fits. There is no organic disease of the affected part.

Hysterical fits occur only in the presence of other people. The patient shrieks (to attract attention), falls to the ground (carefully) then kicks and screams. The attacks are unlike epilepsy, the tongue is not bitten (but onlookers may be!). The hysteric is indifferent to the symptoms whereas a patient with genuine organic disease is anxious.

Treatment is difficult. It is not possible to change the patient's personality. Removal from the stress; sedation, suggestion and hypnosis may help. The nurse should gain the confidence of the patient, be firm, kind and tactful, but ignore the symptoms and avoid sympathising with the patient's 'disabilities'. Splashing cold water on the face may cure a hysterical fit. The underlying conflict must be discussed with the patient.

Obsessional–Compulsive Neurosis

Obsessions are thoughts which repeatedly present themselves into the patient's consciousness in spite of his awareness of their senselessness. Compulsions are unnecessary repeated acts.

Clinically: patients and their parents usually have obsessive personalities and are neat, tidy and conscientious. The neurotic repeatedly checks that the door is locked, rewashes the hands although he has just washed them, repeats certain phrases, or may have to touch things twice or step over certain paving stones. Obsession combined with anxiety causes fears such as claustrophobia (fear of closed spaces), or agoraphobia (fear of open spaces).

Treatment: the obsessional personality cannot be changed but psychoanalysis may be tried and a tranquilliser given if there is anxiety. One in two patients recover spontaneously.

Psychosomatic Disorders

These are organic (physical) disorders due to emotional disturbance. They should be distinguished from emotional disorders due to organic disease, e.g. anxiety in hyperthyroidism due to a toxic adenoma of the thyroid, or anxiety and depression in chronic diarrhoea or cancer.

Clinically: emotional factors may produce headache or vague aches in the body (due to muscular tension), dizziness, palpitations, sweating, itching, indigestion, flatulence, nausea, vomiting and anorexia.

Treatment is to determine the cause and apply psychotherapy.

Anorexia Nervosa This is severe anorexia and loss of weight, usually in young women, due to emotional stress (e.g. fear of pregnancy or fear of obesity). There is overactivity (despite the emaciation), anaemia and constipation. Complications are of malnutrition, e.g. tuberculosis, death from starvation.

Treatment: admission to hospital. The patient must be made to eat and precautions must be taken to make sure that she swallows food, since she may go to great lengths to hide it or throw it away. Chlorpromazine (Largactil) 25–200 mg t.d.s. orally is often effective, and insulin may be given to stimulate appetite.

Psychopathic Personality
A psychopath is a person who has no moral or ethical standards and is antisocial, irresponsible, and aggressive, who may attack others without provocation, is unaffected by punishment and cannot be disciplined. His abnormal behaviour begins in childhood and he is often from a broken home. He fails to learn by experience but is of normal intelligence. He is cold, resentful, selfish, irritable, a pathological liar, often unemployed, sponging on others and stealing, or going from one job to another. He blames others and not himself. The electroencephalogram is abnormal.

Treatment: occupational and group therapy may help.

Drugs: tranquilliser, anticonvulsant.

Schizophrenia
Schizophrenia ('split mind') is a disturbance of perception, thought, emotion and behaviour which has an hereditary basis but is influenced by the environment.

Clinically: the pre-psychotic personality is of an introvert, with timidity, shyness and self-preoccupation.

In the normal person thoughts, emotions and actions are co-ordinated. In schizophrenia they may be unconnected, i.e. there is incongruity between them. This may be shown as laughter in a serious situation or odd behaviour with purposeless acts such as grimacing and peculiar gestures. The patient withdraws from the normal world and prefers to be alone; lacks drive, initiative and affection. He develops ideas of de-realisation (unreality) such as the world seeming unreal; ideas of depersonalisation (he feels that he has changed) such as a feeling that his limbs do not belong to him; delusions (false beliefs which are not corrected by reasoning with him) such as delusions of persecution, e.g. that he is being poisoned, followed, or talked about; or delusions of grandeur, e.g. that he is rich or God. There are hallucinations (sensory impressions without external stimuli to cause them) of voices, shapes and smells.

Simple Schizophrenia. The patient gradually withdraws into a world of unreality and steadily deteriorates.

Paranoid Schizophrenia. Delusions, commonly of persecution, and hallucinations predominate. The course is a progressive deterioration.

Hebephrenic Schizophrenia. Outbursts of anger, laughter, weeping or violence occur, and hallucinations are common.

Catatonic Schizophrenia is usually of acute onset at age 20–30 years. There are phases of excitement (overactivity) and of stupor. In stupor the patient refuses food and resists attention. Negativism (doing the opposite to what he is told), hallucinations and delusions are common. The patient may hold peculiar attitudes or show automatic obedience or echolalia (repeating what has been said to him).

Treatment: delusions and hallucinations are reduced by phenothiazines, e.g. chlorpromazine (Largactil) 25–200 mg q.i.d. orally. The patient should be encouraged in interesting activities, rehabilitated and given suitable employment.

Affective Disorders

Disorders of affect (mood) include mania and depression. There are three types of depression: i.e. that associated with mania, involutional depression, and reactive depression.

Manic-depressive Psychosis is hereditary and develops in the cyclothymic (mood-swinging) personality who is sociable, optimistic, energetic and extrovert at one time and gloomy and irritable at another.

Hypomania is mild mania. **Mania** is an abnormal elation with overactivity and lack of insight. The patient talks continuously, makes puns, has euphoria and insomnia, is cheerful, arrogant and interfering, and has flights of ideas, one idea running into the next, but is easily distracted and seldom finishes anything she starts. Overactivity and restlessness lead to loss of weight. Lack of control may lead to alcoholic and sexual excesses, obscene conversation and attacks on others. There may be delusions of grandeur.

Treatment: sedation; lithium carbonate 0·5 g t.d.s..

Depression. The patient feels tired; has anorexia, weight loss, headache, or indigestion; feels a failure; is self-reproaching and has guilt feelings. Delusions are common, e.g. the patient feels he cannot breathe, has a snake in the stomach, or is wicked or dead. Suicide is common. Thought may be slow (retardation), or the patient may be agitated and apprehensive, wring the hands and continuously moan (agitated depression, i.e. depression with anxiety). Insomnia may be a difficulty in getting to sleep (anxiety) or awaking early and depressed but improving later in the day.

Endogenous depression (involutional melancholia) arises from within and begins at age 50–65 years. The patient thinks the best of life is over and regrets what has not been done. Health is reduced.

Exogenous (reactive) depression is due to external circumstances such as bereavement, loss of money or unemployment.

Treatment: precautions against suicide. Reassurance. History to find the cause and treat it. Maintenance of nutrition and hygiene. Electroconvulsive therapy.

Antidepressant Drugs:

1 *Tricyclic Group*, e.g. Imipramine (Tofranil), amitriptyline (Tryptizol) or nortriptyline (Allegron, Aventyl) 25–75 mg t.d.s. orally, beginning with the small dose. Side-effects: hypotension causing dizziness or syncope, drowsiness, dry mouth, blurred vision, constipation, the neutralisation of the antihypertensive action of guanethidine, bethanidine and clonidine, and interaction with adrenaline and noradrenaline to produce hypertension.

2 *Monoamine Oxidase Inhibitors (M.A.O.I.)* e.g. phenelzine (Nardil) 15 mg t.d.s. orally. M.A.O.I. interact with many foods (e.g. cheese) and drugs (amphetamines, levodopa; ephedrine, as in cough medicines) to produce hypertension which may cause headache or cerebral haemorrhage. The patient must be warned not to take these foods and drugs within 10 days of taking a M.A.O.I.

Dementia

Dementia is a progressive decline in mental faculties due to degeneration or death of cells in the cerebral cortex.

Cause: it may be idiopathic (of unknown cause) or due to known organic disease affecting the brain, such as atherosclerosis, which reduces the blood supply to the brain; Huntington's chorea; syphilis (general paralysis); multiple sclerosis; cerebral tumour; metabolic, endocrine and nutritional disorders; or trauma.

Clinically: there is loss of memory for recent events and subsequently for remote events, impairment of intelligence and judgement, emotional instability, irritability, agitation, anxiety, insomnia, and loss of interest and initiative. The patient becomes self-centred and intolerant of change and has delusions, e.g. of being poisoned or neglected, and hallucinations, and may wander about or leave water- or gas-taps on.

Elderly patients with dementia (senile dementia) usually die, within two years, of infection or fractures. Patients with dementia occurring before old age (presenile dementia) may live five to 10 years. Presenile dementia tends to be due to rare metabolic disorders or specific virus infection. In atherosclerotic dementia there may be paralysis and the outlook is variable.

Treatment is of the cause if possible, e.g. of hypothyroidism syphilis, hypertension, cerebral tumour, malnutrition. The patient should be looked after at home if possible since sudden change is disturbing and familiar surroundings are reassuring to him. Admission to hospital is necessary if he lives alone or is unmanageable at home. The patient is nursed by as few people as possible so that he gets to know their faces, and is placed where ward activities will not disturb him. He needs reassurance and should be told where he is and what day it is, and have a regular daily routine. Attention is paid to the bowels, bladder and skin (to prevent bedsores) and adequate nourishment and exercise is ensured. The patient should be kept as ambulant as possible.

Sedation: chloral hydrate for insomnia or a phenothiazine for disturbed behaviour.

Mental Retardation (Mental Deficiency)
Mental deficiency is mental subnormality due to defective development of the mind during childhood and is legally divided into two grades:

1 Subnormality. The patient is unable to look after himself or his affairs and cannot be taught to do so; the intelligence quotient (I.Q.) being between 50 and 70 (normal average = 100; genius may be 150).

2 Severely subnormal (imbecile, idiot). The I.Q. is below 50. These subjects require help from other people for their survival

Cause:

Genetic—Down's syndrome (mongolism), phenylketonuria, Turner's syndrome, some cretins (hypothyroidism).

Acquired during pregnancy—maternal chronic alcoholism, German measles, toxo-plasmosis, some drugs, trauma during childbirth.

Clinically: the child is inert, lacking curiosity, alertness and movement, and slow in learning to walk and talk.

Treatment is of the cause. Thyroxine for cretinism; special diet for phenylketonuria. Education according to ability, occupational training—some patient's may be able to perform a routine job. Admission to hospital only if there are behavioural difficulties.

Personality Disorders
These include alcoholism, drug addiction and sexual deviation.

Alcoholism and Drug Addiction are psychological dependencies due to lack of self-confidence. The social drinker or therapeutic drug taker may insidiously develop into an habitual drinker or drug addict and become dependent on alcohol or drugs. Symptoms include morning nausea and vomiting, hallucinations, character changes, e.g. lying, and social and intellectual deterioration with loss of employment. Treatment requires total abstinence and begins in hospital with psychotherapy, sedation and vitamins.

Sexual Deviation. Homosexuality ('same sex') and transvestism (sexual pleasure derived from wearing clothing of the opposite sex) result from distorted experiences during adolescence.

15   THE MUSCULOSKELETAL SYSTEM AND CONNECTIVE TISSUES

Anatomy

The skull rests on the first cervical vertebra and consists of the cranium and the face (*Fig. 15.1*). The cranium consists of one frontal, two parietal, one occipital, one sphenoid, one ethmoid and two temporal bones. The face consists of two zygomatic

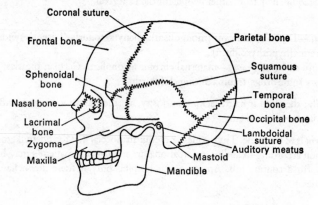

FIG. 15.1   The bones of the skull, lateral view

(cheek) bones, two maxillae (upper jaw), two nasal bones, one vomer, two lacrimal bones, two palatine bones, two inferior conchae and one mandible (lower jaw). Each maxilla contains eight, and the mandible contains 16, sockets for the teeth.

The vertebral column consists of seven cervical, 12 thoracic, five lumbar, five fused sacral and four fused coccygeal bones. A vertebra (*Fig. 15.2*) typically consists of a cylindrical body in front, and a neural arch behind. The vertebral foramen between them contains the spinal cord. The neural arch consists of pedicles which are attached to the posterolateral aspects of the vertebral body and project backwards to continue as the laminae. At the junction of pedicles with laminae are the transverse processes which project laterally, and the superior and inferior articular processes which articulate with the vertebrae above and below. Where the laminae meet in the middle a spinous process arises and projects backwards. The vertebrae, as are all bones, are held together by ligaments. The bodies of adjacent vertebrae are joined by the intervertebral discs (*Fig. 15.3*) which consist of a tough outer layer (the annulus fibrosus), and an inner elastic nucleus (the nucleus pulposus). The nucleus pulposus absorbs mechanical shocks. It is slowly replaced with fibrous tissue with age and becomes more rigid. Each transverse process of the cervical

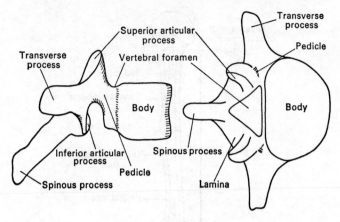

FIG. 15.2 A typical vertebra

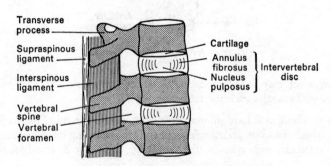

FÍG. 15.3 A portion of the vertebral column

vertebrae contains a foramen (opening) through which the vertebral artery passes on each side.

The thoracic cage (*Fig. 6.1*) consists of the sternum, 12 pairs of ribs and their costal cartilages, and the 12 thoracic vertebrae. The spaces between the ribs (intercostal spaces) contain the intercostal muscles.

The shoulder girdle consists of a clavicle (collar bone) and a scapula (shoulder blade). The bones of the upper limb are the humerus (upper arm), radius and ulna (forearm), eight carpals (wrist), five metacarpals and 14 phalanges (two to the thumb and three to each of the fingers).

The pelvic girdle consists of the sacrum and, on each side, an ilium, ischium and pubis. Where the last three join is a hollow (the acetabulum), the socket for the head of the femur. The lower limb consists of the femur (thigh bone), the tibia and fibula (leg bones), patella (knee cap), and the foot which consists of seven tarsals, five metatarsals and 14 phalanges.

Bone may be compact or cancellous. Compact bone is hard and dense and forms the outer layer of each bone. Cancellous bone is honeycombed and contains bone

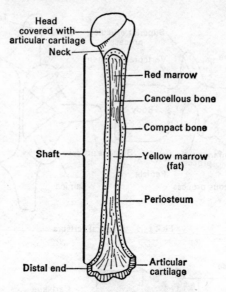

FIG. 15.4 A typical long bone (humerus)

marrow which may be red (producing blood cells) or yellow (fat). Each bone is covered with a tough membrane, the periosteum (*Fig. 15.4*).

Joints are classified as fixed (fibrous, immobile), e.g. the sutures of the skull and the teeth in their sockets, as cartilaginous (slightly movable), e.g between the bodies of the vertebrae, or as synovial (freely movable, *Fig. 15.5*). Synovial joints are

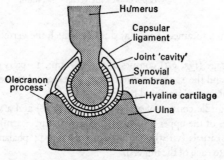

FIG. 15.5 A synovial joint (the elbow)

lubricated by sticky secretions from the synovial membrane which lines them. The parts of the bones forming the synovial joint are lined with articular (hyaline) cartilage and each joint is surrounded by a capsular ligament. The movement of the joint is produced by contraction or relaxation of muscles attached to the bones on each side of the joint.

Function

The bones form a supporting framework for the body; protect certain organs, e.g. the ribs protect the heart and lungs; provide attachment for the voluntary muscles through the periosteum, thus provide for movement; store calcium; and produce blood through the red marrow they contain.

The movements which can occur at a joint are: flexion (bending), extension (straightening or bending backward), adduction (movement towards the midline of the body), abduction (movement away from the midline of the body), rotation (movement around the long axis of a part), supination (turning the palm of the hand or front of the trunk to face upwards), pronation (turning the palm of the hand or front of the trunk to face downwards), inversion (turning the sole of the foot towards the midline), eversion (turning the sole of the foot outwards).

The Muscles

The muscles which concern us here are those receiving intramuscularly injected (i.m.) drugs. The best sites for the injection of irritant solutions or volumes greater than 1 ml are thick muscles such as the glutei, the thigh muscles, or the deltoid muscles over the outer aspect of the shoulders. The glutei ('buttocks) are injected only in the upper and outer quadrants (*Fig. 15.6*) since the sciatic nerve runs beneath the lower

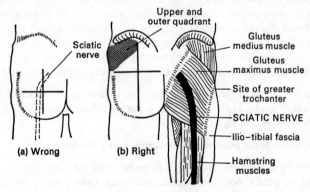

FIG. 15.6   (*a*) Incorrect and (*b*) correct sites for intramuscular injection (the sciatic nerve must be avoided)

half of the gluteus maximus and is easily damaged, with disastrous effects, such as permanent paralysis of the leg. It must be noted that the buttock is not merely the area, used for sitting on, above the crease of the thigh (*Fig. 15.6*); indeed this is the lower part which must never receive injections. The buttock extends from the crease in the thigh up the the iliac crest.

INVESTIGATIONS OF THE MUSCULOSKELETAL SYSTEM

Blood. The E.S.R. is raised in active rheumatoid arthritis, rheumatic fever and infections. The latex fixation test for rheumatoid factor is positive in rheumatoid arthritis (and also in, e.g. pulmonary tuberculosis and liver disease). The serum alkaline phosphatase is increased if there is destruction of bone, e.g. osteomalacia, hyperparathyroidism, myelomatosis, or secondary malignant deposits in bone. The serum uric acid is increased in gout. Electrophoresis of serum proteins is abnormal in myelomatosis and in rheumatoid arthritis.

X-ray of bones to show fractures, tumours, or osteoporosis.

Synovial Fluid is examined for pus and organisms in infections of joints, for crystals of uric acid in gout, and for lymphocytes in rheumatoid arthritis or tuberculosis.

Electromyography is a record of the electrical changes in the muscles and is abnormal in muscular diseases.

Biopsy of Synovium or Muscle may be taken for microscopic examination.

DISEASES OF BONES, JOINTS AND MUSCLES

Osteoporosis
Osteoporosis is reduction in bone density. It is caused by oestrogen or androgen deficiency, hyperparathyroidism, acromegaly, excess of corticosteroids as in Cushing's sydrome and corticosteroid therapy for various conditions such as asthma or rheumatoid arthritis (corticosteroids cause protein breakdown, i.e. loss of bone matrix), malabsorption syndrome (calcium deficiency), and disuse, e.g. prolonged immobilisation (disuse removes the mechanical stress stimulus to bone formation).

Clinically: weakness of the vertebrae produces collapse of the vertebral bodies, causing loss of height, kyphosis, and pain in the back. Fractures are likely to occur especially in the neck of the femur.

Investigations: X-ray of bones shows rarefaction, collapse or fracture.

Treatment: Treat fractures. *Diet*—high in protein and calcium. *Drugs*—calcium gluconate 1·2 g t.d.s. orally for calcium deficiency; oestrogen is given to postmenopausal women; analgesic for pain.

Paget's Disease of Bone (Osteitis Deformans)
This is a degeneration of bone with excessive repair, producing a deformed, thickened but weak bone. It is of unknown cause, and affects one or more bones.

Clinically: it begins after middle age and commonly affects the vertebrae, pelvis, skull, ribs and long bones but not usually the hands and feet. There may be no symtoms, or there may be headaches and a slow enlargement of the skull, or backache (spine involved). Affected bones are deformed and thick, and the soft tissues over them are swollen, hot and red. One or more long bones of the leg may become bowed and the patient loses height.

Complications include pathological fracture, which heals normally, osteogenic sarcoma (rare), deafness from pressure on the auditory nerve, paraplegia from compression of the spinal cord caused by the collapse of vertebral bodies, heart failure due to the high vascularity of the affected part acting as if it were an arterio-venous shunt.

Investigations: X-ray shows the bony abnormality. The serum alkaline phosphatase is raised.

Treatment: mithramycin infusion. Porcine calcitonin 1 mg i.m. daily (or salmon calcitonin 12·5–50 μg i.m. 3–7 times weekly) for 3–6 months then reduced according to the response, prevents bone resorption. Side-effects: rash, diarrhoea, nausea, flushing. Diphosphonates, e.g. disodium etidronate, orally. The patient should remain mobile as long as possible.

Achondroplasia
This is an inherited shortness of long bones due to faulty formation of bone in cartilage, which results in a short stature but a normal-sized trunk and skull. Infants often die *in utero.*

Osteogenesis Imperfecta (Fragilitas Ossium)
This is an inherited disease of bone and fibrous tissue, the bones being fragile. The sclerae of the eyes are blue. Otosclerosis and deafness later occur.

Infective (Septic) Arthritis
Infection of a joint may be due to pus-forming organisms (staphylococci. strepto-cocci, pneumococci, gonococci), when the joint will be red, hot, swollen, painful and tender, or to tuberculosis when the joint will be swollen but is often not inflamed and may be referred to as a 'cold' swelling or 'cold' abscess.

Treatment: antibiotic.

Rheumatoid Disease (Rheumatoid Arthritis)
Rheumatoid arthritis is a chronic polyarthritis, with exacerbations and remissions. It affects mainly the smaller joints. There is a familial incidence. The cause is unknown. It may be an autoimmune disease since the blood contains an abnormal globulin (rheumatoid factor) which is a macroglobulin (IgM) which combines with plasma IgG antibody and complement to damage the connective tissues. Granulation and fibrous tissue form in the joints and limit movement.

Clinically: 70% of patients are female. It begins, commonly at age 20–50 years, with malaise, fatigue, mild pyrexia, tachycardia, sweating, and weight loss. Stiffness and pain in the joints are worse in the morning. It first affects the proximal inter-phalangeal joints which become spindle-shaped, then involves the wrists, elbows, shoulders, ankles and knees. The joints are kept flexed to relieve the pain. There is ulnar deviation of the fingers, muscular wasting, and swelling of bursae. Sub-cutaneous nodules may form. The hands and feet become cold and blue due to a poor blood supply caused by vasculitis. The patient may be prevented from doing things for herself because of deformity, but less than 10% become severely crippled. 20% recover completely.

Complications: pleurisy, pericarditis, pulmonary fibrosis, peripheral neuropathy, and episcleritis may occur, and anaemia is common.

Investigations: blood count (anaemia), E.S.R. (raised), latex test for rheumatoid factor (positive), synovial fluid or biopsy.

Treatment: the aim is to relieve pain and minimise disability. Rest in bed in the acute stage, using a firm mattress, a firm backrest so that the back is kept straight, a cage to take the weight of the bedclothes off the feet, and sandbags or a footrest so that the feet are kept dorsiflexed. The knees are kept straight (no pillows behind them). Splints are used to hold the affected joints in a good position and may need to be worn only at night. The temperature is charted while pyrexial. After the acute phase has passed the muscles are exercised. Radiant heat or paraffin wax baths reduce the stiffness in the hands and feet. Occupational therapy.

Diet: vitamins B and C are given. Diet high in milk (calcium) since calcium is lost from the bones during immobility. A high fluid intake prevents renal calculi from forming.

Drugs: iron for anaemia, sedative for insomnia.

Antirheumatic drugs: aspirin 4–6 g daily. Side-effects: gastric bleeding. Phenylbutazone (Butazolidine) 100–300 mg orally daily. Side-effects: nausea, vomiting, rash, fluid retention, gastric ulcer, agranulocytosis, aplastic anaemia, thrombocytopenia. Indomethacin (Indocid) up to 100 mg daily. Side-effects: nausea, vomiting, headache, vertigo, depression. Ibuprofen (Brufen) 300 to 400 mg b.d. Chloroquine is contraindicated since it causes retinopathy.

Gold (Myocrisin, sodium aurothiomalate) 10–50 mg i.m. weekly to a total of 1 g. Side-effects: renal damage, dermatitis, agranulocytosis, aplastic anaemia, thrombocytopenia. The platelet count is done and the urine is examined for albumin before each injection. Improvement is slow. Corticosteroids, e.g. prednisolone up to 10 mg daily, used for short periods, produce rapid relief of pain and inflammation but have no long-term benefit and produce side-effects (hypertension, fluid retention, peptic ulceration, diabetes mellitus, infection). Intra-articular hydrocortisone is useful.

Orthopaedic surgery, e.g. arthrodesis, tenotomy to correct deformities, or synovectomy (removal of excessive synovial membrane). Spa treatment helps some patients.

Assistance with aids such as shoe horns with long handles, modified door-handles and furniture, ramps instead of steps. Live on the ground floor.

Still's Disease is rheumatoid arthritis in children, associated with splenomegaly and enlarged lymph nodes.

Felty's Syndrome is rheumatoid arthritis in adults, with splenomegaly, enlarged lymph nodes, and pigmentation of the skin.

Sjögren's Syndrome is rheumatoid arthritis associated with deficiency of salivary and lacrimal secretions, producing a dry mouth and dry eyes.

Osteoarthrosis ('Osteoarthritis')
Osteoarthrosis is a degeneration of the articular cartilage and adjacent bone, usually of large joints, followed by outgrowths of new bone (osteophytes) at the margins of the joint. It is due to excessive wear and tear caused by, e.g. obesity; or by injury such as a fracture or repeated minor injuries, as in certain occupations and in neuropathic joints, e.g. syringomyelia. It affected the great reptiles of 180 million years ago.

Clinically: there is pain and stiffness in the joint and, later, restriction of movement; crepitus (a grating sensation) may be felt on movement of the joint. Surrounding muscles may waste and an effusion may occur.

Treatment: prevent further degeneration by reducing bodyweight if the spine, hips and knees are involved, and by discontinuing traumatic occupations. Periods of rest. Rubber heels on footwear to reduce jarring. Walking caliper. Analgesic for pain, e.g. aspirin, paracetamol, phenylbutazone. Physiotherapy, e.g. warmth to the joint (short wave or infra-red therapy) and exercises to strengthen the muscles and give stability to the joint.
Operation, e.g. arthrodesis, osteotomy, replacement with an artificial joint.

Ankylosing Spondylitis
This is an inherited progressive arthritis of the joints of the spinal column, producing gradual fusion of the vertebrae and rigidity of the spine ('poker back', 'bamboo spine'), often with kyphosis. 90% are males aged between 20 and 40 years. If the ribs fuse with the vertebrae because of inflammation of the costovertebral joints, respiration is impaired. Aortitis may occur and cause aortic incompetence. The E.S.R. is increased.

Treatment: analgesics, e.g. phenylbutazone, aspirin. Radiotherapy to the spine in the active phase. Physiotherapy to improve chest movement.

Prolapsed Intervertebral Disc
This is a tear in the annulus fibrosus with protrusion of the nucleus pulposus through the tear (*Fig. 15.7*), usually affecting the fourth or fifth lumbar discs. It is due to sudden twisting or a severe strain such as lifting a heavy weight. It causes back-

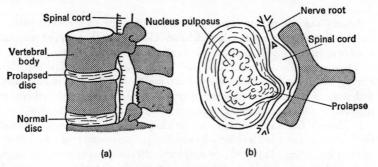

15.7   Prolapsed intervertebral disc: (*a*) side view; (*b*) from above

ache. The protruding material may press on nerve roots supplying the sciatic nerve, causing pain in the buttocks, thigh, or leg (sciatica), depending upon which nerve root is affected. The pain is worse on bending, coughing or sneezing. Flexion of the hip with the leg straight causes pain (Lasègue's sign, straight-leg raising). Symptoms clear up in a few weeks, but may recur. An X-ray of the spine shows narrowing of the disc space.

Treatment: analgesic and rest in bed (reduces the pressure on the disc) on boards in the acute stage. A plaster jacket over the trunk, a surgical belt, traction on the spine, or manipulation may help. Laminectomy (removal of the herniated portion of the disc) if conservative treatment fails.

Gout

Gout is an hereditary disorder of purine metabolism which results in a high level of uric acid in the blood and deposition of sodium urate crystals in and around joints. Purines are present in cell nuclei and are derived from food (meat) and tissue breakdown, and from the rapid turnover of nuclei in polycythaemia and leukaemia. Certain drugs increase the blood uric acid and precipitate gout, e.g. frusemide and thiazide diuretics prevent the excretion of uric acid. Gout usually affects middle-aged males.

Clinically:

Acute Gout: deposition of urate crystals causes the sudden onset of severe pain, swelling and redness of one or more joints, especially of the great toe, but ankles, knees, hands and elbows may be involved. There is pyrexia and leucocytosis. Treatment relieves symptoms in a few days. If untreated, further attacks occur, more urates are deposited and the condition becomes chronic.

Chronic Gout causes arthritis and deformity of joints. 'Chalky' deposits (tophi) of urates are present in joints (articular cartilage and bone), ligaments, and the cartilage of the ears. Tophi may ulcerate and discharge whitish urates through the skin. Urate stones may form in the kidneys and lead to renal failure.

Investigations: the blood uric acid (normal = 0·12–0·36 mmol/l, 2–6 mg%) and E.S.R. are increased.

Treatment:

Acute Gout: the patient stays in bed, painful joints are supported on pillows, and a cradle takes the weight of the bedclothes. The foot may be wrapped in cotton wool or gamgee tissue. The nurse should be careful not to jar the limb.

Drugs: phenylbutazone (Butazolidine) 600 mg orally on the first day, then 100 mg t.d.s., or indomethacin (Indocid) 200 mg the first day then 100 mg daily, with food, or colchicine 0·5 mg orally every two hours until the pain is relieved or toxic effects (vomiting, diarrhoea) appear, then 0·5 mg t.d.s. for several days.

In **Chronic Gout** and between acute attacks (so as to prevent chronic arthritis) the formation of uric acid is reduced by avoiding purines (sweetbread, liver, kidney, fish roe, brain, duck) and the excretion of uric acid is promoted by giving uricosuric drugs: sulphinpyrazone (Anturan) 100 mg t.d.s. orally, or probenecid (Benemid)

500 mg t.d.s. orally, and the urine kept alkaline. Uricosuric drugs are antagonised by salicylates. Allopurinal (Zyloric) 100 mg t.d.s. orally decreases purine synthesis. Abundant fluids should be taken to prevent the formation of renal calculi.

Surgical removal of large or ulcerating tophi.

Muscular weakness occurs in myopathy, hypokalaemia, and myasthenia gravis, and when there is muscular atrophy or paralysis.

Atrophy of Muscles
Muscular atrophy may be part of a general wasting disease, e.g. malnutrition, cancer, tuberculosis; or due to disuse, disease of the nerve supply (poliomyelitis, motor neuron disease, polyneuritis), or myopathy.

Myopathy may be due to an hereditary defect, e.g. pseudohypertrophic muscular dystrophy; inflammation, e.g. polymyositis; or metabolic abnormality, e.g. thyrotoxicosis, corticosteroid excess.

Myasthenia
Myasthenia is excessive fatiguability of voluntary muscles. It occurs in myasthenia gravis and myopathies and in some cases of thyrotoxicosis, carcinoma of the bronchus, and polymyositis.

Myasthenia Gravis is the rapid tiring of muscular movements due to an inadequate response to acetylcholine released by the nerve endings at the neuromuscular junction. The cause is unknown but 20% of cases are associated with a tumour of the thymus. It may be an autoimmune disease.

Clinically: it usually begins in young adults. A group of exercised muscles rapidly tire but recover with rest, e.g. those involved in chewing, swallowing, speaking and vision. The eyelids droop (ptosis) towards evening. Infection, emotional stress, and some drugs (streptomycin, quinine, morphine, barbiturates) make it worse.

Treatment: neostigmine bromide (Prostigmin) prolongs the action of acetylcholine by destroying cholinesterase. Dose: 15 to 45 mg orally 2–4 hourly. Pyridostigmine (Mestinon) 60–240 mg orally q.i.d. In emergencies neostigmine methylsulphate (Prostigmin inj.) 0·5–2·5 mg i.m. or s.c. Atropine 0·6 mg s.c. is given 15 minutes before the neostigmine to diminish its side-effects. Slow i.v. injection of edrophonium (Tensilon) 10 mg immediately increases muscular power. Tracheostomy and assisted ventilation is required if the respiratory muscles are involved. Removal of a thymic tumour. Protection from infection.

'Rheumatism' ('Fibrositis')
These are words used by the public for any pain in muscles, joints and soft tissues. 'Lumbago' is pain in the back. Pain may be due to poor posture or obesity, which

stretch ligaments; draughts; sudden movement causing minor injury such as small tears of ligaments; or general infections, especially viral ones, e.g. influenza.

Treatment: analgesic, local warmth, massage, gradually increasing exercises, correction of faulty posture; lose weight if obese, avoid chills and draughts. Local anaesthetic (1% procaine) may be injected into tender areas.

Collagenoses
These are diseases of the connective tissues.

Systemic Lupus Erythematosus (S.L.E.) is a diffuse disorder of connective tissue of unknown cause. The plasma contains an abnormal globulin (antinuclear factor) which attacks cell nuclei and gives a positive L.E. test. It is an autoimmune disease; i.e. the body is producing antibody (globulin) against its own tissues. 75% are women, usually aged 20–50 years.

Clinically: there is fever, anorexia, weight loss; fatigue, malaise, arthralgia, haemolytic anaemia and an erythematous rash over the hands, and over the face in a 'butterfly' distribution, i.e. over the cheeks and nose. There may be leucopenia, renal damage (proteinuria), endocarditis, pericarditis, pleurisy, pneumonitis, lymph node enlargement, alopecia and hepatitis. The E.S.R. is high. Death is often from renal failure.

Treatment: prednisolone 15 mg q.i.d. at first, reducing slowly to the smallest dose which suppresses symptoms. Chlorambucil for nephritis.

Polyarteritis Nodosa is an allergic disease, usually in young men. Tender nodules are present on small arteries due to degeneration of the wall which may cause clotting. There is fever, tachycardia, eosinophilia and hypertension. Corticosteroid therapy may provide benefit. Most patients die within five years.

Scleroderma is a swelling and hardening (sclerosis) of collagen (connective tissue). It affects the skin, lungs, oesophagus, myocardium and kidneys. There is no specific treatment but deformities are prevented by splinting.

Dermatomyositis is an inflammation of the voluntary muscles, myocardium and skin causing muscular pain and tenderness, skin rashes and death, often from myocarditis of associated malignant disease. Corticosteroids suppress acute, but not chronic, disease.

16 THE SKIN

The skin consists of two main layers. The outer layer is the epidermis and beneath this is the dermis. Beneath the skin is the subcutaneous fatty tissue (*Fig. 16.1*).

The epidermis consists of stratified squamous epithelium which is thickest over the palms of the hands and the soles of the feet. The deepest layer of the epidermis

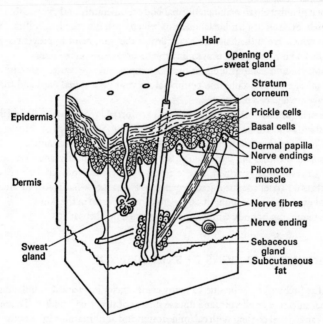

FIG. 16.1   The structure of the skin

is the germinative layer of basal cells which continually divide and produce prickle cells which push towards the surface. The prickle cells develop granules (stratum granulosum) which may be the first stage in the formation of keratin. In the stratum lucidum the granules become colourless and the cell cytoplasm appears to be clear.

The cells of the stratum lucidum lose their nuclei and flatten to become keratin (stratum corneum) which is shed from the surface of the skin. Where it clings to the skin it forms dandruff.

Within the basal cell layer there are melanoblasts (cells containing granules of melanin, the pigment which colours the skin brown).

The surface of the epidermis is rough. This ridging forms the fingerprints and increases friction and the ability to grip. The epidermis does not contain blood vessels and is nourished by diffusion from the dermis.

The dermis consists of white fibrous tissue containing strands of yellow elastic fibres. The superficial layer of the dermis is irregular and forms projections called papillae, which indent the epidermis. The dermis contains blood vessels, lymphatic vessels, sensory nerve endings, hair follicles, hairs and their muscles (arrectores pilorum), and sebaceous and sweat glands. The ducts of the sweat glands pass through the epidermis to the surface of the skin. Hair follicles are downgrowths from the epidermis. At the base of the follicle a cluster of cells, the bulb, produces the hair. As the cells of the bulb grow they are pushed along the follicle and changed into keratin. The colour of the hair is due to its melanin content. White hair does not contain melanin.

Sweat glands help to maintain normal body temperature and excrete some waste materials. Sebaceous glands, the ducts of which open into the hair follicles, secrete sebum which keeps the hair soft, waterproofs the skin, helps to prevent drying of the skin, and is bactericidal, thus killing micro-organisms on the skin.

Sensory nerve endings are sensitive to temperature, pressure, pain and touch, and convey impulses along the peripheral nerves to the spinal cord and thence to the thalamus and cerebral cortex.

The nails (or claws or hooves in animals) are formed from basal cells which form extra thick and hard keratinised dead cells which protect the tips of the fingers and toes. The root of the nail is embedded in skin and covered by the cuticle.

The skin protects the underlying tissues both mechanically and because of its sensory nerve endings which initiate reflex withdrawal from unpleasant stimuli, and acts as a barrier against micro-organisms. From the skin is absorbed vitamin D formed by the action of sunlight on 7-dehydrocholesterol in the skin.

The regulation of body temperature is discussed in Chapter 4.

SYMPTOMS AND SIGNS IN SKIN DISEASE

Pruritus (itching) may be due to many causes including parasites, inflammation, whether infective or allergic, and disease such as obstructive jaundice. Treatment is of the cause, local cooling with calamine lotion and antihistamine by mouth.

Vesicles are small blisters. They occur in certain infectious diseases, e.g. smallpox, chickenpox, and allergies.

Bullae are larger blisters and are due to burns and allergy.

Macules are small round spots, not raised.

Papules are small raised spots (pimples).

Pustules are vesicles containing purulent fluid.

Crusts are dried exudates.

Wheals are local white areas of oedema with a surrounding erythema and are due to injury or allergy.

An Ulcer is loss of surface tissue.

Petechiae are tiny red spots of haemorrhage into the tissues.

Ecchymoses are small flat bruises.

Haematomas are swellings due to blood in the tissues.

DISEASES OF THE SKIN

Infectious diseases causing skin rashes are described in Chapter 4.

Pruritus

Pruritus is itching. Generalised pruritus is due to diabetes mellitus, renal failure, obstructive jaundice, leukaemia, Hodgkin's disease, lice, scabies, dirt, eczema, drugs such as cocaine and codeine, and certain soaps, detergents and clothing (e.g. wool next to the skin).

Localised pruritus: pruritus ani is due to threadworms, piles, anal fissure, candida albicans, sensitivity to local applications such as antihistamines or from phenolphthalein taken orally, or to general causes. Pruritus vulvae may be due to vaginal discharge due to *Trichomonas* or *Candida albicans*, or to broad-spectrum antibiotics, threadworms, lice, glycosuria, lichen planus, or psoriasis.

Treatment is of the cause, adequate cleanliness (but overbathing can cause pruritus) and oily cream for a dry skin.

Dermatitis (Eczema)

Dermatitis is non-infective inflammation of the skin.

Causes: heredity, drying, maceration, radiation, friction, plants (primula, chrysanthemums), occupational (paint, plastics, oils, cement), insecticides, household detergents, soaps, soap powders, rubber gloves, cosmetics such as deodorants or lipstick, hair dyes, nickel (watch-buckles), drugs applied to the skin such as penicillin or antihistamines, especially in nurses who handle drugs frequently.

Atopic eczema is due to allergy and there is a family history of allergy, e.g. hay fever, asthma or eczema.

Contact dermatitis is due to external irritants. Dermatitis artefactae are lesions within easy reach, deliberately produced by the patient, a hysterical female or a psychopath.

Clinically: any part of the body may be affected. If it affects only the folds in the skin, e.g. the axillae, groins or under the breasts, it is called intertrigo. If the skin is also greasy due to overactivity of the sebaceous glands (seborrhoea) it is called seborrhoeic dermatitis. Redness, oedema, itching, vesicles and papules are present. In exfoliative dermatitis the epidermis is shed in large flakes, the skin becoming red and tender, with great heat loss.

Treatment: remove the cause, or wear protective clothing in industry. Apply calamine lotion or hydrocortisone lotion or cream. Soap and detergents are avoided and the skin is cleansed with water or saline. Antihistamine orally to relieve itching. Sedation at night.

Infections of the Skin

Boils, carbuncles, erysipelas, scabies, pediculosis, herpes zoster (shingles) and herpes simplex are described in Chapter 4.

Impetigo Contagiosa is a staphylococcal or streptococcal infection of the skin which is very contagious. It may be due to a purulent discharge from the nose or ear, debility, or to parasites (scabies, lice). Pink macules 1 cm across develop vesicles, then papules in their centres, then become crusts. They affect the face, chest and limbs. Fissures develop at the corners of the mouth and nose. Local lymph nodes enlarge and may suppurate.

Treatment: removal of crusts by bathing in warm water. The hair must be cut if the scalp is involved. Antibiotics, e.g. neomycin cream locally, and treatment of the cause. Splint the arms of children to prevent scratching, since scratching spreads the infection. Precautions must be taken against spread of infection to others. The patient's pillowslips and towels should be boiled.

Sycosis Barbae is a staphylococcal infection of hair follicles (folliculitis) which are the site of papules and pustules. Treatment is with local antibiotics.

Molluscum Contagiosum is a virus infection which is spread by direct contact. It produces small umbilicated (depressed centre) pink nodules.

Treatment: a probe is dipped into carbolic acid (phenol) and inserted into each molluscum. The skin is re-inspected after three weeks in order to treat lesions missed previously.

Lupus Vulgaris is human or bovine tuberculosis of the skin. Smooth yellow semi-transparent ('apple-jelly') nodules appear on the face, mucous membranes of the mouth, nose, pharynx and larynx, and sometimes on the neck, limbs, and anus, spread slowly, ulcerate and cause scarring. There is often tuberculosis elsewhere.

Treatment is as for pulmonary tuberculosis.

Tinea (Ringworm) is a fungus infection.

Tinea capitis is ringworm of the scalp. It is spread by direct contact or by sharing headwear. On the scalp there are circular scaly areas which contain broken hairs. In Wood's light (ultraviolet rays passed through a nickel glass filter) affected hairs show a green fluorescence.

Treatment: all contacts are given griseofulvin 250 mg q.i.d. orally daily after a fatty meal, for four to six weeks. The child has a close haircut, a shampoo, and wears a linen cap. The brush, comb, pillowcase and clothing must not be used by others.

Tinea barbae is ringworm of the beard spread from infected animals, especially cattle. Treatment is with griseofulvin orally.

Tinea pedis is ringworm of the feet ('athlete's foot') spread by walking with bare feet, especially in swimming baths and sports dressing-rooms. The skin between the toes itches, is sodden and shows vesicles.

Treatment is by washing the feet and changing the socks twice daily, and fungicidal cream such as zinc undecanoate (tineafax) or Whitfield's ointment applied locally.

Tinea circinata is ringworm of the skin, a ring of itching scaly red skin showing vesicles.

Treatment is with fungicidal cream.

Tuberculides
Tuberculides are lesions, such as erythema nodosum and erythema induratum (Bazin's disease), due to hypersensitivity of the skin to tuberculin produced by tuberculosis elsewhere in the body.

Treatment is of the tuberculosis. Erythema nodosum has several causes.

Erythema Nodosum
Erythema nodosum is a hypersensitivity to toxins produced by tuberculosis, leprosy, sarcoidosis, streptococci (as in rheumatic fever) and to drugs.

Treatment is of the cause, an adequate diet and vitamins.

Lichen Planus
The cause is unknown but may be a virus. Itching, violet flat shiny papules appear over the skin and coalesce to form plaques. White papules appear on the mucous membranes of the mouth, throat, rectum and vagina. Scarring of the scalp may cause patchy baldness.

Treatment: drugs suspected of activating the condition are discontinued. Fluocinolone or betamethasone cream is applied and covered with an occlusive polythene film.

Urticaria
Urticaria is an allergic reaction of the skin due to certain foods, e.g. strawberries, shell-fish, eggs; drugs such as serum, penicillin or barbiturates; insects, e.g. the hairy caterpillar; nettle or jellyfish stings; or plants. Itchy pink papules and wheals (elevated pink areas with blanched centres) develop in the skin. Treatment is by removal of the cause, local calamine or hydrocortisone to allay irritation and an antihistamine orally (warning the patient that it causes drowsiness and to avoid driving a vehicle).

Alopecia (Baldness)
Alopecia may be genetic, as in the normal male, or acquired. It may be due to hyperthyroidism, hypothyroidism, infection such as secondary syphilis, or drugs such as cytotoxins.

Treatment is of the cause. There is no effective treatment for male or genetic baldness apart from the use of a wig.

Psoriasis

Psoriasis is a common inherited disease precipitated by infection or by trauma to the skin. Thickened reddish patches in the skin are covered by silvery-grey scales. It seldom itches and is not infectious. The nails are pitted, thickened and discoloured, if affected.

Treatment does not cure. Ultraviolet rays, 0·1-1% dithranol ointment, coal tar or corticosteroid (fluocinolone or betamethasone) ointment produce short remissions.

Acne Vulgaris

Acne is overactivity and blocking of the sebaceous glands, especially of the face, chest, shoulders and back. Oxidation of the sebum forms a comedone ('blackhead'). Inflammation develops, pustules appear and may be followed by scarring. Acne begins at the age of 13 years and subsides between 20 and 30 years of age.

Treatment is by frequent washing with soap and water. Woollen underclothing is avoided. The patient should be outdoors in all weathers as much as possible, since ultravoilet light helps.

The diet should contain adequate protein and vitamins. Local zinc sulphate lotion or resorcinol and sulphur paste may be used but creams and ointment are likely to make the condition worse. For pustular acne oxytetracycline 250 mg orally b.d. is given for weeks or months. Pustules may be punctured. Females may be given oestrogens.

Pityriasis Rosea

Pityriasis means scaling. Following an upper respiratory virus infection macules, followed by scaling, develop over the trunk. The rash clears in about six weeks and treatment is unnecessary.

Tumours (Neoplasms) of the Skin

Warts are of different types. Verrucae are warts due to a virus and are common on the fingers, hands and soles. They are infectious and tend to disappear within a few months.

Treatment is with caustics such as silver nitrate, phenol, podophyllin or by electric cautery or carbon dioxide ice, or by surgical excision.

Papillomas are benign tumours which occur commonly on exposed skin such as the face. They are also found on other surfaces e.g. on the mucosa of the colon and bladder.

Treatment is by curettage.

Naevi (birth marks) are congenital tumour-like abnormalities and may be removed surgically or with carbon dioxide ice.

Carcinomas. Basal cell carcinoma (rodent ulcer) is locally malignant but does not metastasise.

Treatment is by excision or radiotherapy and gives a high cure rate.

Epidermoid (Squamous Cell) Carcinoma often affects the face. It spreads to lymph nodes.

Treatment is by excision or radiotherapy and gives a high cure rate if treated before lymphatic spread occurs.

Melanomas are pigmented patches and may be benign or malignant.

Treatment is by excision.

Corn

A corn is a thickening of the keratin layers of the skin produced by repeated pressure, especially tight shoes. It may be painful.

Treatment is by shaving off the thickened part or the application of salicylic acid, and avoiding tight shoes.

Sunburn

Sunburn is due to ultraviolet light. The affected part is red and itches and may form vesicles and ulcers. The patient may feel ill, vomit and be dehydrated.

Treatment: blisters are left intact or opened aseptically and dehydration is treated. Calamine lotion may be used on erythematous areas.

Bedsores

Bedsores are gangrenous ulcers due to ischaemic death of the skin.

Causes: exclusion of blood from the skin by prolonged pressure caused by immobility (paralysis, stiff joints, sedation), lying or sitting on creases in linen, crumbs, or hard pads; or a moist skin, e.g. incontinence of urine or faeces, local sweating (sitting on plastic). Rough handling easily damages skin which is inelastic (elderly patients), has a poor circulation (atheroma) or is poorly nourished.

Friable skin, due to radiotherapy or oedematous conditions (cardiac failure, renal failure). Oedema and congestion embarrass the exchange of metabolites between the blood and the tissues.

Prevention: the use of flowform heel pads, flowform cushions, 'ripple' mattress, tilting bed, water bed, or frequent turning. The use of a hoist, and early mobilisation. The treatment of pressure areas as described under nursing procedures.

Treatment: dead tissue is removed. Local antiseptic should not be used since it damages newly growing tissue. Systemic antibiotic is given if the ulcer is infected. Ultraviolet light may be used. The area is kept clean and dry. Plastic surgery may be needed for large ulcers.

17 THE SPECIAL SENSES (EYE, EAR)

THE EYE (*Fig. 17.1*)

The wall of the eye consists of three layers: the sclera and cornea, the choroid and ciliary body, and the retina. The sclera is the tough outer white layer covered with conjunctiva in front and is continuous with the cornea. The choroid is vascular and pigmented, lines the sclera and becomes the ciliary body in front. The ciliary body

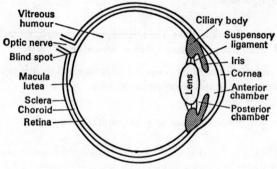

FIG. 17.1   The eye

contains the ciliary muscle, supports the lens through suspensory ligaments and extends forwards over the edge of the lens as the iris. The iris contains pigment and circular and radiating muscle fibres which control the size of the pupil, the opening in the centre of the iris. Bright light entering the pupil causes contraction of the circular fibres of the iris and constricts the pupil, thus reducing the amount of light reaching the retina and preventing retinal damage. In dim light the pupil is dilated by the contraction of the radiating muscle fibres, thus letting in more light. The colour of the iris depends upon the amount of pigment present. Pigment is absent in the albino (pink iris), present in small amounts in blue eyes, and in large amounts in brown eyes.

The lens is transparent, circular and biconvex. It is elastic and its thickness is controlled by the ciliary muscle which adjusts (accommodates) to bend (refract) light waves, reflected from objects, to focus onto the retina, particularly onto the macula lutea. It is surrounded by a capsule.

The retina consists of layers of nerve cells and nerve fibres. The most important nerve cells are the rods and cones. The rods are sensitive to dim light, the cones to bright light and colour. Colour vision is due to different colours having different wavelengths. A white object reflects all wavelengths, a green object absorbs all wavelengths except the green, which it reflects. The nerve fibres converge to form the optic nerve and where this leaves the eye is a blind spot, the optic disc.

Between the cornea and the lens is a space containing clear watery fluid, the aqueous humour, which drains into the circulation through small ducts in front of the ciliary body. The space in front of the iris is the anterior chamber, and that between the iris and the lens is the posterior chamber. Behind the lens is the jelly-like vitreous humour. An image must be projected onto the same part of the retina in each eye, otherwise two objects will be seen (diplopia). A single image is achieved by convergence of the eyes, i.e. the eyeballs are turned by the extrinsic muscles of the eyes (*Fig. 17.2*).

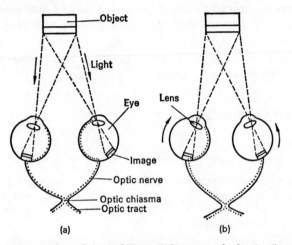

FIG. 17.2   (a) Diplopia due to the image falling on different parts of each retina; (b) convergence produces one image

The Accessory Organs of the Eye. The eyes are protected by the eyebrows, eyelids, eyelashes and lacrimal apparatus. Threat of danger to the eyes causes the eyelids to close (corneal reflex). The lacrimal glands lie above the sides of each eye and secrete tears which contain lysozyme, a bactericidal enzyme. The tears wash over the fronts of the eyes and drain via the nasolacrimal ducts into the nasal cavity.

DRUGS USED IN DISEASES OF THE EYE

Drugs may be used topically in eyedrops, ointments, lotions or in gelatin discs. An antibiotic may be injected subconjunctivally in intraocular infection, or given systemically.

Eyedrops. The lower lid should be everted and a drop expelled from a sterile dropper into the lower conjunctival fornix, not onto the cornea. Contact with tissues or lashes contaminates the dropper and should be avoided.

Ointments are inserted into the fornix using a sterile glass rod with the patient looking upwards. The patient closes the eye and the rod is withdrawn laterally, leaving the ointment in the conjunctival sac. If a tube is used, in order to prevent cross-infection, it must be used by only one patient.

Antibiotics are used in blepharitis (inflammation of the eyelids), bacterial conjunctivitis and in corneal ulcer.

Corticosteroids have an anti-inflammatory effect and are used locally in iritis, iridocyclitis, keratitis or allergic conditions but not in corneal ulceration as they increase the risk of corneal perforation and bacterial infection.

Mydriatics are drugs which dilate the pupil, but may precipitate glaucoma, e.g. atropine, homatropine, cyclopentolate (Mydrilate). They are used in iritis and iridocyclitis.

Miotics narrow the pupil and are used in glaucoma and to counteract mydriatics, e.g. pilocarpine, physostigmine (eserine).

DISEASES OF THE EYE

Conjunctivitis
Conjunctivitis is inflammation of the conjunctiva.

Bacterial Conjunctivitis produces inflammation and a discharge which causes the eyelids to stick together. A swab should be taken and the sensitivity of the organism to antibiotics tested. Penicillin, chloramphenicol or framycetin eyedrops are used two-hourly, plus systemic penicillin.

Viral Conjunctivitis may be due to herpes simplex.

Treatment is with idoxuridine (I.D.U.) 0·1% drops one- to two-hourly for 48 hours, and 1% atropine eight-hourly. The eye is covered with a pad and bandage. Corticosteroids must never be used in herpes simplex infection of the eye, since they stimulate wide spread of the virus and corneal perforation, with loss of the eye. Herpes zoster may involve the eye and treatment is with analgesic and local atropine to prevent synechiae.

Trachoma is an ocular infection by certain intracellular bacteria (chlamydiae), once thought to be a virus. Corneal scarring may cause blindness.

Treatment is with tetracycline.

Allergic Conjunctivitis may be due to local antibiotics, hair dyes, cosmetics, or hay fever (pollen allergy).

Treatment is avoidance of the cause or corticosteroid eye drops.

Uveitis
This is inflammation of the choroid or iris. It may be due to sarcoidosis, injury, or infection (gonococci, syphilis, tuberculosis). In iridocyclitis the inflamed iris adheres to the anterior surface of the lens to form posterior synechiae. This is prevented by dilatation of the pupil with 1% atropine eye drops t.d.s.

Exophthalmos
Exophthalmos (protrusion of the eyeball) is discussed under 'hyperthyroidism'.

Glaucoma
Glaucoma is an increased intraocular pressure due to obstruction to the outflow of aqueous from the eye by inflammation, congenital abnormality, a narrow angle at the root of the iris in long-sighted eyes, or of unknown cause (chronic simple glaucoma). Chronic glaucoma leads to optic atrophy and loss of vision.

Treatment is with eye drops of pilocarpine 2% t.d.s. and physostigmine (eserine) 1% t.d.s. Acetazolamide (Diamox) 500 mg stat. then 125–250 mg six-hourly orally. If these fail surgical iridectomy is performed.

Amblyopia
Amblyopia (dull vision) may be due to beriberi, vitamin B_{12} deficiency, tobacco, or methyl alcohol.

Cataract
Cataract is opacity of the lens of the eye. It is caused by corticosteroids, diabetes mellitus, injury, iridocyclitis, and ionising radiations, and occurs in the elderly.

Treatment is surgical.

Corneal Ulceration
This is usually due to trauma. There is a danger of panophthalmitis, i.e. widespread infection of the eye.

Treatment: antibiotic.

THE SENSE OF SMELL

The nose is discussed under 'Respiratory system'. Odours are due to particles of the odorous substance in the air. The particles dissolve in the secretions of the mucous membrane and stimulate the olfactory nerve endings in the mucosa of the roof of the nose. Nerve fibres pass through the cribriform plate of the ethmoid bone to the olfactory bulb, then backwards to the temporal lobes. Repeated exposure to an odour decreases its perception. Many 'tastes' are really odours.

THE SENSE OF TASTE

The nerve endings for taste are present in taste buds on the tongue, soft palate and pharynx. Taste sensation from the anterior two-thirds of the tongue is received by the chorda tympani branch of the facial (seventh) nerve, and from the posterior one third of the tongue and the pharynx by the glossopharyngeal (ninth) nerve. There are four tastes: sweet, sour, bitter and salt. Impulses pass to the thalamus then to the taste area in the cerebral cortex.

THE EAR

The ear consists of the external ear (the auricle or pinna, and the external auditory canal), the middle ear (tympanic cavity) and the inner ear (*Fig. 7.2*). The pinna helps to cut off sound from behind and to collect sound from in front and the side and to direct it along the external canal to the middle ear. The external canal contains ceruminous glands which secrete cerumen (wax) which waterproofs and protects it. At the end of the canal is the tympanic membrane separating the external ear from the middle ear.

The middle ear lies in the temporal bone and air reaches it through the auditory (pharyngotympanic, Eustachian) tube to balance the air pressure on the outside of the tympanic membrane (*Fig. 7.2*). The tympanic membrane transmits sound vibrations through three minute bones (auditory ossicles), the malleus, the incus, and the stapes, to the cochlea, which is in the inner ear and which contains the auditory nerve endings. The three semicircular canals are also within the inner ear. They signal changes in the position of the head along the vestibular nerve to the brain stem and thence to the cerebellum. The cerebellum also receives impulses of proprioception from muscles and joints and thus co-ordinates body balance.

Deafness
Deafness is of two types:

1 Nerve (perceptive) deafness, due to cochlear disease or to a damaged auditory nerve, e.g. hereditary deaf-mutism, congenital rubella, tumours, persistent loud sound (boiler-makers, discotheques), Ménière's disease.

2 Conduction deafness, due to otosclerosis (fusion of the ossicles), otitis media, obstruction of the external auditory canal (wax, foreign body) or Eustachian tube (upper respiratory infections).

Treatment: deaf children must be educated and learn to speak and to lip read. Hearing aid for the partially deaf.

Pain in the Ear
This may be due to infection of the external auditory canal (otitis externa), middle ear (otitis media), inner ear (labyrinthitis), or mastoid bone (mastoiditis), or to injury, e.g. barotrauma. Symptoms such as vertigo, tinnitus and headache are discussed in Chapter 13.

Otitis Externa
This may be due to plugging with wool and retention of secretions or to bacteria or fungi, and is predisposed by eczema or poking into the ear with hairclips or matchsticks.

Treatment is by cleaning using a probe tipped with non-fluffing wool, and by instilling local antibiotic.

Otitis Media

Otitis media (infection of the middle ear) is usually due to spread of infection along the Eustachian tube from the pharnyx. There is fever, rapid pulse rate, deafness and intense earache. The eardrum becomes inflamed and oedematous. If the drum perforates pus discharges from the ear, with relief of pain.

Treatment is with local heat, ephedrine inhalation or nasal drops, systemic antibiotic and analgesic. If pus is present, incision of the drum (myringotomy) to drain the pus. A discharging ear should be mopped out and kept covered. Inadequate therapy leads to mastoiditis, chronic otitis media and deafness. Other complications are facial palsy and lateral sinus thrombosis. Pain behind the ear (mastoiditis) or headache, vomiting and photophobia (meningitis, brain abscess) should be reported.

Wax

A small amount of soft wax is normally present in the external auditory canal. Large amounts cause deafness and may be removed by softening with drops of olive oil or with forceps. Syringing with warm water (35°C) may be used (but not if there is a perforation of the drum), but there is the danger of rupturing the drum if the jet hits the drum directly.

18   GERIATRICS

Gerontology is the study of old age. Geriatrics is the study and care of the elderly and their diseases. The proportion of old people in the community is slowly rising owing to increased survival, especially of women.

Many of the elderly are quite healthy, socially and intellectually active, and independent.

In normal old age there is a decrease in strength, loss of body height due to osteoporosis, and poor memory for recent events.

The old have the same diseases as the young, but have a higher incidence of degenerative diseases, and accidents are more likely to have serious consequences; e.g. a fractured femur may turn a person, previously self-supporting, into an invalid reliant on others. Since they are old they have outlived their friends, and often their relatives cannot look after them for social reasons such as overcrowding or financial difficulties forcing the relatives to work, leaving nobody at home to look after the infirm.

Working with geriatric patients may give the impression that most elderly people end up in geriatric hospitals suffering from strokes, dementia, incontinence and immobility. This is not true since only one in every 1,000 of people over the age of 65 years go into hospital, and 60% of these are discharged home. 20% will die, but this has to be accepted since there is a limit to all life. 20% become long-term patients.

DISORDERS ESPECIALLY AFFECTING THE OLD

The causes, symptoms, signs, and treatment of these conditions have been described in the earlier chapters.

Atheroma causes cerebrovascular lesions (thrombosis, embolism), dementia, coronary arterial disease, and peripheral vascular disease causing nocturnal cramp in the legs or intermittent claudication. Hemiplegic patients can use their 'good' hand to feed themselves if the food does not need cutting up. Large pieces of food will be left uneaten. A non-slip table mat is useful.

Hypertension. The blood pressure tends to rise naturally with age. Hypertension may lead to cardiac failure or cerebral haemorrhage.

Ankle Oedema is common. It is often postural and results from immobility and a poor venous return, but may be due to cardiac failure.

Postural Hypotension is often associated with drugs, especially sedatives, tranquillisers, antidepressants and diuretics, with vasodilatation, e.g. a hot bath, and with cerebrovascular disease. It occurs in 30% of people over the age of 75 years owing to delayed vasomotor response to standing up suddenly.

Heart Failure and Arrhythmias are common, and may have multiple causes in the elderly. Dyspnoea on exertion is often not a complaint owing to inactivity.

Anaemia is usually due to iron deficiency but may be normochromic, due to chronic renal failure or burnt-out rheumatoid arthritis.

Falls, 'Blackouts' and Giddiness may be due to cardiac arrhythmias, epilepsy, transient ischaemic attacks, postural hypotension, or pneumonia.

Pulmonary Tuberculosis has its highest incidence in elderly men.

Bronchopneumonia is a common complication of cardiac failure, but pyrexia may be absent.

Hypothermia may be due to hypothyroidism, to immobility which prevents the patient from making fires for heating, or to mental deterioration, the patient forgetting adequate clothing, heating and feeding.

Osteoporosis is mostly due to reduced activity but is partly due to deficiency of sex hormones, especially of oestrogen in women. It predisposes to fractures from minor injury. The fractures heal normally.

Loss of Teeth causes changes in the jaw bones, so that dentures do not fit, chewing is painful or difficult, and malnutrition may follow unless food is taken in small portions so that chewing is not necessary.

Deficiencies of vitamins and minerals is common in those living alone who live on 'tea and toast'.

Osteoarthrosis ('osteoarthritis') is usually present. It affects weight-bearing joints (spine, hips, knees), prevents mobility, and may prevent bathing through difficulty in getting out of the bath. Arthritis often leads to feeding difficulties because of deformity, pain, or poor grip. It is easier for the disabled to eat food that can be picked up with the fingers.

Nocturnal frequency, producing insomnia is often due to incipient or actual cardiac failure.

Urinary Incontinence may be due to urinary infection, prolapsed uterus, or confusion. In aphasia the patient is unable to ask for a urinal and may appear to be incontinent. The cure is to offer a urinal at frequent intervals. Large volumes of fluids and diuretics should be avoided near bedtime.

Bowel Disorders. Constipation is common and is due to neglect of the call to stool, a diet low in roughage (the old tend not to eat vegetables), and to intestinal obstruction, e.g. carcinoma of the large bowel. Diarrhoea is due to the causes found at any age, but it is often due to faecal incontinence due to impacted faeces caused by constipation, detected by digital rectal examination.

Failing Vision is common. It reduces mobility and interests, e.g. reading. 20% are improved by glasses (a magnifying lens may help); others have senile cataract, retinopathy (diabetic, hypertensive), or glaucoma.

Glaucoma can be detected by routine screening. Early treatment may prevent visual loss.

Deafness is common. It causes difficulty in communication, in making friends, and in hearing the radio and television, thus causing a loss of active interests. Hearing may be improved by removal of excess wax from the ears or with a hearing aid which must be correctly adjusted. Lip-reading can be facilitated by speaking slowly and clearly, facing the patient.

Psychiatric Disorders include depression, paranoia, dementia (senile and arteriosclerotic) and acute confusional states. Confusion is often due to drugs, and sometimes to urinary or respiratory infection, cerebral ischaemia or hypoxia. Assistance may be needed at meal times. The depressed do not bother to eat, and the demented may not be capable of feeding.

Insomnia is often a complaint but the old need less sleep than the young. Waking early or lying awake for an hour or so is common in the old and this should be explained to them. Drugs should be avoided if possible, and barbiturates should not be used in treating insomnia since they cause confusion in the elderly. Nitrazepam (Mogadon) 2·5–10 mg o.n. or chloral hydrate are suitable. Activity during the day is prophylactic.

Cancer accounts for 16% of deaths over the age of 65 years. Cancers in the elderly are often slowly growing and they can often be alleviated.

Drug therapy in the elderly

Adverse drug reactions are more common in the elderly than in younger people. This is because excretion by the kidneys, and metabolism by the liver, is diminished with ageing. Reduced renal excretion predisposes to ototoxicity and nephrotoxicity with aminoglycosides, hypoglycaemia with chlorpropamide, neuropathy with nitrofurantoin, and intoxication with digitalis. The reduced efficiency of hepatic metabolism leads to higher concentrations and a more prolonged effect of certain drugs, e.g. 20 mg of propranolol ('Inderal') in an old person may produce a similar plasma concentration as 40 mg in a younger individual.

Retention of urine may be precipitated by drugs which relax bladder tone, such as sympathomimetic drugs (e.g. ephedrine) and anticholinergic (atropine-like) drugs (e.g. propantheline, tricyclic antidepressives, antihistamines, antiemetics, and the antiparkinsonian agents benzhexol and orphenadrine).

Incontinence of urine can be precipitated by drugs which depress central control (sedatives, tranquillizers) or increase urine flow (diuretics).

When possible, drugs should be avoided in the elderly and alternatives tried first, e.g. a hot milk drink instead of a hypnotic. If drugs are necessary, the fewest possible should be used.

Before a new drug is given it is advisable to know what other drugs the patient is having so that drug interactions can be avoided. Certain drugs should be given in smaller doses than usual (e.g. digoxin, corticosteroids, streptomycin).

The old are more likely to fail to take drugs, owing to forgetfulness or dementia or may take the wrong dosage due to poor eyesight or hearing. Supervision is required under these circumstances. Time should be spent explaining the effects of the drug, and of omitting it, since a patient who understands why he is taking tablets will appreciate the consequences of omitting a dose. Elderly patients may not be able to read the instructions on the label of the container and should, therefore, be told verbally the reason for the drug, its name, its dose, its timing, and any serious side effects.

If a patient is on long term therapy, regular visits should be made by the district nurse, health visitor or doctor, to check that the patient is taking the drug correctly and to look for complications.

Care of the Elderly

In order to maintain activity and happiness in the old, and to reduce the demands on the social services, it is important to protect the old from injury, infection and malnutrition with advice and help from the family doctor, health visitor, district nurse, medical social worker, and the priest or minister. It is better if advisors work together in a common centre so that the exchange of information is rapid and adequate, and medical records are easily available. Delays mean that help is often too late. A common cause of delay in attending to the needs of the old is that the elderly take deterioration in health for granted and do not report it.

It is preferable that the elderly live in their own homes since they prefer independence, and institutionalising old people causes loss of independence, some loss of personal identity, and loss of routine work, which increases apathy. Further lack of interests is caused by inability to read or watch television (cataract, glaucoma), or to hear (wax in the ears, nerve deafness) and by being ignored by others. Apathy leads to neglect of clothing, personal appearance and diet. To retain interest hospital patients should be given small tasks to perform; the nurse should talk to the patients, stimulate them to talk to each other, and encourage relatives to visit, frequent brief visits being better than infrequent long ones. The life of the elderly can be improved by treating not only those diseases which may be totally incapacitating, such as angina, cardiac failure, and hemiplegia, but also those conditions which have pronounced social disadvantages, such as cataract, constipation, and wax in the ears, and by providing aids and assistance.

Dangers in the home should be avoided such as unguarded fires, gas fires and ovens that need lighting with matches, slippery floors, and loose mats. To prevent falling in the dark the light switch should be near the bed, or a bedside lamp used.

Old people should be visited frequently, especially in cold weather, to make sure they are warmly clothed and that their diet is adequate and balanced. The social services provide home help, laundry services, meals on wheels, aids (commodes, bed rests, disposable bedding, plastic covers for mattresses, aids for walking, wheelchairs), chiropody services, and financial help.

Local councils may provide individual bungalows or flats with an inter-communicating system so that the old people can talk to their home warden who lives in the centre.

If the person cannot manage at home, residential accommodation in a hostel is offered, and this may be temporary; e.g. when a relative or friend, who is looking after the patient, goes on holiday.

Day-care centres provide meals, physiotherapy, occupational therapy, and contact with others, the patient returning home each evening and thus retaining some independence.

Hospital services for the elderly provide treatment, and rehabilitation for ward patients and day cases. They sometimes provide holiday relief for relatives, but this is not the function of the hospital but of the hostel or day-care centre.

If the patient attends clinics, physiotherapy or other centres, appointments should be given in writing, otherwise they may be forgotten, and the mode of transport should be suitable for the patient's abilities.

The type of service and treatment required is decided after a geriatric assessment has been made. Assessment includes the detection of physical disabilities such as inability to dress, eat or walk—can the patient do these at all? with help? or unaided? urinary incontinence; faculties of speech, sight and hearing; and mental condition, whether normal, confused or demented. Full physical examination, a blood count, urinanalysis and chest X-ray should be performed.

Confinement of the elderly to bed should be avoided if possible, since it leads to contractures, bedsores, osteoporosis, incontinence, apathy, and the permanently bedridden state.

19 THE CONTROL AND ADMINISTRATION OF DRUGS, POISONING, ALCOHOL

Acts of Parliament control the sale and distribution of drugs and poisons. Certain drugs require a prescription. Drugs previously known as 'Dangerous Drugs' are now included, with certain other drugs, under the heading of 'Controlled Drugs'.

Prescription
The prescription for controlled drugs must be indelible, must show the address of the prescriber (except N.H.S. or social health authority prescriptions), and in the prescriber's own handwriting must show the name and address of the patient, the date, the dose and the total amount of medicine to be supplied.

In prescribing drugs for in-patients there should be a prescription sheet on which prescriptions and a record of administration ONLY are written. The sheet must be available to the doctor whenever he is seeing a patient, and to the nurse whenever medicines have to be given. Not more than one prescription sheet should be in use at one time for a patient. A new sheet must not be started merely because the first is not immediately available. Full sheets should be cancelled and retained with the patient's notes.

The sheet should show the name and age of the patient, his unit number and ward. Drugs are written preferably in CAPITAL letters, giving the quantity, form, time and route of administration, and signed by the prescriber. Drug cancellations are shown by being crossed out, initialled and dated.

Storage of Drugs
Ward stocks must be appropriate for the needs of the ward, regularly checked by the pharmacist, and ordered by the ward sister or charge nurse or their deputy, on a printed requisition form. All drugs must be kept in locked containers, including drugs in transit. Drugs regularly administered may be kept in a lockable container permanently fixed to a trolley which can be securely parked either in a lockable cupboard or by locking it to the wall or floor. The key to controlled drugs is kept by a qualified person.

Administration of Drugs
Hospital staff should be aware of all the drugs a patient has been having prior to admission to hospital (these drugs are legally the property of the patient), especially steroids, insulin and digoxin, and beware of drug incompatibility.

Medicine rounds should be at the same time each day and should be taken when possible by two nurses, excluding nursing auxiliaries. When the medication is a controlled drug one of the nurses must be qualified.

No medication is given to a patient unless it is prescribed by a medical officer. Treatment may be cancelled only by the medical officer.

Procedure for Checking Drugs

1 Before administration of a drug the patient must be identified correctly, using the identity band/bed card AND by addressing the patient by name.

2 The written prescription is read and the dose, time and route of administration must be clearly understood by both nurses.

3 The label of the appropriate container is checked with the drug treatment sheet.

4 The correct amount of the drug is placed in the appropriate measure and the contents of the measure re-checked with the drug treatment sheet and the container.

5 The container is returned to the cupboard and the cupboard is locked if it contains a controlled drug.

6 The nurse checking the procedure observes the administration of the medicine.

7 The nurse giving the drug records its administration on the prescription sheet at the time the drug is given to the patient. In the case of a controlled drug this is also recorded in the Controlled Drugs register, *signed* (not initialled) by both nurses (one of whom must be qualified), and the remaining stock checked.

The dose of the drug should not be set out in advance of the medicine round.

Injections

The skin is cleaned with antiseptic and allowed to dry. The drug is checked against the patient's name. Air is emptied from the syringe by holding it vertically and forcing fluid into the needle, holding a swab at the end of the needle to prevent the drug from spraying into the air. The skin is drawn taut and the needle inserted at 30° for subcutaneous injection, or at 90° for intramuscular injection. The plunger is withdrawn to make sure the needle is not in a blood vessel. The drug is injected fairly quickly and the area massaged with a swab. For frequent injections the site is changed each time. Care must be taken not to inject near nerves.

Intradermal (i.d.) injection is painful and can be used for only small amounts of solution. It is used in sensitivity testing.

Subcutaneous (hypodermic, s.c.) injection is the injection of up to 2 ml of solution just under the skin, usually on the outer aspect of the thigh or arm or on the abdomen. The drug becomes effective in about 20 minutes.

Intramuscular (i.m.) injection is injection into the deltoid, quadriceps (thigh), preferably the outer aspect, or the upper and outer quadrant of the buttock (*Fig. 15.6*) for up to 10 ml of fluid.

DRUG INTERACTIONS

Certain drugs alter the actions of other drugs. Thus the anticoagulant action of warfarin is increased by sulphonamides, nalidixic acid, salicylates or phenylbutazone; the antihypertensive action of adrenergic blockers is lost if amphetamine, sympathomimetics, or tricyclic antidepressants are given; barbiturates decrease the action of several drugs by increasing their inactivation by the liver; and the hypoglycaemic action of the sulphonylureas is increased by sulphonamides, salicylates and phenylbutazone.

Antacids containing magnesium, aluminium or calcium reduce the absorption of tetracyclines by chelation. Tetracyclines and chloramphenicol are inactivated by lactate solution. Penicillins are inactivated in solutions containing tetracyclines, hydrocortisone or vitamin C. The activity of the penicillins and kanamycin is reduced if added to dextrose solution, which is slightly acid.

POISONING

Poisons may be inhaled (carbon monoxide, sprays, dusts), swallowed, injected, or absorbed through the skin. Treatment is of three types, general, the use of antidotes (specific and non-specific), and symptomatic. General treatment is required in most cases since there is usually no specific antidote.

Ingested Poisons

These may be corrosive (acids, caustic soda, ammonia) or non-corrosive. Corrosives damage the tissues they contact, causing blistering or ulceration of the mouth, dysphagia, abdominal pain, tachycardia, and vomiting, often of blood and shreds of damaged tissue.

Further absorption of poison is prevented by immediately emptying the stomach by inducing vomiting or by gastric aspiration and lavage, except after paraffin oil and petroleum ingestion since even a small amount of these entering the lungs causes severe pneumonitis.

Vomiting is induced by stimulating the fauces, e.g. with the fingers, or by giving an emetic, e.g. syrup of ipecacuanha 20 ml orally, within four hours of ingestion of the poison. Apomorphine 2–8 mg s.c. may be given, neutralising with nalorphine (lethidrone) 5–10 mg i.v. after vomiting. Vomiting may be induced after four hours if drugs which delay gastric emptying have been taken e.g., salicylates, tricyclic antidepressants, atropine. Vomiting should not be induced after corrosive ingestion since corrosives burn the tissues.

Gastric lavage: false teeth are removed and the procedure is briefly explained to the patient, emphasising that although it is uncomfortable, with the patient's co-operation it does not take long. The patient is placed semi-prone on the left side with the head-end of the table tilted 15° below the hips to reduce the risk of inhalation of fluid. A cuffed endotracheal tube may be introduced to reduce the risk of inhalation and must be used in corrosive poisoning or in the comatose patient. A stomach tube, lubricated with water or with the minimum amount of liquid paraffin, is passed; its position is verified by aspiration of gastric contents with a syringe, and the stomach is emptied. If the stomach is not emptied, lavage may force gastric contents into the duodenum and promote absorption. Lavage is performed by attaching a funnel to the stomach tube and pouring in 300 ml of tap water with the funnel raised above the patient, then lowering the funnel below the level of the patient to aspirate, tilting the funnel to pour into a container. This is repeated, using 300–600 ml of tap water each time, until the washings are clear. The initial aspirate and the first washing are kept for examination, suitably labelled. The stomach tube is passed with special care after corrosive ingestion since it may perforate the oesophagus or stomach (the benefits of lavage outweigh the dangers).

Gastric lavage should be performed up to six hours after ingestion of poison. After this time the stomach will have emptied unless there is gastrointestinal stasis, as in severe poisoning, and in salicylate poisoning when pylorospasm prevents gastric emptying and the drug can be aspirated up to 24 hours after ingestion.

After lavage for salicylates 10 g sodium bicarbonate is left in the stomach to combat acidosis, and a diuresis is forced with 200 ml 25% mannitol i.v. or with a diuretic such as frusemide 40 mg i.v., and abundant oral or i.v. fluid is given.

If corrosives cannot be aspirated, for acids give magnesia, chalk or whitewash in 500 ml water. For alkalis give citric acid (or the juice of six lemons), tartaric or acetic acid (vinegar 50 ml in 500 ml water). After neutralising a corrosive a demulcent (such as whites the of three eggs in 300 ml water), or milk, is given. For **bleach** give sodium thiosulphate 5 g in 200 ml water orally.

Paracetamol overdosage of more than 15 g in a single dose or a plasma level exceeding 200 mg/l at four hours and 70 mg/l at 12 hours after ingestion, is likely to cause liver damage. *Treatment:* gastric lavage (or syrup of ipecacuanha 10–15 ml in children under 5 years).

Haemodialysis or haemoperfusion removes free paracetamol from the blood. The formation of toxic metabolites is reduced by cysteamine 2 g i.v. in 5% dextrose over 10 minutes then 800 mg in the next four hours and 800 mg in the next 16 hours, or by methionine 2·5 g four hourly orally for four doses or by i.v. acetylcysteine.

Poisoning by Sedatives and Tranquillisers, e.g. Barbiturates cause respiratory depression, cardiac failure, shock and coma. The airway is cleared by suction and positioning of the neck, and the stomach is washed out. Severe respiratory depression requires artificial respiration, urinary retention needs catheterisation. Irregularity of the pulse and other evidence of heart failure is watched for, and the blood pressure is recorded. For shock, the foot of the bed is elevated, and if necessary metaraminol 2–5 mg i.m. is given to raise the blood pressure. In severe poisoning a forced alkaline diuresis is obtained by giving 500 ml 1·26% sodium bicarbonate i.v. then 200 ml 25% mannitol i.v., each in 30 minutes. Haemodialysis may be used. Naloxone (Narcan) 0·4 mg i.v. or i.m. is given for poisoning with morphine, pethidine, methadone, or pentazocin.

Mushroom or Parathion (Insecticide) Poisoning. Atropine 2 mg i.v. is given every 10 minutes until signs of atropinisation appear. Pralidoxime mesylate 1 g i.v. slowly may be given in addition to atropine.

Paraquat (Weedkiller) produces ulceration of the buccal cavity and fauces. More than 10 ml leads to liver, renal and cardiac damage and death within hours or days from pulmonary oedema and haemorrhage. Smaller amounts produce pulmonary fibrosis and respiratory failure. *Treatment:* gastric lavage, purgative and Bentonite (aluminium silicate) or 30% Fullers earth orally to prevent absorption.

Acute Iron Poisoning. Children may take coloured tablets if left within reach. Iron poisoning causes shock and haemorrhagic gastro-enteritis. After gastric lavage using desferrioxamine 2 g in 1 l of warm water, 10 g desferrioxamine in 100 ml water is left in the stomach to chelate iron left in the gut and 2 g is given 12-hourly i.m. or i.v.

Heavy metals. Poisoning with arsenic, antimony, bismuth, gold or mercury is treated with dimercaprol (BAL) 2·5 mg/kg six-hourly deeply i.m., then b.d. for three days, then once daily until recovery or with D-penicillamine 300 mg t.d.s. Lead poisoning is treated with calcium disodium edetate (Versenate) 20 mg/kg slowly i.v. b.d. as 2% solution in 5% dextrose or normal saline, or with D-penicillamine.

Inhaled Poisons. Carbon monoxide is present in coal gas and car exhausts, and has an affinity for haemoglobin which is 200 times that of oxygen, thus causing hypoxia, with headache, dyspnoea, giddiness and weakness. 0·2% in air may be fatal. Complications include arrhythmias and cardiac failure.

Treatment: move the patient into fresh air, make sure the airway is clear; give artificial respiration and oxygen. Oxygen with 5% carbon dioxide is better since it stimulates the respiratory centre. Hyperbaric oxygen displaces carbon monoxide from haemoglobin, and is used in severe poisoning if it can be given within 30 minutes.

Poisons on the Skin or Conjunctiva should be washed off.

Symptomatic treatment of respiratory failure, shock, renal failure, and coma has been described earlier.

Psychiatric Help should be given on recovery.

ALCOHOL

Alcohol is both a poison and a drug of addiction. It is rapidly absorbed from the stomach, and is metabolised to water and carbon dioxide, supplying energy (calories). It is a diuretic, vasodilator, and central nervous system depressant. The apparent initial stimulating effect is due to inhibition of the normal control of the higher centres of the brain, thus removing inhibitions. Larger amounts cause disturbed behaviour, muscular inco-ordination and coma.

Alcohol may precipitate a fit in an epileptic. It increases the actions of sedatives, such as barbiturates.

Acute intoxication is treated by making the patient vomit or by gastric lavage, and by giving vitamin B_1 i.m., and copious fluids. Spontaneous vomiting in the semiconscious patient may cause asphyxia by inhalation of vomit.

Gastric contents should be observed and saved for examination. Signs of injury should be looked for. Chronic alcoholism causes muscular inco-ordination ('the shakes'), chronic gastritis, hepatic cirrhosis, cardiomyopathy, neuropathy (peripheral neuritis and optic atrophy), mental deterioration, hallucinations, delirium tremens and dementia. Treatment is reduction of alcohol intake, with sedation to prevent withdrawal symptoms; aversion therapy and psychotherapy.

Alcohol has no medicinal use except in terminal disease such as cancer, and possibly in peripheral vascular disease. Its use as a sedative may lead to addiction. It should not be used as 'first aid' in shock since it causes vasodilatation which increases the shock.

Everybody has to die. Most people hope that it will be later rather than sooner, but to a few death is a merciful release from chronic illness or depression.

One problem, in a patient with fatal incurable disease, is what to tell the patient; and this depends on each individual since each patient's needs differ. There is an occasional patient who prefers not to discuss his illness although subconsciously he guesses, and fears, the truth but does not wish to face it consciously. It would be wrong to say anything which might bring the truth to this patient's conscious mind. Another person will phrase his questions to show that he is seeking reassurance rather than the truth; thus any direct answer that might suggest death should be avoided. The attendant should never lie since the patient may detect the lie, will no longer trust the attendant, and will have guessed the truth. Others wish to know the truth and should be told it in time for them to make a will and put their affairs in order, but should not be told in one sudden blow. The blow should be soft and gradual so that the patient can adjust to it more easily. Tact and kindness should be used. The patient with incurable cancer should first be told, e.g., that one possible cause of his symptoms may be cancer, but that in any case many cancers are curable (which is true). Several days, or perhaps weeks, later (depending on how near is death) he is told that he does have cancer but that the treatment he is having is hoped to be effective, which is true for many cancers and is true if the treatment is for pain or secondary infection.

Unpleasant information should be given by a person who is experienced and tactful.

Near relatives must be informed of the diagnosis and prognosis, and may need sympathetic support.

The patient should not be left on his own, but should receive full attention, which will be appreciated by both the patient and his relatives. During his last hours the patient should not be left in anxious loneliness, but should be comforted, preferably by a close relative.

Last Offices

After death the bedclothes are removed, except for a sheet and a pillow, and the pyjamas are taken off. A record of rings and jewellery is entered into the ward record book; the items are removed and given to the hospital administrator, except for the wedding ring if the relatives wish it to be left on the finger. The nurse should not give them to the patient's friends since they may pass to the wrong person. The mouth is cleaned and any dentures replaced.

Rigor mortis, a stiffening of the muscles, begins soon after death. Before this the eyes should be closed and if necessary the lids are held in place with pads of damp wool. The limbs are straightened, the mouth is closed, and the lower jaw supported by a roll of bandage beneath the chin or passed around the head and jaw, split in the centre where the chin rests on it. The support is removed when rigor mortis sets in.

About an hour after death the nurse and an assistant should 'lay out' the body. It is washed with soap and water, the nails are trimmed, the nostrils and ears are cleaned with moist swabs, and small wool plugs inserted using forceps. The rectum and vagina are plugged with absorbent wool to prevent the escape of discharges. The ankles are tied together with bandage, the hair is combed, the face of a male is shaved, clean dressings placed on wounds, and a nightgown or shroud is put on. The hands are placed behind the buttocks or across the chest.

The patient's name, the ward and the hour and date of death are recorded on a slip of paper attached to the case notes. The patient's full name is written on the leg or on a tape tied around the ankle.

The body is covered with a clean sheet and removed to the mortuary. Linen and blankets are sent to the laundry, plastic-covered mattresses, bed-frames and lockers are washed with soap and water or wiped with antiseptic.

21 IONISING RADIATIONS

Ionising radiations are rays produced by special machines or given off from radio-active isotopes, e.g. X-rays from high-voltage machines or gamma (γ) rays from radioactive elements such as radium or radioactive iodine.

Note: Non-ionising radiations include ultraviolet and infrared rays which are used in physiotherapy.

Use: small amounts of X-rays are used in taking X-ray films, and traces of radioactive isotopes are used to show the function of an organ, e.g. the radioactive iodine uptake by the thyroid in thyroid disease, radioactive phosphorus and iron in the measurement of blood volume.

Large amounts of X-rays or radioisotopes are used to kill tumour tissue. Radio-isotopes may be selectively taken up by certain tissues, e.g. iodine by the thyroid, phosphorus by the bone marrow.

Radioisotopes may be used in sealed containers (radium, gold, radon) which cannot leak, or may be given as unsealed liquids or powders which may accidentally spill. They are excreted in the urine or faeces, and may be present in vomit and cause contamination (radioiodine, phosphorus, gold).

Effects of Radiation

Therapeutic doses of radiation damage the tissues and produce a reaction similar to that of a burn. The patient has a burning feeling in the irradiated area. The tissues through which the radiations pass are also damaged. The skin through which X-rays enter and leave becomes erythematous or may dry and desquamate. In more severe burns the skin blisters and becomes moist, or the whole thickness of the skin may be destroyed. Hair may fall out. On healing the area becomes pigmented or leaves thin white scars which break easily and ulcerate on minor injury. Small dilated blood vessels (telangiectases) may appear. Radiation also produces sickness; the patient feels tired, has nausea and may vomit.

Nursing Care

Before radiotherapy the patient should take a well-balanced diet containing protein and vitamins. After therapy at least 2·5 l of fluid should be taken daily to prevent dehydration and to remove toxins. Patients with lesions of the mouth, throat and oesophagus need encouragement to take fluids; feeding by a Ryle's tube may be necessary, and a fluid balance chart should be kept. Radiation to the abdomen may cause dehydration from diarrhoea, and i.v. fluid may be needed.

The patient is susceptible to infection because he is already ill and has a low resistance. Radiation reduces this resistance still further. Prevention of cross-infection, especially if the white cell count is low, is by barrier nursing (Chapter 4). The patient should be in a side ward labelled 'Caution, radioactivity'. The nurse should keep at least 3 m (10 ft) away from the patient, except when this is impossible and should wear a film badge which indicates radiation dosage. Visitors' stay near the patient should be brief and those under 16 years or who are pregnant are not allowed to visit, owing to the possibility of radiation damage to growing tissues.

The skin must be kept dry and powdered with starch; not with heavy metals, such as zinc oxide, which increase burning. The skin where the X-rays enter and leave must not be washed. Shaving, heat, draughts and tight clothes are avoided since they may injure the sensitive skin. Sterile crusts may be left, but infected ones are removed.

An antiemetic, e.g. chlorpromazine, is given for radiation sickness.

Sealed radioactive containers should be inspected four-hourly to ensure that they have not been displaced. Containers of radium are removed with long-handled forceps and special rubber gloves are worn. They are placed in a second container (of lead) for transfer to the radium safe, and the removal slip is signed.

Unsealed radioactive isotopes may accidentally cause contamination. Internal contamination follows their ingestion or inhalation. To prevent this eating, drinking and smoking are prohibited in the room containing radioactive material. If there is external contamination the part should be washed immediately and thoroughly with detergent, and examined with a Geiger–Muller counter.

Disposal of Radioactive Waste

The excreta (urine and faeces) from the patients tested or treated with radioisotopes should be collected and stored in protected containers until monitoring by the Geiger–Muller counter shows that the radioactivity has decayed to a safe level, when it can be flushed down the sewage system.

Bedpans are cleaned by flushing with water for five minutes. Contaminated glassware, linen, clothing and the ashes from material which has been burned, are also stored and monitored. If radioactive material (e.g. urine) is spilt, it is mopped up with blotting paper held in forceps while wearing special rubber gloves; all contaminated material is put in a plastic bag which is placed in the lead-lined container.

The reasons for all precautions should be explained to the patient so as to obtain his understanding and co-operation.

Specific Isotopes

Radioactive Iodine (^{131}I) therapy may be used in thyrotoxicosis or in carcinoma of the thyroid with metastases. The patient is in a cubicle and has his own crockery. Rubber gloves are worn while crockery is being handled. All urine is collected for 48 hours, since iodine which is not taken up by the thyroid is excreted in the urine, and is kept in bottles in a lead-lined container. The patient's sweat may contain iodine and contaminate newspapers, books and clothing. Rubbish is placed in plastic bags and checked with a Geiger–Muller counter before disposal. Clothing is checked before the patient is sent home. Staff wear rubber gloves and aprons kept just outside the room.

Radioactive Colloidal Gold (^{198}Au) may be injected into a cavity, e.g. pleural, if there is a malignant effusion. To distribute the gold over the whole cavity the patient should have 20-minute periods lying on the back, the right side, the left side, and then the abdomen over about three hours. Leakage from the site of injection must be watched for, wearing special rubber gloves to inspect the dressing. Urine and faeces do not need special precautions.

Radioactive Phosphorus (^{32}P) is used in polycythaemia. It is excreted in the urine, which should be collected for 48 hours and its radioactivity measured to make sure it is low enough for safe disposal.

APPENDIX 1   THE GENERAL CARE OF THE PATIENT

The patient admitted to hospital enters a strange world and is apprehensive in case he has cancer or is to undergo an operation, and worries about his family at home. The nurse should introduce herself and deal with the patient calmly, tactfully, pleasantly and reassuringly.

The patient should be made comfortable. His name, age, address and religion; the name, address and telephone number of next-of-kin; and the name of his family doctor, should be recorded.

Rest in bed helps to combat disease but predisposes, especially in the elderly, to stiff joints, weak muscles, bedsores, constipation, and venous thrombosis, which must all be prevented. Noise disturbs rest and should be avoided. Cupboards, doors, bedpans and trolleys should not be allowed to bang, and nurses' shoes should have rubber soles and heels.

Daily Routine

Each morning the patient should be bathed and the bed made. The hands are washed in the middle of the day; after defaecation; and at night; and the hair is brushed (observing discreetly for parasites and nits). The mouth, skin and bowels are cared for. The patient is assessed for the intensity of treatment required on the grounds of age, general condition, degree of arterial disease, and the disease causing admission. Thus an elderly, poorly nourished patient with paralysis will need frequent turning and care to pressure areas, whereas a young fit person with appendicitis will need less intensive nursing.

Note: in the interests of both patients and staff, procedures of an intimate nature should not be performed by a male nurse on a female patient.

Feeding

The patient should be positioned comfortably and be allowed to wash his hands. The nurse washes her hands before handling crockery or cutlery or serving food. Everything should be within easy reach of the patient. Helpings should be small; more being given later if required. Only one course should be served at a time. Plates, glasses and cups should not be too full.

For recumbent patients a serviette is placed under the chin and the head is raised by placing the hand beneath the pillow, not under the neck. The patient is fed at his own pace. Liquids may be taken through a straw or from a feeder with tubing attached. The patient should be advised to place his tongue on the opening of the straw or tube to stop the flow of fluid when desired. A liquid diet may be given via a Ryle's tube passed through the nose.

The diet should be adequate in calories, fat, protein, vitamins and minerals.

Moving the Patient

The patient who is weak or unable to move should be lifted, not dragged, into position in bed. Dragging causes friction between the skin and the sheet and predisposes to bedsores. Before lifting, the pillows should be tidied and the bedclothes loosened. The nurse should not attempt to lift a heavy patient without assistance, either from the patient, if permitted, or from a second nurse. There are several ways of lifting. In the Australian lift each nurse places her shoulder under the patient's axilla and the arm below the thigh, grasping the other nurse's wrist. The nurse should keep her back straight, bending from the hips so as to prevent injury to her back.

To turn a patient the nurse stands at the side to which the patient is to be turned; places his arm across his chest and crosses his legs; reaches over him; and with one hand around the pelvis and the other below the shoulder, turns him towards her.

To move a patient from a trolley to a bed, the two are placed at right angles to each other, the head of one near the foot of the other. Three persons stand on the same side of the patient and lift together.

Bathing in Bed ('Blanket Bath')

Procedure. Explain the procedure to the patient. Screen the bed. Ask the patient if he wishes to use a bedpan or urinal. Place clean nightwear on a nearby radiator to warm. Turn the bedclothes back, leaving the patient covered with his top sheet. A large bath towel is placed beneath him to prevent the bedding from getting wet. Remove the patient's nightwear, drape a blanket over him if he is likely to feel cold, and wash him with soap and hot water, starting with the face and neck, using the face flannel and towel, allowing the patient to wash and dry his own face if able. A second (body) flannel is used for the remainder of the body, only exposing those parts of the patient which are being washed. When the arms, chest and abdomen have been washed and dried the water in the bowl is changed and the lower limbs, genitals and buttocks are washed. The patient should wash and dry his own pubic area, if able. If possible, the feet should be placed in the bowl of water.

During bathing the patient is unobtrusively examined, and any skin rashes, bruises, sacral oedema or other abnormality reported. The pressure areas are massaged during the bed bath, the patient dressed in the warmed nightwear, the nails trimmed if necessary, and the hair brushed or combed. The teeth or dentures are cleaned (the patient may do this) and a mouthwash is given.

The bed is made with clean linen and the patient repositioned and asked if he is comfortable.

Female patients may be helped with their cosmetics.

Care of the Skin (Pressure Areas)

The causes of 'bedsores' are discussed in Chapter 13. The areas to be treated are the elbows, shoulder blades, tips of the shoulders, occiput, vertebrae, iliac crests, buttocks, knees, ankles and heels.

Reassure the patient and explain the reason for the procedure. Close the windows and screen the patient. Turn back the bedclothes, leaving a sheet covering the patient. Clean the area with a damp 'inco' wipe, especially the buttocks if the patient is incontinent. Wash with soap and water, and at the same time massage gently but firmly with the palm of the hand, using a circular kneading movement so that the superficial tissues move over the deeper parts. Dry the area thoroughly. Sparingly apply fine talcum powder. Remake the bed.

Barrier creams or sprays do not prevent bedsores, but if they are used the area must be thoroughly washed and dried before they are applied or re-applied.

Pressure areas are treated two-hourly if the patient is confined to bed or is incontinent. The patient is encouraged to move in bed and his position should be regularly altered by turning. The sheet must be free from creases and crumbs.

Ripple beds, tilting beds and decubitus pads are aids to the prevention of pressure sores, but the above procedure must also be used.

Any indication of a pressure sore commencing must be reported immediately to the sister in charge. The first sign is a reddening of the skin, a burning feeling or irritation.

Care of the Nails and Hair

Fingernails should be trimmed with scissors to the shape of the fingertips. Toenails should be cut straight across (if cut short and curved, the free margin of the nail may dig into the tissues as it grows, producing an 'ingrowing toenail'. Nails cut more easily after soaking in warm water. The hair should be brushed or combed daily and washed weekly, observing for parasites and nits. If a man is too ill to shave himself, he may be shaved by a visiting barber, convalescent patient, or the nurse.

FIRE

If a fire occurs the nurse must sound the alarm, remove patients from near the fire, and try to put the fire out, e.g. disconnect electrical equipment if it is on fire. Doors and windows must be kept closed to avoid fanning the flames and spread of smoke to the rest of the hospital. More people die from smoke than burns and there is least smoke near the floor.

APPENDIX 2
VENEPUNCTURE (PHLEBOTOMY)

Explain the procedure to the apprehensive patient. The skin is allowed to dry if cleaned with a swab and spirit, the arm is held straight and steady. A large vein in the antecubital fossa is distended, if necessary, by blocking the venous return with a blood pressure cuff or tourniquet. The needle and syringe is held with the bevel of the needle upwards, the thumb of the free hand is used to stretch the skin to be punctured and the needle is pushed rapidly through the skin and into the vein, the wall of which is felt as a slight resistance. Blood is aspirated into the syringe, being careful not to withdraw the needle from the vein. The tourniquet is released to prevent leakage of blood into the tissues and bruising. The needle is then removed and pressure applied over the puncture with a clean swab (the patient can do this with his free hand) until bleeding stops. The blood sample is put into the appropriate bottle and mixed if anticoagulated.

APPENDIX 3   UNITS OF MEASUREMENT

Prefixes applied to symbols for various units:

T = tera = 10^{12}	1×10^{12} = one million million
G = giga = 10^{9}	1×10^{9} = one thousand million
M = mega = 10^{6}	1×10^{6} = one million, 1,000,000
k = kilo = 10^{3}	1×10^{3} = one thousand, 1000
c = centi = 10^{-2}	1×10^{-2} = one hundredth, 0·01
m = milli = 10^{-3}	1×10^{-3} = one thousandth, 0·001
μ = micro = 10^{-6}	1×10^{-6} = one millionth, 0·000001
n = nano = 10^{-9}	
p = pico = 10^{-12}	
f = femto = 10^{-15}	
a = atto = 10^{-18}	

Mass (weight) gram, g

1 g = 1000 mg = 1,000,000 μg = 15·4 grains = 0·035 ounces.   1 ounce = 28·4 g
1 kg = 1000 g = 2·2 lb.   1 lb = 453·6 g = 0·4536 kg   1 grain = 65 mg

Length metre, m   Angstrom unit, Å

1 m = 100 cm = 1000 mm = 1,000,000 μm = 10^{10} Å = 1·094 yard = 39·37 inches
1 km = 0·62 mile = 3281 ft   1 yard = 0·914 m   1 Å = 10 nm
1 inch = 2·54 cm   1 mile = 1760 yd = 5280 ft = 1·609 km

Area square metre, m^2

1 m^2 = 1·196 sq yd = 10·76 sq ft   1 sq yd = 0·836 m^2
1 acre = 4840 sq yd = 4047 m^2 1 sq mile = 640 acres = 2·59 km^2

Volume cubic metre (cu m), m^3 litre, l

1 cubic millimetre = 1 mm^3 = 1 cu mm
1 pint = 568 ml = 0·568 litre = 20 fl ounces
1 litre = 1000 ml = 35·2 fluid ounces = 1·76 pint
1 fluid ounce = 28·4 ml   1 gallon = 4·55 litre   1 ml = 1000 μl
1 cubic inch = 16·4 cm^3 1 cu ft = 0·028 m^3

Pressure Pascal Pa

1 atmosphere = 760 mm Hg (mercury) = 760 torr = 29·92 in Hg = 1033 g weight
per cm^2 = 1013 millibars = 1,013,250 dyn/cm^2 = 14·7 lb/in^2 = 101·3 kPa

Heat calorie (cal.), joule

1000 cal. = 1 kcal. = 1 C = 4·187 J (joule).

Temperature: each °C (Celsius, Centigrade) = 1·8°F, 1°C = 32+1·8°F

°C = (°F−32)×$\frac{5}{9}$

°C	0	10	20	30	35	37	40	45	100
°F	32	50	68	86	95	98·6	104	113	212

A mole (mol) is the molecular or atomic weight, in grams, of a substance (whether atoms, molecules or ions), and it contains a standard number of particles.

APPENDIX 4 MAXIMUM DESIRABLE BODY WEIGHTS OF ADULTS

HEIGHT (no shoes)			Men		WEIGHT (naked)	Women
cm	ft	in	kg Medium frame	lb + for large frame − for small frame	kg Medium frame	lb + for large frame − for small frame
150	4	11	53 ± 5	117 ± 11	50 ± 5	111 ± 11
153	5	0	54 5	119 11	52 5	114 11
155	5	1	55 5	121 11	53 5	117 11
158	5	2	56 5	124 11	54 5	120 12
160	5	3	58 5	128 11	56 5	123 12
163	5	4	60 5	132 12	57 6	126 12
165	5	5	62 5	136 12	59 6	130 12
168	5	6	63 6	140 12	61 6	134 12
170	5	7	65 6	144 13	62 6	138 12
173	5	8	67 6	148 13	64 6	141 12
175	5	9	69 6	152 13	66 7	145 13
178	5	10	71 6	157 13	68 7	149 13
180	5	11	73 6	162 13	70 7	154 13
183	6	0	76 6	168 13	72 7	159 13
186	6	1	79 6	174 14	74 7	164 13
188	6	2	81 7	179 14	76 7	169 13

(for shoes and clothes add 10 lb in men and 6 lb in women)

APPENDIX 5   DIETS

1   Semifluid Diet

Milk, custard, junket, Benger's food, jellies, eggs, chocolate, plain toffee, ice cream, sugar, soft bread and butter, mashed potatoes, minced meat, purée vegetables and liquidized foods. Used in very ill patients e.g. typhoid, dysphagia, and E.N.T. disorders.

2   Low Roughage (Low Residue) Diet

Allowed: tea, coffee, cocoa, milk, Horlicks, Ovaltine, baked custard, ice cream, yoghurt, sugar, Cornflakes, Rice Krispies, white bread, sponge or milk pudding, mashed potatoes, flower of cauliflower, marrow, sieved vegetable juice, vegetable extract, bacon, ham, meat, poultry, fish, cheese, jelly, fruit purée, butter, margarine, honey.

Not allowed: brown or wholemeal breads or biscuits, coarse cereals, roast or chipped potatoes, peas, beans, onions, leeks, radishes, cress, cucumber, celery, parsley, skins and pips in tomatoes, jam or marmalade, fruit, nuts, pickles, mustard, curry powder, sauces, chutney, spices, duck, kippers, sardines.

Used in ulcerative colitis and sometimes in carcinoma of the bowel.

3   High Residue Diet

Add bran and vegetables such as cabbage and carrots. Take salads, fruit with skins, wholemeal bread, coarse marmalade.

4   Fluid Diets

(i) Milk 1·14 l (2 pints), skimmed milk powder 114 g (4 oz), sugar 170 g (6 oz), and 1 teaspoonful Marmite (for vitamin B), provides 2000 kcal. (8·4 MJ), 50 g fat, 290 g carbohydrate, and 80 g protein, For extra protein add two eggs, milk, skimmed milk, Casilan or Complan. For extra calories add sugar, milk or glucose. Water is added to provide the required daily fluid intake, e.g. adding 1·86 l provides a total of 3 l fluid.
(ii) Complan 150 g, Caloreen (glucose polymer) or glucose 75 g, cellevac granules 3 g, Becosyn syrup 5 ml, made up to 1 l. 3 l daily (as 125 ml/hour) supply 10·7 MJ.
(iii) 'Clinifeed' (Roussel). Food supplements: 'Complan', 'Nutrament', 'Build-up' (Carnation), 'Two-shakes' (Kelloggs).

5   Low Fat Diet (25 g)

Allowed: fruit, sugar, tea, coffee and cereals with skimmed milk from allowance (total = 1 pint 0·57 l), jelly, jams, honey, meat extracts, kidney, chicken, liver, tripe (steamed, boiled or grilled without fat), white fish, lean meat, egg white, boiled potatoes, vegetables, boiled sweets.

Not allowed: fried foods, dripping, oils, fats, salad creams, fatty meat, duck, sausages, pork, tongue, fatty fish, cheese, milk, cream, ice cream, butter, margarine, pastry, cakes, nuts, chocolate.

Used in gall bladder disease or steatorrhoea.

6 Weight-reducing Diet

1000 kcal., 4·2 MJ daily, containing fat 40 g, protein 50 g and carbohydrate 100 g.

Allowed: tea or coffee, black or with milk from a total allowance of 284 ml (0·5 pint) daily, tomato juice, meat or vegetable extract, unsweetened fruit juice, grapefruit or melon (no sugar), four thin slices of bread which may be toasted, with butter from an allowance of 7 g (0·25 oz) daily. Average helpings of lean meat, white fish, salmon or kippers (not fried), boiled or poached egg, fresh or stewed fruit without sugar. Large helpings of tomato, lettuce, runner beans, cress, cucumber, celery, onions, brussels sprouts, spinach, cabbage, cauliflower, marrow. Saccharin for sweetening. Unlimited soda water, clear soup, black tea or coffee.

Not allowed: fat—fried food, oils, cream, dripping, salad cream; flour—thickened soups or gravies, pastry, cereals, cakes, scones, bread, biscuits; sugar or glucose—sweets, chocolates, syrup jam, honey, marmalade, packet jelly; starch—peas, broad beans, parsnips, turnips, swedes, beetroots, potatoes.

Note: Each thin slice of bread may be replaced by 60 g (2 oz) of potatoes.

7 Low Protein Diet (40 g daily)

Breakfast	Tea or coffee with milk from allowance. Sugar allowed. Porridge or cereal with stewed fruit and sugar, or dairy (double) cream, but no milk. Mushrooms on fried bread, tomatoes or fruit. Bread, two slices of large thin cut, or one thick slice. Butter or margarine. Syrup, marmalade, honey.
Mid-morning	Black coffee, tea with lemon or milk from allowance, or fruit juice and sugar, or meat or vegetable extract.
Lunch	Tomato juice, fruit juice, or clear soup. 45 g (1½ oz) meat, chicken, liver, ham or 60 g (2 oz) fish. Potatoes, vegetables, fruit (fresh, stewed or tinned), dairy cream.
Tea	Tea with milk from allowance. Bread, two thin slices, butter or margarine, jam, honey, syrup, Marmite. Sponge cake, jam tart.
Dinner	One egg or 30 g (1 oz) cheese or meat or 45 g (1½ oz) fish. Salad or vegetables. Bread, one slice, or potatoes. Fruit as for lunch.
Bedtime	Fruit juice and sugar, or tea or coffee with milk from allowance.

Daily allowance is 142 ml (¼ pint) of milk. If more milk is preferred 230 ml (8 oz) may be used instead of meat or cheese.

Used in acute and chronic renal failure.

Low Protein Dishes: fruit pie, jam tart, fruit jelly, fruit crumble, tomato, onion, vegetable pie, spaghetti, macaroni, rice, clear soups. May have cream and glucose polymer ('Caloreen').

8 High Protein (110 g), Low Salt (30 mmol = 0·7 g Na)

Breakfast Tea or coffee with milk from allowance. Sugar allowed. Porridge without salt, shredded or puffed wheat. Boiled, poached, scrambled or fried egg without salt, or white fish without salt. Salt-free bread, unsalted butter, jam, marmalade or honey.

Mid-morning Fruit drink with sugar, or coffee with milk from allowance.

Lunch Liver or meat 90 g (3 oz), or white fish (130 g 4½ oz) without salt. Gravy, vegetables and potatoes without salt. Stewed or fresh fruit, jelly or milk pudding or custard with milk from allowance.

Tea Tea with milk from allowance, with sugar. Salt-free bread. Unsalted butter or margarine. Jam. Meat or chicken 60 g (2 oz) unsalted. Salt-free cake or jam tart.

Dinner Meat or chicken 90 g (3 oz) or fish 130 g (4½ oz) without salt. Salad or vegetables unsalted. Salt-free bread and unsalted butter, or unsalted potatoes. Fresh or stewed fruit and milk pudding.

Bedtime Remainder of milk, with tea or coffee if required, or fruit juice.

Daily allowance is 568 ml (1 pint) of milk, with 15 g (½ oz) Casilan added to milk puddings and drinks. No salt is used in cooking or added at the table.

Used in nephrotic syndrome, malnutrition.

9 Low Sodium Diet (30 mmol = 0·7 g Na)

Avoid salt, butter or margarine containing salt, self-raising flour, bread containing salt, biscuits, cakes, baking powder and soda, meat and vegetable extracts, bacon, ham, sausages, tinned meat, cheese, salted or tinned fish, pickles, chutneys, sauces, tinned vegetables, tinned soups, dried fruit (except prunes), meat and fish pastes, chocolate, cocoa, malted milk.

The following may be taken: unsalted bread, unsalted butter or margarine, plain flour, fruit juices or squashes, boiled sweets, sugar, jelly, cream, vinegar, pepper, mustard, curry powder, meat pies, fruit pies and tarts.

Note: an ordinary diet with salt omitted from the cooking and at the table, contains 130 mmol (130 mEq, 3 g) of sodium providing that salty food (bacon, ham, cheese) are avoided.

10 Diabetic Diet
See Table 12·2 page 317.

APPENDIX 6 NATIONAL HEALTH SERVICE

The theoretical aim is to prevent disease where possible, and to provide the best treatment where prevention fails.

The Organisation of the National Health Service (NHS)

Since April 1974 (NHS reorganisation Act) all branches of the NHS have been controlled by a single administration, i.e. the Secretary of State for Social Services who controls the Department of Health and Social Security (D.H.S.S.). The D.H.S.S. controls the Regional Health Authorities (R.H.A.), each of which in turn is in control of up to eleven Area Health Authorities (A.H.A.). The R.H.A. carries out regional policies and priorities within the framework directed by the D.H.S.S., submits plans, e.g. of major building programmes, to the D.H.S.S., and checks that the A.H.A. has implemented agreed plans. The members of the R.H.A. are appointed by the Secretary of State. The members of each A.H.A. are a chairman appointed by the Secretary of State, four members appointed by the Local Authority, one university nominee, and others appointed by the R.H.A.

Each A.H.A. controls the District Management Teams (D.M.T.) which implement the plans of the A.H.A., control all the District Health Services, and are responsible for improving services and the use of resources, guided by health care planning teams which have responsibility for one aspect of health care, such as the elderly, children, maternity or the mentally ill.

The D.M.T. consists of the following ex officio members: District Community Physician; District Nursing Officer; District Finance Officer; District Administrator and two medical representatives, one a consultant and one a general practitioner. The district medical committee co-ordinates the medical aspects of health care. The district administrator manages all administrative, institutional and support services, assisted by sector administrators who control the local hospital and other administrators.

In each district the nursing service is managed by the District Nursing Officer. The District Dental officer and public health doctors are co-ordinated by the District Community Physician, and all are accountable to their Area counterparts. This scheme gives each officer in the chain specific responsibility in his own speciality and ensures that orders given by the Central Office of the D.H.S.S. will be carried out. This central government control was not seen previously when each local group, whether hospital, public health or district nursing, was able to use its own discretion in local matters. In theory there is better co-ordination between the different services, and suggestions for improvements in the service may be made by local teams and passed on to the higher authorities.

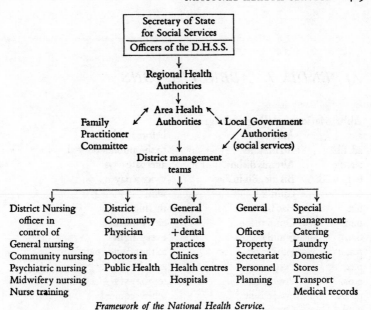

Framework of the National Health Service.

APPENDIX 7   ABBREVIATIONS

Abbreviations relating to drugs

a.c.	Ante cibum	before food
ad. lib.	Ad libitum	to the amount desired
alt. die.	Alternis diebus	alternate days
b.d., b.i.d.	Bis die, Bis in die	twice a day
c̄	Cum	with
h.n.	Hac nocte	this night
o.m.	Omni mane	every morning
o.n.	Omni nocte	every night
p.a.	Parti affectae	to the affected part
p.c.	Post cibum	after food
p.oc.	Pro oculis	for the eyes
p.r.n.	Pro re nata	when required
q.i.d.	Quater in die	four times a day
stat.	Statim	at once
t.i.d., t.d.s.	Ter (in) die (sumendum)	three times a day
i.d.	Intradermal(ly)	into skin
i.m.	Intramuscular(ly)	into muscle
i.v.	Intravenous(ly)	into a vein
s.c.	Subcutaneous(ly)	into subcutaneous tissue

Other Abbreviations

A.C.T.H.	Adrenocorticotrophin
A.D.H.	Antidiuretic hormone
A.H.G.	Anti-haemophilic globulin
A.S.O.	Antistreptolysin O
B.C.G.	Bacille Calmette-Guérin
B.M.R.	Basal metabolic rate
B.P.	Blood pressure
B.S.P.	Bromsulphalein
°C	Degree Celsius (centigrade)
Ca	Calcium
C.C.K.	Cholecystokinin
C.I.	Colour index
Ci	Curie
Cl	Chloride
C.K.	Creatine kinase
C.N.S.	Central nervous system
CO_2	Carbon dioxide

C.R.F., C.R.H.	Corticotrophin-releasing factor or hormone
C.S.F.	Cerebrospinal fluid
C.V.S.	Cardiovascular system
D.C.	Direct current
D.N.A.	Deoxyribonucleic acid
E.C.F.	Extra-cellular fluid
E.C.G., E.K.G.	Electrocardiograph
E.D.T.A.	Edetic acid
E.E.G.	Electroencephalograph
E.S.R.	Erythrocyte sedimentation rate
°F	Degree Fahrenheit
Fe	Ferrum, iron
F.F.A.	Free fatty acids
F.S.H.	Follicle-stimulating hormone
G.C.F.T.	Gonococcal fixation test
G.H., S.T.H.	Growth hormone, somatotrophin
G.I.T.	Gastro-intestinal tract
G.P.I.	General paralysis of the insane
G.U.S.	Genito-urinary system
h	Hour
H	Hydrogen
Hb	Haemoglobin
HCl	Hydrochloric acid
HCO^-_3	Bicarbonate
I	Iodine
I.C.F.	Intracellular fluid
I.N.H.	Isoniazid (Isonicotinic acid hydrazide)
I.Q.	Intelligence quotient
i.u.	International units
I.V.P.	Intravenous pyelogram
I.Z.S.	Insulin zinc suspension
K	Kalium, i.e. potassium
L.A.T.S.	Long-acting thyroid stimulator
L.D.H.	Lactic dehydrogenase
L.H.	Luteinising hormone
L.T.H.	Luteotrophin
M.A.O.I.	Monoamine oxidase inhibitors
M.C.H.C.	Mean corpuscular (red cell) haemoglobin concentration
M.C.V.	Mean corpuscular volume
Mg	Magnesium
Na	Natrium, i.e. sodium
N.P.H.	Isophane insulin (Neutral protamine zinc insulin, Hagedorn)
N.P.N.	Non-protein nitrogen
O_2	Oxygen
O.P.	Osmotic pressure
O.T.	Old tuberculin

P	Partial pressure
P.A.S.	Para–amino salicylic acid
P.B.I.	Protein–bound iodine
P.T.H.	Parathyroid hormone
P.U.O.	Pyrexia of unknown origin
P.Z.I.	Protamine zinc insulin
R.B.C.	Red blood cell
R.C.F.T.	Reiter's complement fixation test
R.S.	Respiratory system
S.G.	Specific gravity
S.G.O.T.	Serum glutamic oxaloacetic transaminase (aspartate aminotransferase)
S.G.P.T.	Serum glutamic pyruvic transaminase (alanine aminotransferase)
S.I.	Soluble insulin
T_3	Tri-iodothyronine
T_4	Thyroxin
T.A.B.	Typhoid, paratyphoid A and B vaccine
T.B.G.	Thyroxine binding globulin
Tm	Maximal tubular reabsorption
T.S.H.	Thyroid-stimulating hormone (thyrotropin)
u.v.	Ultraviolet
W.B.C.	White blood cell
W.R.	Wassermann reaction
$<$	Less than
$>$	Greater than

INDEX

British Library Cataloguing in Publication Data

Harrison, Roger James
    Textbook of medicine with relevant physiology and
    anatomy. – 2nd ed. – (Modern nursing series).
    1. Medicine
    I. Title   II. Series
    610   R130

    ISBN 0-340-25164-6
    ISBN 0-340-25165-4 Pbk

First published 1977, Reprinted 1979
 Second edition 1980, Reprinted 1981

Printed in Great Britain for
Hodder and Stoughton Educational,
a division of Hodder and Stoughton Limited,
Mill Road, Dunton Green, Sevenoaks, Kent
by Hazell Watson & Viney Ltd,
Aylesbury, Bucks